# ANIMAL MODELS IN AIDS

# ANIMAL MODELS IN AIDS

International TNO Meeting,
Maastricht, The Netherlands, 23–26 October 1989

*Editors:*

H. SCHELLEKENS
TNO Primate Center, Rijswijk, The Netherlands

M.C. HORZINEK
Department of Virology, Veterinary Faculty, State University, Utrecht, The Netherlands

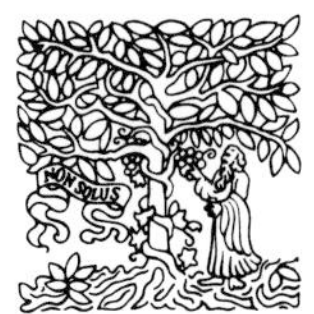


1990
ELSEVIER
Amsterdam – New York – Oxford

This book is printed on acid-free paper.

ISBN 0-444-81264-4

Published by:
Elsevier Science Publishers B.V.
(Biomedical Division)
P.O. Box 211
1000 AE Amsterdam
The Netherlands

Sole distributors for the USA and Canada:
Elsevier Science Publishing Company, Inc.
655 Avenue of the Americas
New York, NY 10010
USA

**Library of Congress Cataloging-in-Publication Data**

International TNO Meeting (1989: Maastricht, Netherlands)
Animal models in AIDS/International TNO Meeting, Maastricht, the Netherlands, 23-26 October 1989; editors, H. Schellekens and M. Horzinek.
p. cm. -- (Animal models; vol. 1)
Includes bibliographical references.
Includes index.
ISBN 0-444-81264-4 (alk. paper)
1. AIDS (Disease)--Animal models--Congresses. I. Schellekens, Huub. II. Horzinek, Marian C. III. Nederlandse Centrale Organisatie voor Toegepast-Natuurwetenschappelijk Onderzoek. IV. Title. V. Series.
[DNLM: 1. Acquired Immunodeficiency Syndrome--congresses.
2. Disease Models, Animal--congresses. 3. Retrovirus Infections--veterinary--congresses. WD 308 I6104a 1989]
RC607.A26I63 1989
616.97'92'0072--dc20
DNLM/DLC
for Library of Congress

90-3617
CIP

Printed in The Netherlands

# PREFACE

About one year ago an international meeting on 'Animal Models in AIDS' took place in Maastricht, The Netherlands. The convention was organized by the Netherlands Organization for Applied Research (TNO), acting upon an initiative of the editors of this volume. More than 150 scientists from 18 countries travelled to this charming city on the Maas river, situated in the southernmost province of Limburg and enjoyed its hospitality and medieval atmosphere. In the splendid Congress Center, the participants experienced a lively dialogue between all those scientists for whom lentiviruses have become the focus of research: physicians, veterinarians, molecular biologists.

The written accounts of this meeting are assembled in the present volume. The reader will find an exhaustive compilation of experimental results obtained with retroviral, specifically lentiviral systems in apes and monkeys, cattle, sheep, horse, cat, rabbit and the mouse. It was the editors' aim to present the whole array of currently available animal models as well as their possible application in vaccine development and antiviral chemotherapy. We think that the stage is set for a comparative evaluation of the different virus-host systems and for a rational selection of the suitable model to solve a specified problem.

H. SCHELLEKENS
M.C. HORZINEK

# CONTENTS

## SIMIAN RETROVIRUSES



## FELINE RETROVIRUSES

## LARGE ANIMAL MODELS



## MOUSE MODELS

**OUTLOOK**

# LIST OF CONTRIBUTORS

N. ALMOND
AIDS Collaborating Centre, National Institute of Biological Standards and Control, Blanche Lane, Potters Bar EN6 3QG, U.K.

M. BABA
Department of Bacteriology, Fukushima Medical College, Fukushima 960–12, Japan

M. BAIER
Paul Ehrlich Institute, 6070 Langen, F.R.G.

J. BALZARINI
Rega Institute for Medical Research, Katholieke Universiteit Leuven, B-3000 Leuven, Belgium

A. BARNARD
AIDS Collaborating Centre, National Institute of Biological Standards and Control, Blanche Lane, Potters Bar EN6 3QG, U.K.

A. BASKERVILLE
PHLS Centre for Applied Microbiology and Research, Division of Pathology, Porton Down, Salisbury SP4 0JG, U.K.

J.K. BATTLES
Laboratory of Cell and Molecular Structure, Program Resources, Inc., National Cancer Institute-Frederick Cancer Research and Development Center, Frederick, MD 21702–1201, U.S.A.

M. BENDINELLI
Department of Biomedicine, Section of Virology, University of Pisa, Pisa, Italy

R. BENTHIN
SBL Primate Research Center, Karolinska Institute, Stockholm, Sweden

Z. BENTWICH
R. Ben Ari Institute of Clinical Immunology, Kaplan Medical Center, Hebrew University Medical School, Rehovot, Israel

L. BERGMANN
J.W. Goethe University, 6000 Frankfurt, F.R.G.

G. BIBERFELD
Department of Immunology, National Bacteriological Laboratory, S-10521 Stockholm, Sweden

K. BREUGELMANS
N.V. INNOGENETICS Research Laboratories, B-2000 Antwerp, Belgium

H. BURKHARDT
Sektion Tierproduktion und Veterinärmedizin, Humboldt Universität, DDR-1040 Berlin, G.D.R.

S. CHAMARET
Unité d'Oncologie Virale, Institut Pasteur, Paris, France

S.C. CLABOUGH
Veterans Administration Medical Center and University of Maryland at Baltimore, Baltimore, MD, U.S.A.

N. COOK
PHLS Centre for Applied Microbiology and Research, Division of Pathology, Porton Down, Salisbury SP4 0JG, U.K.

T. CORCORAN
AIDS Collaborating Centre, National Institute of Biological Standards and Control, Blanche Lane, Potters Bar EN6 3QG, U.K.

R.M. COZENS
Research Department, Pharmaceutical Division, Ciba-Geigy Ltd., CH-4002 Basel, Switzerland

M.P. CRANAGE
PHLS Centre for Applied Microbiology and Research, Division of Pathology, Porton Down, Salisbury SP4 0JG, U.K.

E. DE CLERCQ
Rega Institute for Medical Research, Katholieke Universiteit Leuven, B-3000 Leuven, Belgium

A. DITTMER
Department of Veterinary Medicine, University of Zurich, CH-8057 Zurich, Switzerland

P.R. DONAHUE
Children's Hospital of St. Paul, St. Paul, MN 55102, U.S.A.

D. DORMONT
Centre de Recherches du Service de Santé des Armées, Commissariat à l'Energie Atomique, DPS/SPE, 92265 Fontenay aux Roses and Unité d'Oncologie Virale, Institut Pasteur, Paris, France

D. DWYER
Unité d'Oncologie Virale, Institut Pasteur, Paris, France

H. EGBERINK
Institute of Virology, Department of Infectious Diseases and Immunology, School of Veterinary Medicine, State University of Utrecht, 3584 CL Utrecht, The Netherlands

J.W. EICHBERG
Department of Virology and Immunology, Southwest Foundation for Biomedical Research, San Antonio, TX 78284, U.S.A.

M. EVERS
Deutsches Primatenzentrum, Abteilung Virologie und Immunologie, D-3400 Göttingen, F.R.G.

T.M. FOLKS
Retroviral Research Branch, CDC, Atlanta, GA, U.S.A.

M. FRANCHINI
Department of Veterinary Medicine, University of Zurich, CH-8057 Zurich, Switzerland

C. FROMHOLC
AIDS Collaborating Centre, National Institute of Biological Standards and Control, Blanche Lane, Potters Bar EN6 3QG, U.K.

M.B. GARDNER
Department of Medical Pathology, University of California at Davis, Davis, CA 95616, U.S.A.

K.J. GARVEY
Laboratory of Cell and Molecular Structure, Program Resources, Inc., National Cancer Institute-Frederick Cancer Research and Development Center, Frederick, MD 21702-1201, U.S.A.

T.J. GATESMAN
Deutsches Primatenzentrum, Abteilung Virologie und Immunologie, D-3400 Göttingen, F.R.G.

H.R. GELDERBLOM
Robert-Koch-Institut, D-1000 Berlin 65, Germany

M.E. GERSHWIN
Department of Internal Medicine, Division of Rheumatology/Allergy/Clinical Immunology, University of California, Davis, CA 95616, U.S.A.

D. GHEYSEN
Smith Kline Biologicals, Rixensart, Belgium

M.A. GONDA
Laboratory of Cell and Molecular Structure, Program Resources, Inc., National Cancer Institute-Frederick Cancer Research and Development Center, Frederick, MD 21702-1201, U.S.A.

P.J. GREENAWAY
PHLS Centre for Applied Microbiology and Research, Division of Pathology, Porton Down, Salisbury SP4 0JG, U.K.

C. GRIEF
AIDS Collaborating Centre, National Institute of Biological Standards and Control, Blanche Lane, Potters Bar EN6 3QG, U.K.

Ch. GRUND
Robert-Koch-Institut, D-1000 Berlin 65, Germany

D. GUETARD
Unité d'Oncologie Virale, Institut Pasteur, Paris, France

S. HARTUNG
Paul Ehrlich Institute, 6070 Langen, F.R.G.

K.-G. HEDSTRÖM
SBL Primate Research Center, Karolinska Institute, Stockholm, Sweden

O. HERCHENRÖDER
Deutsches Primatenzentrum, Abteilung Virologie und Immunologie, D-3400 Göttingen, F.R.G.

U. HERZ
Robert-Koch-Institut, D-1000 Berlin 65, Germany

H.-K. HOCHKEPPEL
Research Department, Pharmaceutical Division, Ciba-Geigy Ltd., CH-4002 Basel, Switzerland

P.M. HOFFMAN
Veterans Administration Medical Center and University of Maryland at Baltimore, Baltimore, MD, U.S.A.

A. HOLY
Institute of Organic Chemistry and Biochemistry, Czechoslovak Academy of Sciences, 16610 Prague, Czechoslovakia

E.A. HOOVER
Colorado State University, Fort Collins, CO 80523, U.S.A.

G. HUNSMANN
Deutsches Primatenzentrum, Abteilung Virologie und Immunologie, D-3400 Göttingen, F.R.G.

T. ISHIDA
Department of Clinical Pathology, Nippon Veterinary and Zootechnical College, 1-7-1 Kyonan-cho, Musashino, Tokyo 180, Japan

C.J. ISSEL
Department of Veterinary Science and Veterinary Microbiology and Parasitology, Louisiana State University, Baton Rouge, LA 70803, U.S.A.

A. JENKINS
AIDS Collaborating Centre, National Institute of Biological Standards and Control, Blanche Lane, Potters Bar EN6 3QG, U.K.

K.-D. JENTSCH
Deutsches Primatenzentrum, Abteilung Virologie und Immunologie, D-3400 Göttingen, F.R.G.

P. JOHNSTONE
PHLS Centre for Applied Microbiology and Research, Division of Pathology, Porton Down, Salisbury SP4 0JG, U.K.

E. KARGE
Staatliches Institut für Epizootiologie und Tierseuchenbekämpfung, DDR-1903 Wusterhausen (Dosse), G.D.R.

K. KARJALAINEN
Basel Institute for Immunology, 4058 Basel, Switzerland

J.R. KEDDIE
Health and Safety Executive, Technology Division, Stanley Precinct, Bootle, Merseyside, U.K.

K. KENT
AIDS Collaborating Centre, National Institute of Biological Standards and Control, Blanche Lane, Potters Bar EN6 3QG, U.K.

T.J. KINDT
Laboratory of Immunogenetics, NIAID, Bethesda, MD, U.S.A.

F. KIRCHHOFF
Deutsches Primatenzentrum, Abteilung Virologie und Immunologie, D-3400 Göttingen, F.R.G.

P.A. KITCHIN
AIDS Collaborating Centre, National Institute of Biological Standards and Control, Blanche Lane, Potters Bar, EN6 3QG, U.K.

A. KONNO
Department of Clinical Pathology, Nippon Veterinary and Zootechnical College, 1-7-1 Kyonan-cho, Musashino, Tokyo 180, Japan

M. KOOLEN
Institute of Virology, Department of Infectious Diseases and Immunology, School of Veterinary Medicine, State University of Utrecht, 3584 CL Utrecht, The Netherlands

B. KOTTWITZ
Department of Veterinary Medicine, University of Zurich, CH-8057 Zurich, Switzerland

G. KRAUS
Paul Ehrlich Institute, 6070 Langen, F.R.G.

H. KULAGA
Neuropsychiatry Branch, NIMH Neurosciences Center at St. Elizabeths, Washington, DC 20032, U.S.A.

R. KURTH
Paul Ehrlich Institute, 6070 Langen, F.R.G.

J.M.A. LANGE
Department of Medicine, AIDS Unit and Human Retrovirus Laboratory, Academic Medical Center, Amsterdam, The Netherlands

O. LAUNAY
INSERM U13, Hôpital Claude Bernard, Paris, France

P. LEBON
Hôpital Saint Vincent de Paul, Paris, France

R. LEHMANN
Department of Veterinary Medicine, University of Zurich, CH-8057 Zurich, Switzerland

C. LING
AIDS Collaborating Centre, National Institute of Biological Standards and Control, Blanche Lane, Potters Bar EN6 3QG, U.K.

J. LIVARTOWSKI
Centre de Recherches du Service de Santé des Armées, Commissariat à l'Energie Atomique, DPS/SPE, 92265 Fontenay aux Roses Cedex, France

P.A. LUCIW
Department of Medical Pathology, School of Medicine, University of California, Davis, CA 95616, U.S.A.

W. LÜKE
Deutsches Primatenzentrum, Abteilung Virologie und Immunologie, D-3400 Göttingen, F.R.G.

H. LUTZ
Department of Veterinary Medicine, University of Zurich, CH-8057 Zurich, Switzerland

B. MAHON
AIDS Collaborating Centre, National Institute of Biological Standards and Control, Blanche Lane, Potters Bar EN6 3QG, U.K.

J.L. MARTIN
Veterans Administration Medical Center and University of Maryland at Baltimore, Baltimore, MD, U.S.A.

D. MATTEUCCI
Department of Biomedicine, Section of Virology, University of Pisa, Pisa, Italy

M.F. McENTEE
Johns Hopkins University School of Medicine, Division of Comparative Medicine, Baltimore, MD 21205, U.S.A.

T.P. McGRAW
Department of Medical Pathology, University of California, Davis, CA 95616, U.S.A.

J. MERREGAERT
Laboratory of Biotechnology, University of Antwerp, B-2610 Wilrijk, Belgium

A. MESHORER
Experimental Animal Unit, The Weizmann Institute of Science, Rehovot, Israel

K. MILLS
AIDS Collaborating Centre, National Institute of Biological Standards and Control, Blanche Lane, Potters Bar EN6 3QG, U.K.

L. MONTAGNIER
Unité d'Oncologie Virale, Institut Pasteur, Paris, France

R.C. MONTELARO
Department of Biochemistry, Louisiana State University, Baton Rouge, LA 70803, U.S.A.

E. MOZES
Department of Chemical Immunology, The Weizmann Institute of Science, Rehovot, Israel

J.I. MULLINS
Stanford University, Stanford, CA 94305, U.S.A.

L. NAESENS
Rega Institute for Medical Research, Katholieke Universiteit Leuven, B-3000 Leuven, Belgium

K. NAGASHIMA
Laboratory of Cell and Molecular Structure, Program Resources, Inc., National Cancer Institute-Frederick Cancer Research and Development Center, Frederick, MD 21702–1201, U.S.A.

O. NARAYAN
Johns Hopkins University School of Medicine, Division of Comparative Medicine, Baltimore, MD 21205, U.S.A.

D. NEUMANN-HAEFELIN
Abteilung Virologie, Institut für Medizinische Mikrobiologie und Hygiene, Universität Freiburg, D-7800 Freiburg, F.R.G.

S. NICK
Deutsches Primatenzentrum, Abteilung Virologie und Immunologie, D-3400 Göttingen, F.R.G.

I. NICOL
Centre de Recherches du Service de Santé des Armées, Commissariat à l'Energie Atomique, DPS/SPE, 92265 Fontenay aux Roses Cedex, France

H. NIPHUIS
TNO Primate Center, 2280 HV Rijswijk, The Netherlands

S. NORLEY
Paul Ehrlich Institute, 6070 Langen, F.R.G.

E. NORRBY
Department of Virology, Karolinska Institute, School of Medicine, Stockholm, Sweden

B. ÖBERG
Department of Virology, Karolinska Institute, Stockholm, Sweden

M.S. OBERSTE
Laboratory of Cell and Molecular Structure, Program Resources, Inc., National Cancer Institute-Frederick Cancer Research and Development Center, Frederick, MD 21702–1201, U.S.A.

J.M. OVERBAUGH
University of Washington, Seattle, WA 98195, U.S.A.

M. ÖZEL
Robert-Koch-Institut, D-1000 Berlin 65, Germany

M. PAGE
AIDS Collaborating Centre, National Institute of Biological Standards and Control, Blanche Lane, Potters Bar EN6 3QG, U.K.

L.A. PALLANSCH
Laboratory of Cell and Molecular Structure, Program Resources, Inc., National Cancer Institute-Frederick Cancer Research and Development Center, Frederick, MD 21702-1201, U.S.A.

G. PAULI
AIDS-Zentrum des Bundesgesundheitsamtes, Berlin, Germany

R. PAUWELS
Rega Institute for Medical Research, Katholieke Universiteit Leuven, B-3000 Leuven, Belgium

N.C. PEDERSEN
Department of Veterinary Medicine, School of Veterinary Medicine, University of California, Davis, CA 95616, U.S.A.

D.Y. PIFAT
Laboratory of Cell and Molecular Structure, Program Resources, Inc., National Cancer Institute-Frederick Cancer Research and Development Center, Frederick, MD 21702-1201, U.S.A.

J.J. POCIDALO
INSERM U13, Hôpital Claude Bernard, Paris, France

F. POLZIEN
Deutsches Primatenzentrum, Abteilung Virologie und Immunologie, D-3400 Göttingen, F.R.G.

M.L. POSS
Colorado State University, Fort Collins, CO 80523, U.S.A.

P. PUTKONEN
Department of Immunology, National Bacteriological Laboratory, S-10521 Stockholm, Sweden

S.L. QUACKENBUSH
Colorado State University, Fort Collins, CO 80523, U.S.A.

P. REISS
Department of Medicine, AIDS Unit, Academic Medical Center, Amsterdam, The Netherlands

R. RENNE
Abteilung Virologie, Institut für Medizinische Mikrobiologie und Hygiene, Universität Freiburg, D-7800 Freiburg, F.R.G.

H. REUPKE
Robert-Koch-Institut, D-1000 Berlin 65, Germany

B.A. RIDEOUT
Department of Veterinary Medicine, School of Veterinary Medicine, University of California, Davis, CA 95616, U.S.A.

D.S. ROBBINS
Veterans Administration Medical Center and University of Maryland at Baltimore, Baltimore, MD, U.S.A.

I. ROSENBERG
Institute of Organic Chemistry and Biochemistry, Czechoslovak Academy of Sciences, 16610 Prague, Czechoslovakia

H.A. ROSENTHAL
Institut für Medizinische Virologie, Bereich Medizin (Charité), Humboldt-Universität, DDR-1040 Berlin, G.D.R.

S. ROSENTHAL
Zentralinstitut für Molekularbiologie, Akademie der Wissenschaften der DDR, DDR-1115 Berlin-Buch, G.D.R.

J. RUBINSTEIN
Experimental Animal Unit, The Weizmann Institute of Science, Rehovot, Israel

E. SAMAN
N.V. INNOGENETICS Research Laboratories, B-2000 Antwerp, Belgium

H. SCHELLEKENS
TNO Primate Center, 2280 HV Rijswijk, The Netherlands

D. SCHREINER
Deutsches Primatenzentrum, Abteilung Virologie und Immunologie, D-3400 Göttingen, F.R.G.

M. SCHWEIZER
Abteilung Virologie, Institut für Medizinische Mikrobiologie und Hygiene, Universität Freiburg, D-7800 Freiburg, F.R.G.

P. SILVERA
AIDS Collaborating Centre, National Institute of Biological Standards and Control, Blanche Lane, Potters Bar EN6 3QG, U.K.

M. SINET
INSERM U13, Hôpital Claude Bernard, Paris, France

J. SLACHMUYLDERS
TNO Primate Center, 2280 HV Rijswijk, The Netherlands

E. SOLDAINI
Department of Biomedicine, Section of Virology, University of Pisa, Pisa, Italy

E.E. SPARGER
Department of Veterinary Medicine, School of Veterinary Medicine, University of California, Davis, CA 95616, U.S.A.

C. STAHL-HENNIG
Deutsches Primatenzentrum, Abteilung Virologie und Immunologie, D-3400 Göttingen, F.R.G.

E.J. STOTT
AIDS Colloborating Centre, National Institute of Biological Standards and Control, Blanche Lane, Potters Bar EN6 3QG, U.K.

J. SWINNEN
Laboratory of Biotechnology, University of Antwerp, B-2610 Wilrijk, Belgium

Z. SZOTYORI
AIDS Collaborating Centre, National Institute of Biological Standards and Control, Blanche Lane, Potters Bar EN6 3QG, U.K.

F. TAFFS
AIDS Collaborating Centre, National Institute of Biological Standards and Control, Blanche Lane, Potters Bar EN6 3QG, U.K.

A. TANIGUCHI
Department of Clinical Pathology, Nippon Veterinary and Zootechnical College, 1-7-1 Kyonan-cho, Musashino, Tokyo 180, Japan

R. THORSTENSSON
Department of Immunology, National Bacteriological Laboratory, S-10521 Stockholm, Sweden

T. TOLLE
Deutsches Primatenzentrum, Abteilung Virologie und Immunologie, D-3400 Göttingen, F.R.G.

I. TOMODA
Department of Clinical Pathology, Nippon Veterinary and Zootechnical College, 1-7-1 Kyonan-cho, Musashino, Tokyo 180, Japan

M. TORTEN
Department of Veterinary Medicine, School of Veterinary Medicine, University of California, Davis, CA 95616, U.S.A.

A. TRAUNECKER
Basel Institute for Immunology, 4058 Basel, Switzerland

M.E. TRUCKENMILLER
Laboratory of Immunogenetics, NIAID, Bethesda, MD, U.S.A.

H. VAN HEUVERSWIJN
N.V. INNOGENETICS Research Laboratories, B-2000 Antwerp, Belgium

P. VARLET
INSERM U152, Hôpital Cochin, Paris, France

M. VOGEL
Paul Ehrlich Institute, 6070 Langen, F.R.G.

G. VOGT
Centre de Recherches du Service de Santé des Armées, Commissariat à l'Energie Atomique, DPS/SPE, 92265 Fontenay aux Roses Cedex, France

B.R. VOWELS
Department of Medical Pathology, University of California, Davis, CA 95616, U.S.A.

T. WASHIZU
Department of Clinical Pathology, Nippon Veterinary and Zootechnical College, 1-7-1 Kyonan-cho, Musashino, Tokyo 180, Japan

Z. WEISMAN
R. Ben Ari Institute of Clinical Immunology, Kaplan Medical Center, Hebrew University Medical School, Rehovot, Israel

A. WERNER
Paul Ehrlich Institute, 6070 Langen, F.R.G.

N.T. WETHERALL
Department of Pathology, Vanderbilt University School of Medicine, Nashville, TN 37232-2561, U.S.A.

Th. WINKEL
Robert-Koch-Institut, D-1000 Berlin 65, Germany

M. WITVROUW
Rega Institute for Medical Research, Katholieke Universiteit Leuven, B-3000 Leuven, Belgium

# A summary of the WHO Informal Consultation on Animal Models for evaluation of drugs and vaccines for HIV infection and AIDS (Geneva, 14–15 September 1989)

J. ESPARZA and S. OSMANOV

Global Programme on AIDS, World Health Organization, Geneva, Switzerland

The pandemic of AIDS calls for the rapid development of effective vaccines and therapies to prevent and to treat HIV infection and disease. The Global Programme on AIDS (GPA) of the World Health Organization (WHO) is committed to play a facilitating role that would accelerate the development and evaluation of safe, effective and affordable vaccines, and treatments for HIV infection and AIDS.

Well-standardized animal models capable of mimicking HIV infection and disease would provide valuable tools for in vivo analysis of candidate anti-HIV drugs and vaccines prior to their clinical evaluation in humans.

With an objective to review the experience with different animal models currently in use, and to develop recommendations to WHO, an Informal Consultation was convened by GPA/WHO (Geneva, 14–15 September 1989), which was attended by six experts from four countries *.

Having reviewed the present state of the art, the group formulated the requirements for the hypothetical 'ideal' HIV animal model for evaluation of candidate drugs and vaccines.

The 'ideal' animal model for drugs: (a) should make use of HIV itself; (b) it should be a small animal with well-known genetics, immunology and metabolism;

* Participants in the consultation: J.M. Dupuy, Rhone Mérieux, Lyon, France; P.N. Fultz, Yerkes Regional Primate Research Center, Atlanta, USA; R. Kurth (Chairman), Paul-Erlich Institute, Frankfurt, Federal Republic of Germany; D. Mosier, Medical Biology Institute, La Jolla, USA; R.M. Ruprecht (Rapporteur), Dana Farber Cancer Institute, Boston, USA; O. Varnier, Institute of Microbiology, Genoa, Italy; and from the Global Programme on AIDS, World Health Organization, Geneva, Switzerland: J. Esparza, S. Osmanov, H. Tamashiro, Y.M. Shao, F. Sonnenburg. Full report of the consultation available from: Biomedical Research Unit, Global Programme on AIDS, World Health Organization, 1211 Geneva 27, Switzerland.

(c) the target cells should be CD4+ lymphocytes and macrophages; (d) target organs should include blood, lymphoid tissues and the brain; (e) the mode of transmission should mimic that of HIV, including perinatal transmission; (f) the induced disease should have a short incubation period and resemble human AIDS.

The 'ideal' animal model for vaccines should have the characteristics mentioned above. In addition it is important that the virus challenges be made with standardized inocula, including virus infected cells, as well as cell-free virus. Mucosal route of challenge, such as vaginal and per-urethra should be previewed and standardized.

Such an ideal model does not exist. Thus, drugs and vaccines need to be evaluated in animal models with various shortcomings, and the ultimate selection of the most appropriate model would depend on a number of different parameters.

The Group discussed the advantages and shortcomings of different animal models currently in use, as well as their suitability for drug and vaccine development in comparison with the formulated hypothetical ideal animal model. The general agreement of the Group was that HIV infection of chimpanzees provides the ultimate model to test efficacy of vaccines in preventing infection, but the fact that chimpanzee is an endangered species in the wild and is a very scarce and costly resource largely limits the use of this model.

There was a consensus that SIV infection of macaques could be considered presently as the 'gold standard' in the development of drugs and vaccines for HIV infection and AIDS. The major advantage of this model is that SIV mimics HIV in its genomic organization, genetic variability, sexual transmission, central nervous system involvement and progression of the infection to disease.

The potentials of other animal models currently in use were also discussed, such as HIV infection of macaques, rabbits or mice (transgenic mice or human/mouse chimerae), models with the use of murine retroviruses and feline leukemia virus.

Against this information the WHO Working Group developed proposed schemes for the optimal use of animal models for the evaluation of drugs and vaccine against HIV.

The recommendations to WHO include the following: WHO should facilitate the use of animal models for the preclinical development of therapeutic agents and vaccines against HIV by: (1) disseminating information on the availability of various animal models for the development of antiviral drugs, immunomodulators and vaccines; (2) providing advice on the use of animal models, particularly those experiments using animals in limited supply; (3) encouraging the use of appropriate small animal models prior to studies in non-human primates; (4) encouraging the gathering of information on safety and efficacy in animal models prior to the initiation of phase 1 trials in humans; (5) facilitating international collaboration between investigators to ensure optimal utilization of animal models; (6) promoting standardization of animal models, viral strains, challenge doses of virus, route of viral challenge, etc., to facilitate comparison of data; (7) maintaining a catalogue of available resources relevant to animal studies (reagents and animals).

*Eds. H. Schellekens and M.C. Horzinek*
*Animal Models in AIDS*



# 1

# Morphogenesis and fine structure of lentiviruses *

HANS R. GELDERBLOM, MUHSIN ÖZEL, DIRK GHEYSEN [1], HILMAR REUPKE, THORSTEN WINKEL, UDO HERZ, CHRISTIAN GRUND and GEORG PAULI [2]

Robert Koch-Institut and [2] AIDS-Zentrum des Bundesgesundheitsamtes, Berlin, Germany and [1] Smith Kline Biologicals, Rixensart, Belgium

## Introduction

### The retrovirus family: classification

Retroviruses comprise a family of structurally and conceptionally related agents which on the basis of biological and morphological criteria are grouped into three subfamilies, the Onco-, Spuma- and Lentivirinae (Matthews, 1982; Fig. 1). Under natural conditions oncoviruses establish persistent, slowly progressive infections, e.g., in wild mice (Gardner, 1978). Under experimental conditions such viruses may ultimately induce malignancies in vivo and cell transformation in vitro. Therefore much scientific effort was concentrated in the late 1960s on this subfamily in order to find a general mechanism for cancer induction. Detailed studies were performed in the early 1970s on the biological and biochemical properties of oncoviruses and their specific interaction with the host cell. From these investigations much has been learned about retrovirus structure and function in general, and normal and malignant cell growth regulation in particular (for reviews, see Frank, 1987a; Weiss et al., 1984). The ultimate goal, however, of the oncovirological studies, finding the key to the human cancer problem, was not reached.

Spuma- or foamyviruses have been encountered as passengers in different species with a still unknown pathogenic potential in vivo (Weiss et al., 1984; Weiss, 1988). They have been isolated from a variety of species including cats, cattle, monkeys, and man, share common subfamily specific antigens, and induce in vitro characteristic cytopathic effects leading to cell death (Gelderblom, 1987;

* Dedicated to Professor Dr. Meinrad A. Koch on the occasion of his 60th birthday.

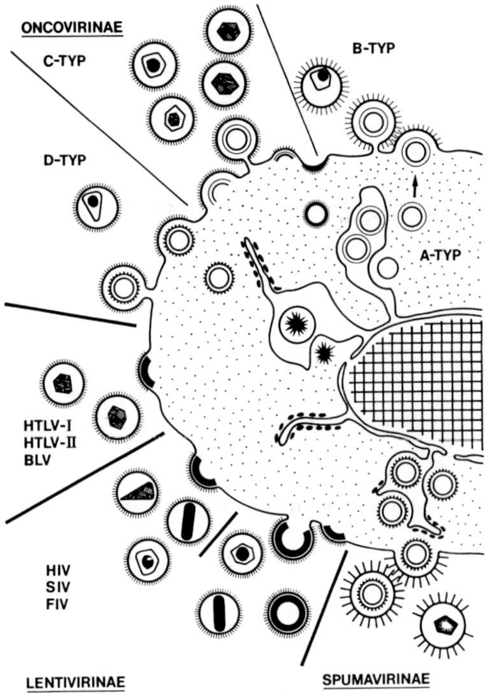


Fig. 1. Morphological classification of the Retrovirus family, modified from Gelderblom et al. (1985a, 1989). The oncovirus subfamily comprises particles of types A–D. Type A structures are morphologically completely assembled cores of the prototype B-type mouse mammary tumor virus, while C-type particles are known to cause sarcomas and lymphomas, e.g., in avian and mammalian species. Their core is formed at cellular membranes concomitantly with the budding process, and after budding condensed to an isometric core. D-type oncoviruses have preformed cores, too, and are known to occur and to cause malignancies in certain primates. HTLV-I and related viruses represent an intermediate group exhibiting morphological features during assembly and after maturation of both onco- and lentiviruses. Members of the lentivirus group are assembled at cellular membranes, similar to the C-type particles. They differ, however, in the distance of the bulging core shell from the plasma membrane, and its thickness. After release from the cell, the *gag* proteins form cone-shaped cores, while the envelope knobs are shed readily. Spumaviruses show envelopment of preformed cores, which never condense fully, and shedding of the envelope knobs, too.

Hooks and Gibbs, 1975; Matthews, 1982). Spumavirus genomic structure has been resolved only recently (Maurer and Flügel, 1988). It was never observed that they transform their target cells in vitro, nor do they induce malignant growth in their specific hosts.

Lentiviruses show a clear cytopathology in vitro and in vivo, and are serologically related, although to different degrees. Primate specific lentiviruses share approximately 60% of conserved proteins (R. Desrosiers, personal communication). Serological cross-reactivities localized mainly to the viral core, but also to the envelope, have also been described between human immunodeficiency virus (HIV) and equine infectious anemia virus (EIAV) (Montagnier et al., 1984; Montelaro et al., 1988; Schneider et al., 1986, 1987).

TABLE 1
Structural criteria for the morphological classification of retroviruses (modified from Gelderblom et al., 1985a)

| | |
|---|---|
| *Morphogenesis* | |
| A | Cores preformed in the cytoplasm |
| B | Core assembly concomitant with budding |
| C | Distance of core shell to prospective envelope |
| D | Dimension of the RNP-core complex |
| *Morphology* | |
| E | Shape of the core (isometric or tubular) |
| F | Site of the isometric core (con- or eccentric) |
| G | Dimension of envelope projections |
| H | Anchorage stability of envelope projections |

Certain lentiviruses, like HIV and simian immunodeficiency virus (SIV), are able to infect a specific subset of lymphocytes in addition to cells of the mononuclear macrophage lineage (Gendelman et al., 1986, 1989; Rozenberg and Fauci, 1989). This dual host range might be an important factor for the induction of progressive immuno-suppression which ultimately leads to a breakdown of the immune system and death of the infected individuum.

Retrovirus classification is based on the pioneering electron microscopic work of Wilhelm Bernhard who introduced morphological criteria to group a number of RNA-containing viruses, known to cause malignancies in mice and chickens, into A-, B-, and C-type particles (Bernhard, 1960). This was a decade before the description of reverse transcriptase, the key enzyme in the life cycle of these viruses. It is based on structural details (Table 1) observed during the assembly of virions, i.e., during budding, and after morphological maturation, after release from the host cell. The classification was expanded whenever new members of the retrovirus family were described (de Harven, 1974; Matthews, 1982; for review, see Gelderblom et al., 1989) and it turned out that the morphological grouping also reflected biological functions. The morphological assignment of a retrovirus isolate to a particular subfamily therefore directly helped in perceiving its functional properties and designing further investigations. Morphogenesis and morphology of retroviruses, especially of the oncovirus subfamily, are described in a number of reviews (Bolognesi et al., 1978; de Harven, 1974; Dubois-Dalque, 1984; Frank et al., 1978; Frank, 1987a–c; Gelderblom and Frank, 1987; Gelderblom, 1987; Sarkar, 1987).

## The lentivirus subfamily

Comprising a well defined subfamily of the retroviruses, the Lentivirinae have long been neglected in favor of the transforming oncoviruses. However, the etiological agent for equine infectious anemia was already described in 1904 as a virus, now grouped as a lentivirus (Vallée and Carré, 1904). In veterinary medicine lentiviruses have long been recognized as the cause of devastating, slowly progressive diseases of some Ungulatae. Sigurdsson in 1954 coined the term "slow infection" for the emerging new clinical syndrome (Sigurdsson, 1954). As the prototype lentivirus, the ovine Maedi-Visna virus (MVV) has been characterized thorougly. MVV causes chronic progressive pneumonia (Maedi) as well as progressive encephalopathy (Visna) (Gendelman et al., 1986; Sigurdsson et al., 1960; for recent reviews, see Haase, 1986; Narayan and Clements, 1989; Perk, 1988; Petursson et al., 1989).

Visna-like viruses, now called bovine immunodeficiency virus (BIV), were isolated from cattle suffering from lymphocytosis and lymphadenopathy (Georgiades et al., 1978; Gonda et al., 1987; Van der Maaten et al., 1972). From horses presenting with hemolytic anemia EIAV was recovered (Gonda et al., 1978; Kobayashi, 1961; Vallée and Carré, 1904; Weiland et al., 1977) and caprine arthritis encephalitis virus was recovered from goats (Belov and Whalley, 1988; Crawford et al., 1980; Dahlberg et al., 1981; Perk, 1988; Weinhold, 1974).

The detection of HIV as the cause of AIDS in 1983/1984 (Barré-Sinoussi et al., 1983; Gallo et al., 1984; Popovic et al., 1984) and its characterization as a lentivirus immediately prompted intensified research efforts and consequently led to the isolation of lentiviruses from a variety of different species. Of major interest is the isolation of SIVs, which usually, in their natural hosts, have only a low pathogenic potential (Benveniste et al., 1986; Daniel et al., 1985; Fultz et al., 1986; Murphey-Corb, 1986; Ohta et al., 1988; Tsujimoto et al., 1988).

In heterologous monkey species, however, SIV might cause immunodeficiencies of different degrees which make them a valuable model for AIDS research (Fultz et al., 1986; Desrosiers and Letvin, 1987; Gardner and Luciw, 1988; Schneider and Hunsmann, 1988). Feline T-lymphotropic virus or feline immunodeficiency virus (FIV), described recently, now serves as a non-primate model in AIDS research (North et al., 1989; Pedersen et al., 1987).

The particular biology of lentiviruses, e.g., the regulatory pathways, the high genetic variability and the virus induced immunodeficiency disorders have been reviewed by Cullen and Green (1989), Dahlberg (1988), Haase (1986), Haseltine (1988, 1989), Narayan and Clements (1989), Perk (1988), and by Weiss and coworkers (1984).

## Molecular anatomy of lentiviruses

Retroviruses are composed of approximately 35% lipid, 60% protein, 3% carbohydrate and 1% RNA. The lipids of the viral envelope are derived from the plasma membrane during particle assembly. Similar to the situation with other enveloped viruses, the lipid composition of HIV resembles that of the plasma membranes of the host cell (Aloia et al., 1988). In the ribonucleoprotein (RNP) portion of the viral core two copies of the positive strand RNA genome are present coding for virus structural and for regulatory proteins, which are believed to be non-structural proteins in most cases.

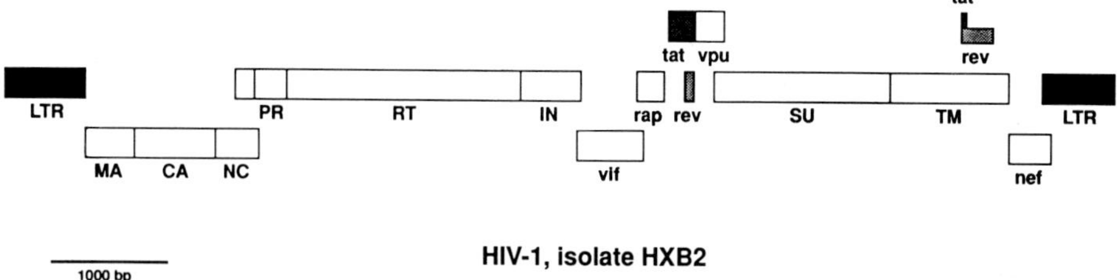


Fig. 2. Genomic structure of HIV-1 indicating the location of the different structural and regulatory proteins on three large precursor proteins as well as the open reading frames of the six functional proteins.

Information for virus structural proteins is arranged in the genome in the order 5′-*gag-pol-env*-3′. They are transcribed as three large precursor proteins which are processed to the final structural proteins of the core and the envelope (Figs. 2, 3). In contrast to oncoviruses, lentiviruses produce several regulatory proteins studied in most detail in HIV. Here, up to now six distinct proteins (vif, rap (vpr), out (vpu), tat, rev, and nef) have been identified regulating virus replication (Cohen et al., 1988; Cullen and Green, 1989; Dahlberg, 1988; Gallo et al., 1988; Haseltine, 1989). These proteins exert a number of intertwined positive and negative regulatory effects on virus production and thus represent important factors for virus latency, activation and production.

Retrovirus structural proteins have been designated since 1974 by the letters "p" or "gp" for (glyco)protein followed by the molecular weight of the protein (August et al., 1974). Recently a simplified nomenclature has been proposed (Leis et al., 1988) which uses a two-letter acronymic code describing either the location in the virion, the enzymatic activity and/or biological function of the protein

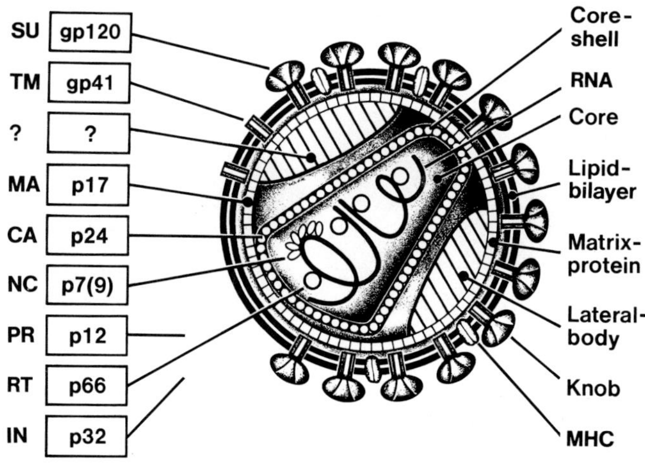


Fig. 3. 2-D diagram of HIV-1, modified from Gelderblom et al. (1987 a,b).

(Fig. 3). Thus MA stands for matrix protein, CA for capsid, NC for nucleocapsid, SU for surface, and TM for transmembrane protein. PR denominates the viral protease, RT reverse transcriptase, and IN the viral integrase. This code is similar to that used for other enveloped viruses and helps to avoid confusion when

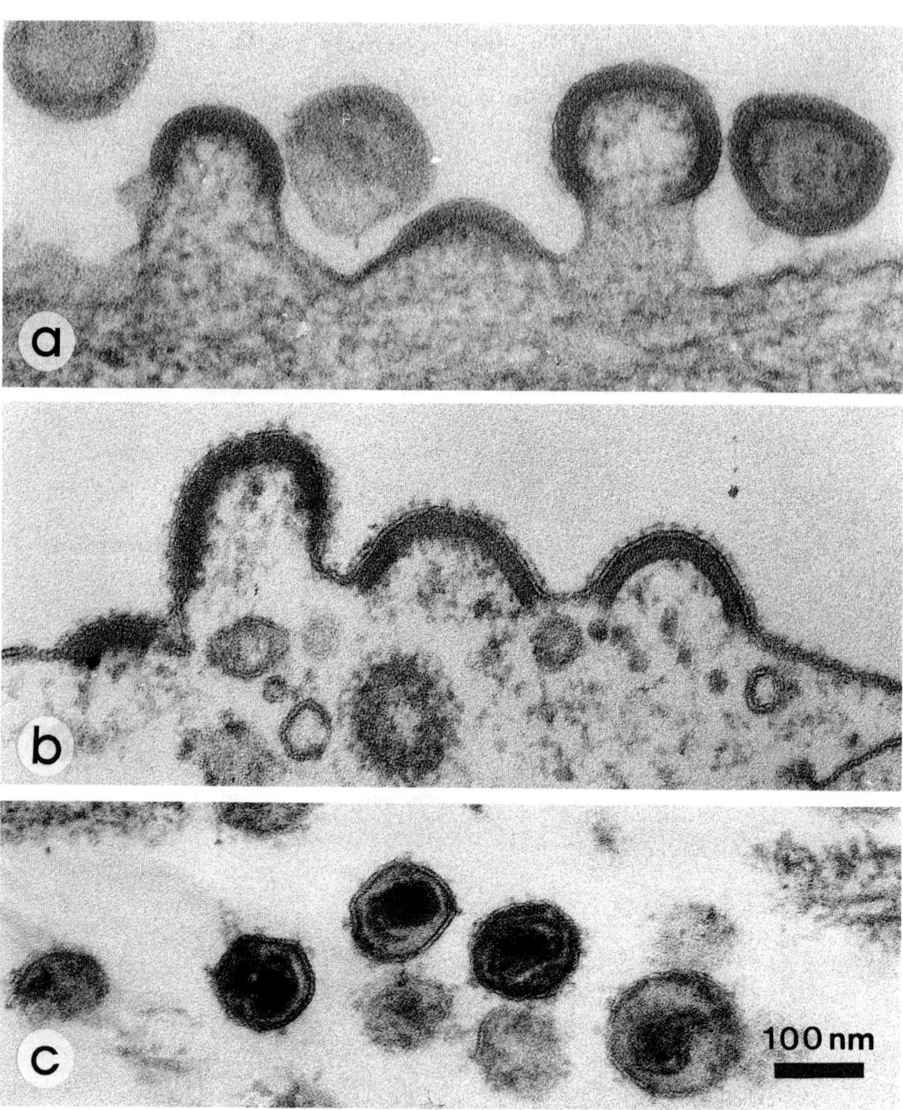


Fig. 4. Thin section micrographs of MVV prepared without (a) and after tannic acid treatment (b and c). TA cytochemistry allows the easy detection of surface projections on budding virions, which show a ribonucleoprotein portion closely attached to the prospective viral envelope. Cell released particles, smaller than the immature virions and showing condensed, elongated cores, have shed most knobs (c). Magnification: ×120,000

denominating proteins of similar function in different retroviruses, which show different molecular weights.

## Morphogenesis of lentiviruses

The assembly of lentiviruses, like that of other retroviruses, takes place as a budding process at cellular membranes. At the site of budding, underneath the lipid bilayer and very closely attached to it, a compact electron dense shell 18–20 nm in thickness can be seen growing. In parallel with the assembly of this *gag* protein layer (MA, CA, NC), envelope surface projections appear on the viral bud (Figs. 4a,b). They are particularly well demonstrated using tannic acid treatment of the cells before embedding followed by conventional heavy metal contrasting (Gelderblom et al., 1987; Schidlovsky et al., 1978). Structural details of the *gag* protein shell, however, are lost to a great extent in the high contrast introduced with this technique. Without tannic acid cytochemistry usually two thin dense lines (Fig. 4a,b) can be differentiated in this layer (Gelderblom et al., 1988, 1989). After completion of the core shell to a sphere of about 120–130 nm, the immature particle with a diameter of 130–150 nm is pinched off the cell surface still retaining its inner spherical organization (Bouillant and Becker, 1984; Filice et al., 1987; Gelderblom et al., 1985a; Hockley et al., 1988; Katsumoto et al., 1987; Nakai et al., 1989; Palmer et al., 1988a).

Later, probably in the course of several minutes or hours, the inner constituents become rearranged to form the condensed core of the morphologically mature lentivirus particle (Figs. 4c, 6c, 7b). This morphological transition is fast, as intermediate steps are observed rarely (Gelderblom et al., 1985a, 1989) and usually accompanied by a decrease in viral diameter to 110–130 nm, as also observed by Bouillant and Becker (1984) and Munn et al. (1985).

The application of recombinant DNA technology made it possible to elucidate some essential steps in virus assembly and maturation. Using baculovirus as a vector for the propagation of HIV and SIV *gag* constructs in the insect *Spodoptera frugiperda* host cell system, selfassembly of precursor *gag* protein into virus-like particles was shown despite the absence of both viral RNA and envelope protein (Delchambre et al., 1989; Gheysen et al., 1989; Overton et al., 1989). The core organization of the particles formed closely resembles that of immature lentiviruses (Fig. 5a). They contain uncleaved p55 *gag* precursor protein molecules which in the budding process bind with their myristilated amino terminus to the protruding lipid envelope of the host cell. Released particles are membrane-bound, measure 120–150 nm in diameter (Fig. 5b,c), and can be harvested for further characterization from cell culture supernatants. Due to the absence of the viral protease in this construct, the p55 particles are not processed further to the final structural proteins. Proteolytic cleavage of the *gag* precursor apparently is the prerequisite for the rearrangement of the inner structural constituents to a state observed in mature lentiviruses (Figs. 6, 7) and it is essential in order to render the particles infectious (Kohl et al., 1988). At present it is not known whether the aspartic type of viral protease exerts its action during the assembly

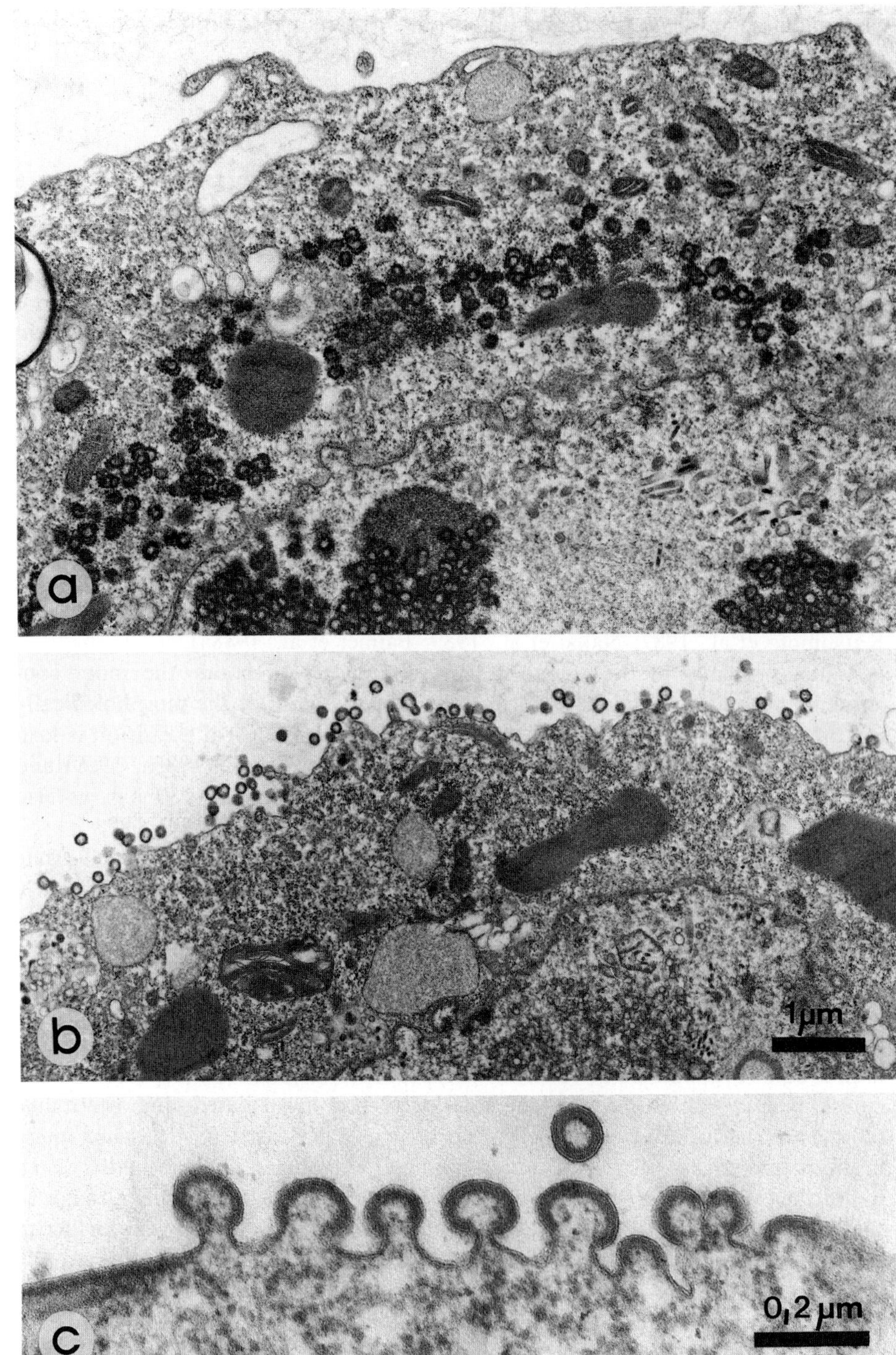
a
b
1µm
c
0,2 µm

process, i.e., during budding, or whether it is active also after release of the newly formed particle. But it is well conceivable that the morphologically immature particles already contain the cleaved polypeptides of the mature virion, however, still in their original position. On the other hand, in HIV and SIV preparations, the p55 *gag* precursor is present in considerable amounts. Under specific preparation conditions, in case of Friend murine C-type oncoviruses, such a preserved so called "native" core has been observed (Frank et al., 1978). If their findings can be generalized, we have to assume that the rearrangement of the processed structural proteins within the virion, leading to a condensation of the NC and RNP portion, needs additional factors, e.g., a change in pH or osmolarity.

Depending on the virus cell system, the numerical relation of budding structures to mature particles varies considerably. With high producer strains of HIV, like HTLV-IIIB, LAV-1, and SBL6669, viral buds are observed only rarely (Gelderblom et al., 1985a, 1988). This contrasts to many fresh isolates, particularly from patients in early stages of HIV infection, which often show multiple buds at the cell surface (Fenyö et al., 1988; Gelderblom, unpublished). This slow particle formation, as shown in Fig. 4 for MVV, indicates that these isolates are restricted in their in vitro growth, probably on the genetic level.

## Myristilation of MA proteins

As shown especially in the baculovirus system myristilation of the *gag* precursor is a prerequisite for particle formation and budding: without myristilation of p55 no membrane targeting occurs, and *gag* precursor proteins are found assembled as extended masses of core-like structures in both the nucleus and the cytoplasm of the transfected Spodoptera cells (Fig. 5). Myristilation, the post-translational attachment of a C14 fatty acid, is commonly observed with the MA of retroviruses (Henderson et al., 1983; Rein et al., 1986; Veronese et al., 1988).

## Organization of the inner structural proteins

### *Matrix protein and "lateral bodies"*

In morphologically mature HIV, MA forms an electron dense layer 5–7 nm in thickness, which is directly attached to the lipid bilayer and clearly separated from the broad end of the core by an electron lucent space (Gelderblom et al.,

Fig. 5. Thin sections of *Spodoptera frugiperda* insect cells after infection with different baculovirus HIV *gag* constructs. (a) Assembly of core-like structures is observed to occur in the nucleus and the cytoplasm when the cell is infected with a construct deleted in its 5′-amino terminus, e.g., in the myristilation site. Cells infected with constructs containing the intact myristilation site (b, c) show particle formation exclusively at the plasma membrane. The particles formed closely resemble immature lentiviruses, even after release from the cell, but do not show envelope knobs (c). Magnifications: (a, b) ×12,000, (c) ×80,000

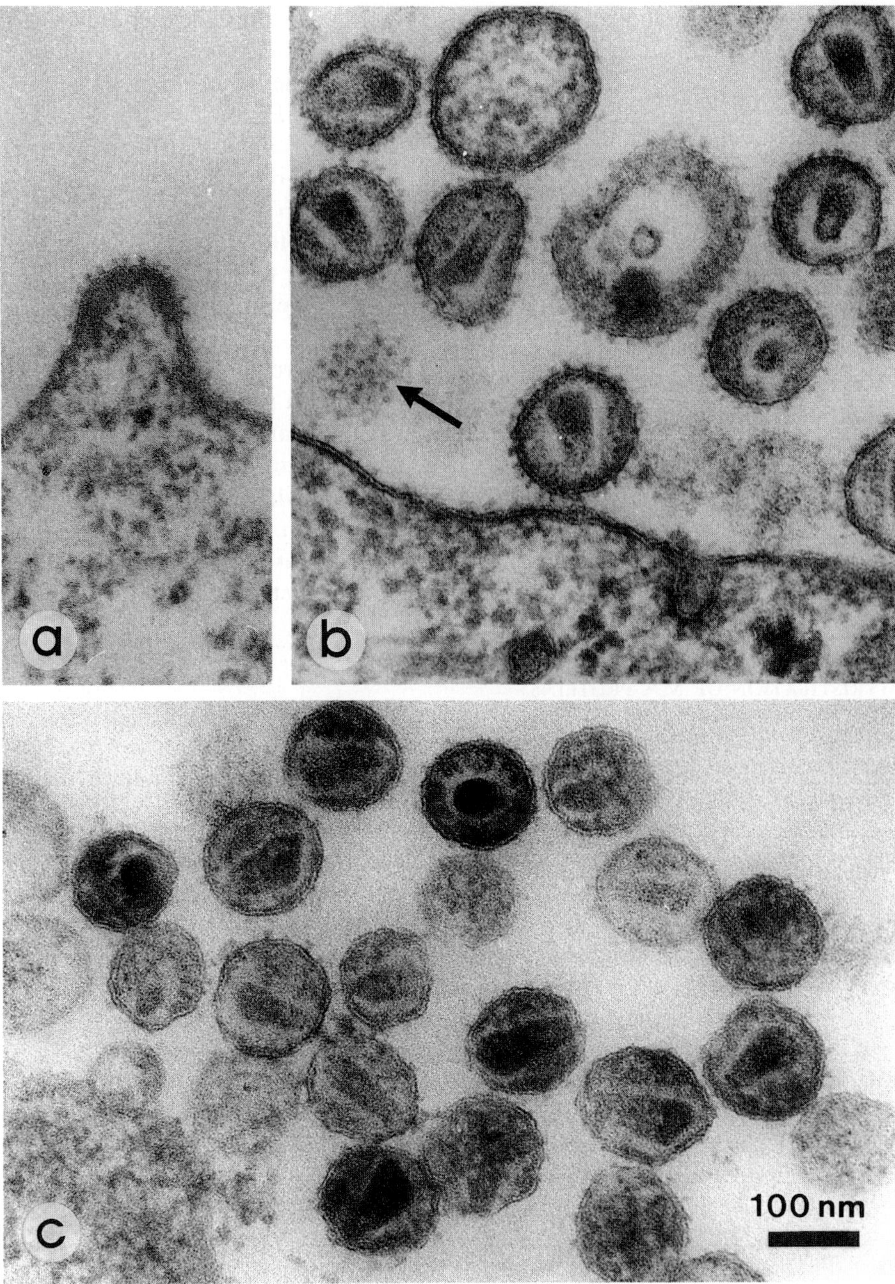


Fig. 6. Thin sections of SIVmac infected H9 cells processed for electron microscopy on day 3 (a, b) and day 6 (c) post infection. The viral bud (a) is studded densely with surface projections and characterized by a ribonucleoprotein shell closely attached to the lipid bilayer. Cell released particles on day 3 showing a variety of core orientations and still a great number of envelope knobs. Occasionally in very tangential section planes, these projections are observed forming a dense pattern (arrow in b). In 6 day old cultures most of the knobs are already shed (c). Magnification: ×120,000

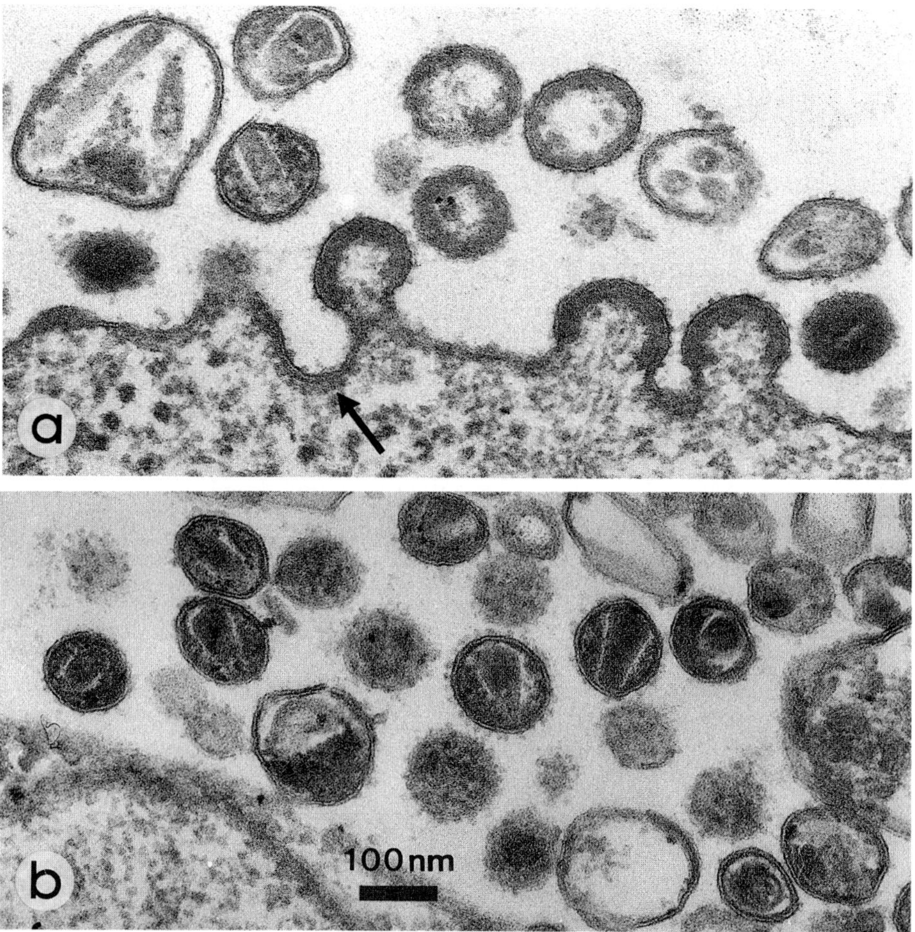


Fig. 7. Thin section of SIVagm showing budding and released particles. Virus formation interestingly often occurs in the direct vicinity of clathrin coated pits (arrow in a) indicating concomitant uptake processes to occur by a receptor mediated process. A grossly enlarged particle with several tubular cores, and another norm-sized SIV with a tubular core are shown in (a), too. Morphologically mature SIV showing cone-shaped cores which in their different orientations are clearly separated from the surrounding electron dense masses ("lateral bodies" in b). Magnification: ×100,000

1987; Marx et al., 1988; Niedrig et al., 1988). HIV, SIV and EIAV exhibit large electron dense masses of an unknown composition, "lateral bodies", along the axes of the viral core and often in direct continuity with MA (Figs. 6, 7). It is not unlikely that these masses represent "non-structural", regulatory viral proteins, e.g., in HIV-2 and SIV preparations a high amount of the regulatory vpx protein was detected associated with the virion (Henderson et al., 1988).

By computer emulation modeling, MA of HIV was shown to form an eicosahedral 60-sided shell with 32 vertices underlying the lipid bilayer (Marx et al., 1988). This shell obviously might play a morphopoietic role both in particle assembly and, as discussed later, in the arrangement of envelope knobs.

*The core structure of mature lentiviruses*

The cores of mature lentiviruses, like HIV, SIV, EIAV, are elongated, cone-shaped structures spanning almost the entire diameter of the virion. The broad end of the core with a maximal diameter of 60–65 nm occasionally shows an angulated outline; it is always separated from the envelope associated MA protein by a clear halo, while the small end of the core in thin sections often appears to be continuous with the envelope associated MA protein layer (Figs. 6c, 7b). The cone-shaped structure of the cores of these viruses has been revealed in both negative staining and thin section electron microscopy (Bouillant and Becker, 1984; Chippaux-Hyppolite et al., 1972; Chrystie and Almeida, 1988, 1989; Dahlberg et al., 1981; Dubois-Dalcq et al., 1976, 1984; Frank, 1987c; Gelderblom et al., 1985a, 1987, 1989; Gonda et al., 1985, 1988; Grief et al., 1989; Hockley et al., 1988; Ladhoff et al., 1986; Munn et al., 1985; Palmer et al., 1988; Palmer and Goldsmith, 1988; Roberts and Oroszlan, 1989; Weiland et al., 1977; Weiland and Bruns, 1980). A less dense outer shell, 4–5 nm in thickness with a periodicity of 4 nm, can be differentiated from the inner electron dense portion of the core. This dense portion, usually confined to the stumpy, broad end of the cone, is assumed to represent the RNP of the virion.

The core capsid is made up of CA, p24 and p26 in case of HIV and EIAV, respectively (Chrystie and Almeida, 1989; Gelderblom et al., 1987; Roberts and Oroszlan, 1989) assembled in a hitherto unknown symmetry. A conical appearance in thin section EM could be explained principally also by the projection of a section which was cut obliquely through a tubular, cylindrical structure (Lecatsas et al., 1984; Takahashi et al., 1989). From high resolution studies and the analysis of serial sections, however, it became clear that the majority of the mature cores are indeed cone-shaped, occasionally showing well defined double cones (Gelderblom et al., 1988).

However, tubular cores occur in released particles (Fig. 7a), though only at a low percentage from less than 1 to up to 5% depending on the virus cell system. Tubular cores are typically longer, measuring often more than 200 nm, compared to the normal more uniform length of 100 nm of the cone-shaped bodies. Tubular cores show a diameter of only 45 nm in contrast to 60–65 nm measured at the broad end of the cone-shaped cores. A tubular mode of assembly of the *gag* proteins is also observed with other retroviruses, and was shown to occur also in the baculovirus HIV/SIV *gag* systems (Delchambre et al., 1989; Gheysen et al., 1989). Occasionally several cores, cone-shaped and/or cylindrical ones, can be observed enveloped within one particle, indicating that budding and release are not necessarily dependent on a stoichiometric interaction of envelope and *gag* proteins.

Besides the obvious structural functions of the *gag* derived MA and CA, and the functional PR, the other structural and the regulatory viral gene products determine lentivirus morphogenesis in a complex way. It was shown, e.g., that a deletion of 19 base pairs in the non-coding region between the HIV-1 5′LTR and the *gag* gene still allowed particle production. However, these particles were unable to incorporate viral RNA, because the packaging signal for the genomic RNA was deleted (Lever et al., 1989). Such packaging sequences have been located to homologous genome regions of other retroviruses, too.

## The envelope glycoproteins

Retroviral envelopes are studded with surface projections or knobs, which measure, depending on the particular virus group, between 5 and 11 nm in length (for reviews, see Frank, 1987a–c; Gelderblom and Frank, 1987; Sarkar et al., 1987; Matthews, 1982).

The knobs of HIV, similar to those of SIV and MVV (Figs. 4, 6, 7), measure 9–10 nm in height and have a broad, slightly convex surface 14–15 nm in diameter (Gelderblom et al., 1987; Grief et al., 1988; Hockley et al., 1988; Palmer et al., 1988). SU and TM of HIV are derived from a common gp160 precursor, which after glycosylation becomes endoproteolytically cleaved (McCune et al., 1988). The knobs of retroviruses are composed of the outer envelope SU glycoprotein, which is heavily glycosylated.

Compared to the surface projections of other enveloped viruses, retroviral knobs are weakly anchored to the viral surface resulting in their easy loss. The extent of loss, however, shows marked differences in the different virus subfamilies, which might be explained by their modes of anchorage to the virion. While oncovirus knobs are covalently linked by disulfide bridges to the TM (Pauli et al., 1978; Pinter and Fleissner, 1977; Schneider and Hunsmann, 1978), the SU projections of HIV are bound only by non-covalent bonds to the TM protein (Modrow et al., 1987). This weak anchorage explains the extensive, spontaneous loss of the viral knobs of HIV, SIV and MVV observed in vitro, which in vivo might have immunopathogenic consequences (Clayton et al., 1989; Gelderblom et al., 1985b, 1987, 1988; Lanzavecchia et al., 1988; Schneider et al., 1986; Rozenberg and Fauci, 1989; Siliciano et al., 1988; Weiland and Bruns, 1980).

The progressive loss of knobs is readily revealed by thin section electron microscopy. In 3 day old cultures knobs are seen evenly spaced on budding particles (Fig. 6a), while cell released virions in the same preparation (Fig. 6b) have already shed many knobs. In 6 day old cultures they are virtually all gone (Fig. 6c).

From image analysis using rotational enhancement techniques a number of 72 knobs was found arranged in a regular T = 7 levo symmetry on the envelopes of HIV and SIV (Gelderblom et al., 1987; Özel et al., 1988; Takahashi et al., 1989). This primarily unexpected regularity might be explained by the MA protein which underneath the viral lipid bilayer forms a scaffold (Marx et al., 1988) for the isometric insertion of the envelope proteins. The SU protein knobs present on fresh virions form a dense cover, which might even inhibit antibodies from reacting with structures underneath and near to the lipid bilayer.

Several lines of evidence suggest that the knobs are not monomers, but oligomeric complexes of TM and SU.

(1) The dimensions of the HIV knobs evidently are too large to account for a single gp120 polypeptide as the morphological entity.

(2) In an analysis of the polypeptide stoichiometry of EIAV a number of about 300 gp90 SU molecules per virion has been determined (Parekh et al., 1980). From the number of 72 knobs per virion it follows that the knobs are oligomeric complexes of SU, consisting of three or probably four structural units.

(3) Evaluating TEM micrographs of thin sections of HIV and of negatively stained SIV, triangular structures can be seen on the viral surface (Gelderblom et al., 1988, 1989; Grief et al., 1989), suggesting a trimeric structure.

(4) Recent biochemical investigations using chemical cross-linking of the SU and TM proteins support an oligomeric, i.e., tri- or tetrameric, structure of the HIV envelope knobs (Pinter et al., 1989; Schawaller et al., 1989).

## Host derived constituents of the viral envelopes

Like other enveloped viruses, lentiviruses acquire a number of host encoded constituents during budding from cellular membranes (Gelderblom et al., 1987; Henderson et al., 1987; Hoxie et al., 1987; Kannagi et al., 1987). The stable insertion of MHC class I and especially class II determinants in the viral bilayer is of particular interest. In the regulation of the immune system the interaction of MHC class II protein with the CD4 receptor is an essential step in the activation of CD4 positive lymphocytes which are the main host cell of HIV. CD4, present on a subset of T cells and on macrophages, also serves as the cellular receptor for HIV (Dalgleish et al., 1984; Klatzmann et al., 1984). The determinants involved in binding of HIV SU have been localized to a small region within the V1 domain of CD4 (Arthos et al., 1989). Binding of MHC class II proteins, in contrast, involves a much larger area of the CD4 molecule comprised of domains I and II (Clayton et al., 1989). CD4 binds SU with a high affinity of $10^{-9}$ (Lasky et al., 1987). Though the MHC class II-CD4 interaction is about four orders of magnitude lower, the cooperative binding of both "viral" envelope proteins, the class II protein and gp120 SU, to the CD4 of the prospective host cell might facilitate virus entry.

Furthermore, MHC antigens on virions might interfere with regulatory events of cells involved in the immune defense. This functional impairment might add to the indirect and direct cytocidal effect of HIV to cells of the immune system.

## Lentivirus cell interaction

The host cell range of HIV and SIV is determined by the high affinity binding of the SU protein to the V1 domain of the cellular CD4 receptor (Arthos et al., 1989; Lasky et al., 1987). The gp120-CD4 interaction is considered essential in initiating virus entry. Whether other cell surface proteins, such as the comple-

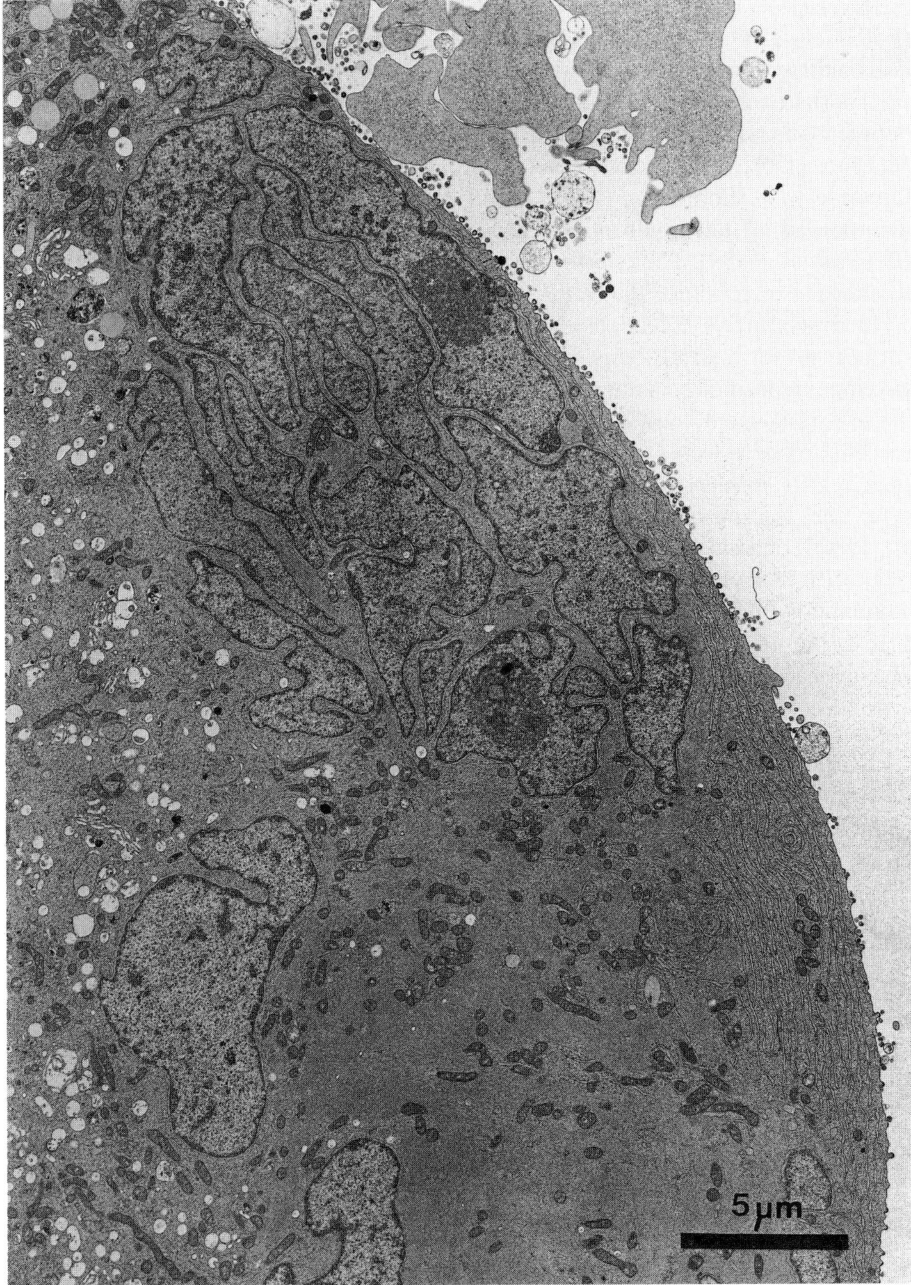


Fig. 8. Thin section showing syncytium formation in SIVagm infected H9 cells. The cell surface is densely covered with budding and immature virions, while in the cell body several nuclei of varying shapes are seen. Cellular organelles, like mitochondria, endoplasmic reticulum and vesicles, are confined to different regions indicating a highly disordered dynamic organization of the syncytium. Magnification: $\times$4,800

ment receptor, might play an additional role in virus uptake is under discussion (Bolognesi, 1989; Sölder et al., 1989). Two mechanisms have been described for virus entry: receptor mediated uptake via clathrin coated pits followed by transport to and processing in the endosomes, as well as pH-independent fusion between the viral envelope and the plasma membrane (Goto et al., 1988; McClure et al., 1988; Pauza et al., 1988; Ribas et al., 1988; Stein et al., 1987; Grewe et al., submitted). The domain responsible for membrane fusion was identified as a highly hydrophobic region near to the amino terminus of TM gp41 (Bosch et al., 1989). The question which of the observed entry mechanisms leads to effective infection of the cell is still unresolved.

In a productive infection virus *gag* precursor proteins migrate to the cell surface to form viral buds in a selfassembly process. Concomitantly, viral envelope molecules become accessible at the plasma membrane, in a particularly dense arrangement over the bud. Exposed envelope glycoproteins can mediate the binding of infected and uninfected CD4 positive cells. TM mediated fusion then results in the recruitment of uninfected T-helper cells into the growing syncytium leading finally to the death of cells (Gelderblom et al., 1988; Lifson et al., 1986; Sodroski et al., 1986; Yoffe et al., 1987).

In such syncytia (Figs. 8, 9) virus assembly takes place mainly at intracellular membranes into grossly enlarged channels of the endoplasmic reticulum rather than at the surface of the syncytia (Dowsett et al., 1987; Gelderblom et al., 1988; Harris et al., 1989).

## Immunopathogenesis

Mechanisms leading to dysfunction and depletion of CD4 positive cells can be deduced also from the shedding of SU from mature virions. Binding of soluble gp120 to CD4 receptors interferes with normal CD4-MHC class II interaction thus blocking normal T cell functions. The CD4-SU complex formed at the cell surface might act as a neoantigen leading to autoimmune phenomena directed against CD4 present on infected as well as on non-infected cells. Bound soluble SU was shown to be processed and presented by MHC class II restricted CD4 positive cells (Lanzavecchia et al., 1988). Thus both the uninfected SU presenting cell as well as the SU decorated T cell can be lysed by SU specific T cell clones (Siliciano et al., 1988).

As clearly demonstrated in the MuLV oncovirus system (Schwarz et al., 1976), in addition to *env* coded proteins, also internal, *gag* derived molecules might become accessible during productive retrovirus infections. Clinical investigations have shown that *gag* and RT specific cytotoxic T lymphocytes were present in HIV infected persons. These findings underline the importance of internal or

Fig. 9. Thin section of an H9 cell syncytium after infection with HIV-1. In syncytia virus budding occurs mainly into large cytoplasmic vesicles containing high numbers of morphologically mature virions. In addition extracellular virus particles are seen at the cell surface and between the cell projections. Magnification: ×40,000

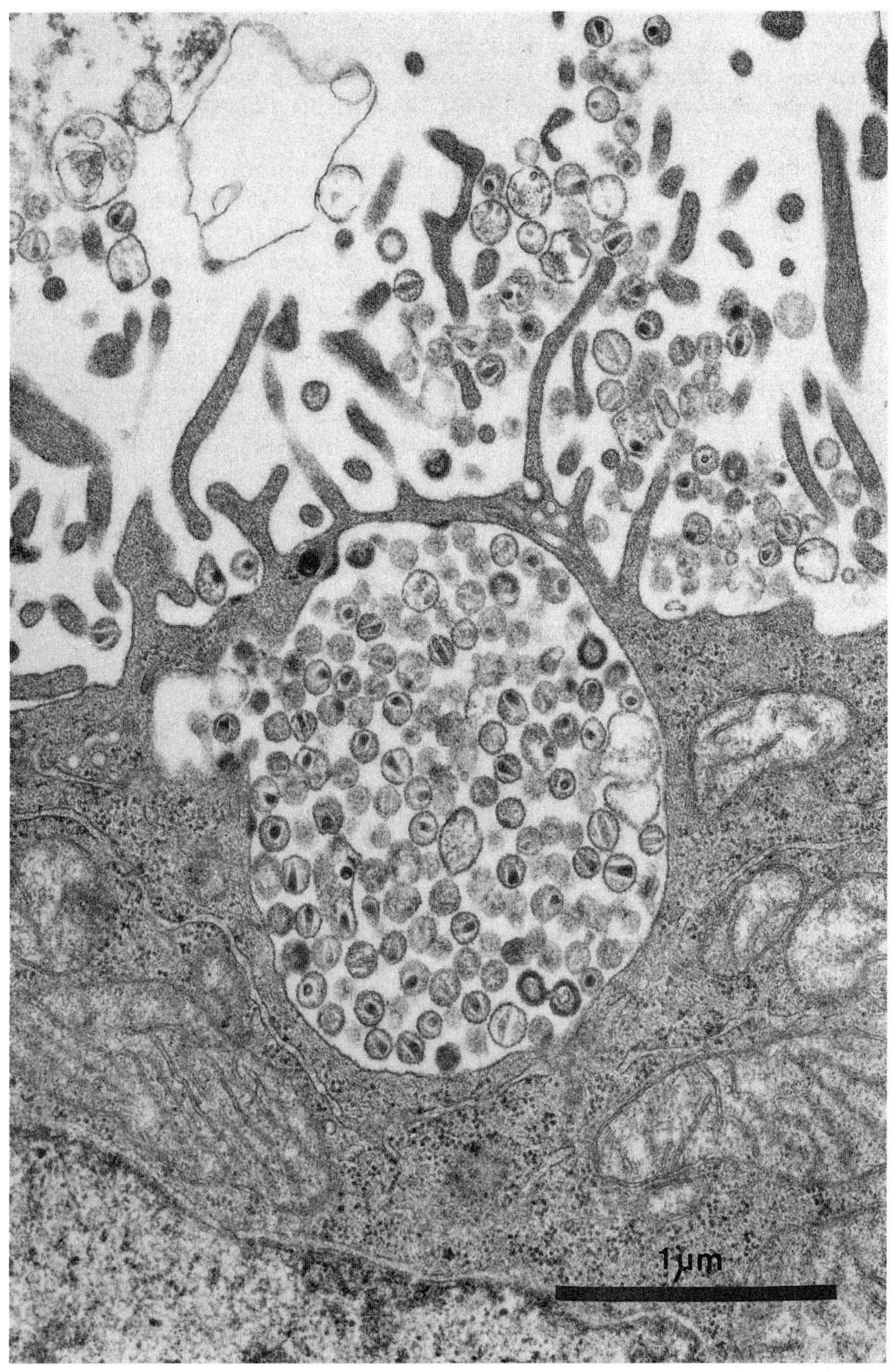
1 µm

possibly also of regulator proteins for the clinical course of the HIV infection. The recently demonstrated cell surface expression of several HIV-1 CA *gag* determinants (Laurent et al., 1989) is in agreement with the role of cytotoxic T cells in immune surveillance (Lusso et al., 1989; Nixon et al., 1988; Riviere et al., 1989; Walker et al., 1988).

Humoral defense mechanisms might have deleterious effects, too. Antibodies directed against the viral SU protein and the inner viral antigens have been demonstrated by immunoelectron microscopy (Hausmann et al., 1987). SU specific antibodies might neutralize HIV, but at the same time they might induce antibody dependent cellular cytotoxicity (ADCC) of SU antigen presenting cells leading to a further diminution of uninfected CD4 positive cells.

The diminishing number of CD4 positive T-helper cells represents a direct parameter for the staging of AIDS as the loss of these immunoregulatory cells generally reflects the progression of the HIV infection to overt AIDS. In MVV, in contrast, the primary host cell is the macrophage. In vitro, however, MVV grows in a variety of ovine cells and does not show the restriction observed for HIV (Pétursson et al., 1989).

Being the primary host cells of HIV besides cells of the macrophage monocyte lineage (Gartner et al., 1986; Knight and Patterson, 1988), the T-helper cells might be eliminated in vivo by two cytopathic mechanisms: (1) the direct cytopathic effect due to virus replication which is induced (at least in part) by the accumulation of "toxic" amounts of unintegrated double-stranded viral DNA in infected cells (Muesing et al., 1985; Somasundaran and Robinson, 1988), and (2) the formation of syncytia, i.e., multinucleated giant cells, due to the fusogenic properties of the TM protein. The continuous recruitment of uninfected CD4 positive cells into the growing multinucleated complex in vitro leads to large syncytia, containing occasionally hundreds of nuclei, and to cell death, because these complexes are no longer viable (Figs. 8, 9). Syncytium formation might be involved in CD4 positive cell depletion in vivo.

HIV in humans can be found replicating both in cells of the monocyte macrophage lineage (Eilbott et al., 1989; Gartner et al., 1987; Knight and Patterson, 1987) and in T-helper lymphocytes. HIV replication in macrophages is usually slow with large masses of virus particles assembled in the dilated endoplasmic reticulum. Since infected macrophages—compared to T-helper cells—are remarkably resistant against the cytopathic effect of HIV they survive for prolonged periods of time and thus might function as a long lasting virus reservoir.

In vitro MVV and CAEV show a broad host cell range growing to high titers in monocytes/macrophages and in a variety of fibroblastoid cell lines derived from sheep or goats, respectively. In vivo, however, MVV replication is obviously restricted in monocytes. This restricted growth seems to be the major factor for the "slowness" of the disease (Pétursson et al., 1989). An answer to the question why MVV is restricted in vivo might help to find out effective regulatory pathways of these viruses and to delineate additional means of virus control in infected persons.

## Acknowledgements

This work would not have been possible without the generous supply of viruses and susceptible cells by many colleagues: we thank Eva Maria Fenyö, Ron Desrosiers and M.D. Daniel, Robert C. Gallo and Mika Popovic, Magret Gudnadottir, Gerhard Hunsmann, Luc Montagnier, and Ron Montelaro for their help. Our thanks are also due to Mrs. Bärbel Jungnickl and Mr. Bernd Wagner for preparing the photographic prints, Dipl. Biol. Wolfgang Weigelt for preparing Fig. 2, the genomic chart of HIV, and Mr. Wolfgang Lorenz for skillful drawing of Fig. 3. The work presented was supported in part by research grant 01 ZR 89018 to H.G. of the Bundesministerium für Forschung und Technologie, Bonn.

## References

Aloia, R.C., Jensen, F.C., Curtain, C.C., Mobley, P.W. and Gordon, L.M. (1988) Lipid composition and fluidity of the human immunodeficiency virus. *Proc. Natl. Acad. Sci.* 85, 900–904.

Arthos, J., Deen, K.C., Chaikin, M.A., Fornwald, J.A., Sathe, G., Sattentau, Q.J., Clapham, P.R., Weiss, R.A., McDougal, J.S., Pietropaolo, C., Axel, R., Truneh, A., Maddon, P.J. and Sweet, R.W. (1989) Identification of the residues in human CD4 critical for the binding of HIV. *Cell* 57, 469–481.

August, J.T., Bolognesi, D., Fleissner, E., Gilden, R.V. and Nowinski, R.C. (1974) A proposed nomenclature for the virion proteins of oncogenic RNA viruses. *Virology* 60, 595–601.

Barré-Sinoussi, F., Chermann, J.C., Rey, F., Nugeyre, M., Chamaret, S., Gruest, C., Daquet, C., Axler-Blin, C., Vézinet-Brun, F., Rouzioux, C., Rozenbaum, W. and Montagnier, L. (1983) Isolation of a T-lymphotropic retrovirus from a patient at risk for acquired immune deficiency syndrome (AIDS). *Science* 220, 868–871.

Belov, L. and Whalley, J.M. (1988) Virus-specific polypeptides of caprine arthritis encephalitis virus recognized by monoclonal antibodies to virion proteins p24 and p14. *J. Gen. Virol.* 69, 1097–1103.

Benveniste, R.E., Arthur, L.O., Tsai, C.-C., Sowder, R., Copeland, T.D., Henderson, L.E. and Oroszlan, S. (1986) Isolation of a lentivirus from a macaque with lymphoma: comparison with HTLV-III/LAV and other lentiviruses. *J. Virol.* 60, 483–490.

Bernhard, W. (1960) The detection and study of tumor viruses with the electron microscope. *Cancer Res.* 20, 712–727.

Bolognesi, D.P. (1989) Do antibodies enhance the infection of cells by HIV? *Nature* 340, 431–432.

Bolognesi, D.P., Montelaro, R.C., Frank, H. and Schäfer, W. (1978) Assembly of type C oncornaviruses: a model. *Science* 199, 183–186.

Bosch, M.L., Earl, P.L., Fargnoli, K., Picciafuoco, S., Giombini, F., Wong-Staal, F. and Franchini, G. (1989) Identification of the fusion peptide of primate immunodeficiency viruses. *Science* 244, 694–697.

Bouillant, A.M.P. and Becker, S.A.W.E. (1984) Ultrastructural comparison of oncovirinae (type C), spumavirinae, and lentivirinae: three subfamilies of retroviridae found in farm animals. *J. Natl. Cancer Inst.* 72, 1075–1084.

Chippaux-Hyppolite, C., Taranger, C., Tamalet, J., Pautrat, G. and Brahic, M. (1972) Aspects ultrastructuraux du virus visna en cultures cellulaires. *Ann. Inst. Pasteur* 123, 409–420.

Chrystie, I.L. and Almeida, J.D. (1988) The morphology of human immunodeficiency virus (HIV) by negative staining. *J. Med. Virol.* 25, 281–288.

Chrystie, I.L. and Almeida, J.D. (1989) The recovery of antigenically reactive HIV-2 cores. *J. Med. Virol.* 27, 188–195.

Clayton, L.K., Sieh, M., Pious, D.A. and Reinherz, E. L. (1989) Identification of human CD4 residues affecting class II MHC versus HIV-1 gp120 binding. *Nature* 339, 548–551.

Cohen, E.A., Terwilliger, E.F., Sodroski, J.G. and Haseltine, W.A. (1988) Identification of a protein encoded by the vpu gene of HIV-1. *Nature* 334, 532–534.

Crawford, T.B., Adams, D.S., Cheevers, W.P. and Cork L.C. (1980) Chronic arthritis in goats caused by a retrovirus. *Science* 207, 997–999.

Cullen, B.R. and Greene, W.C. (1989) Regulatory pathways governing HIV-1 replication. *Cell* 58, 423–426.

Dahlberg, J.E. (1988) An overview of retrovirus replication and classification. In: K. Perk (Ed.), *Immunodeficiency Disorders and Retroviruses. Advances in Veterinary Science and Comparative Medicine,* Vol. 32. Academic Press, London, pp. 1–35.

Dahlberg, J.E., Gaskin, J.M. and Perk, K. (1981) Morphological and immunological comparison of caprine arthritis encephalitis and ovine progressive pneumonia viruses. *J. Virol.* 39, 914–919.

Dalgleish, A.G., Beverly, P.C.L., Clapham, P.R., Crawford, D.H., Greaves, M.F. and Weiss, R.A. (1984) The CD4 (T4) antigen is an essential component of the receptor for the AIDS retrovirus. *Nature* 312, 763–766.

Daniel, M.D., Letvin, N.L., King, N.W., Kannagi, M., Sehgal, P.K., Hunt, R.D., Kanki, P.J., Essex, M. and Desrosiers, R.C. (1985) Isolation of a T-cell tropic HTLV-III-like retrovirus from macaques. *Science* 228, 1201–1204.

Delchambre, M., Gheysen, D., Thines, D., Thiriart, C., Jacobs, E., Verdin, E., Horth, M., Burny, A. and Bex, F. (1989) The *gag* precursor of simian immunodeficiency virus assembles into virus-like particles. *EMBO J.* 8, 2653–2660.

Desrosiers, R.C. and Letvin, N.L. (1987) Animal models for acquired immunodeficiency syndrome. *Rev. Inf. Dis.* 9, 483–446.

Dowsett, A.B., Roff, M.A., Greenaway, P.J., Elphick, E.R. and Farrar, G.H. (1987) Syncytia—a major site for the production of the human immunodeficiency virus? *AIDS* 1, 147–150.

Dubois-Dalcq, M., Holmes, K.V. and Rentier, B. (Eds.) (1984) *Assembly of Enveloped RNA Viruses.* Springer-Verlag, Vienna, New York.

Dubois-Dalcq, M., Reese, T.S. and Narayan, O. (1976) Membrane changes associated with assembly of visna virus. *Virology* 74, 520–530.

Eilbott, D.J., Peress, N., Burger, H., LaNeve, D., Orenstein, J., Gendelman, H.E, Seidman, R. and Weiser, B. (1989) Human immunodeficiency virus type 1 in spinal cords of acquired immunodeficiency syndrome patients with myelopathy: expression and replication in macrophages. *Proc. Natl. Acad. Sci.* 86, 3337–3341.

Fenyö, E.M., Morfeldt-Manson, L., Chiodi, F., Lind, B., von Gegerfelt, A., Albert, J., Olausson, E. and Åsjö, B. (1988) Distinct replicative and cytopathic characteristics of human immunodeficiency virus isolates. *J. Virol.* 62, 4414–4419.

Filice, G., Carnevale, G., Lanzarini, P., Orsolini, P., Soldini, L. and Cereda, P.M. (1987) Human immunodeficiency virus (HIV): an ultrastructural study. *Microbiologica* 10, 209–216.

Frank, H. (1987a) Retroviridae. In: M.V. Nermut and A.C. Steven, (Eds.), *Animal Virus Structure.* Elsevier, Amsterdam, New York, Oxford, pp. 253–256.

Frank, H. (1987b) Oncovirinae: type C oncovirus. In: M.V. Nermut and A.C. Steven, (Eds.), *Animal Virus Structure.* Elsevier, Amsterdam, New York, Oxford, pp. 305–311.

Frank, H. (1987c) Lentivirinae. In: M.V. Nermut and A.C. Steven, (Eds.), *Animal Virus Structure.* Elsevier, Amsterdam, New York, Oxford, pp. 295–304.

Frank, H., Schwarz, H., Graf, Th. and Schäfer, W. (1978) Properties of mouse leukemia viruses XV. Electron microscopic studies on the organization of Friend leukemia virus and other mammalian C-type viruses. *Z. Naturforsch.* 33c, 124–138.

Fultz, P.N., McClure, H.M., Anderson, D.C., Swenson, R.B., Anand, R. and Srinivasan, A. (1986) Isolation of a T-lymphotropic retrovirus from naturally infected sooty mangabey monkey *(Cercocebus atys). Proc. Natl. Acad. Sci.* 83, 5286–5290.

Gallatin, W.M., Gale, M.J., Hoffman, P.A., Willerford, D.M., Draves, K.E., Benveniste, R.E., Morton, W.R. and Clark, E.A. (1989) Selective replication of simian immunodeficiency virus in a subset of CD4+ lymphocytes. *Proc. Natl. Acad. Sci.* 86, 3301–3305.

Gallo, R., Wong-Staal, F., Montagnier, L., Haseltine, W.A. and Yoshida, M. (1988) HIV/HTLV gene nomenclature. *Nature* 333, 504.

Gallo, R.C., Salahuddin, S.Z., Popovic, M., Shearer, G.M., Kaplan, M., Haynes, B.F., Palker, T.J., Redfield, R., Oleske, J., Safai, B., White, G., Foster, P. and Markham, P.D. (1984) Frequent detection and isolation of cytopathic retrovirus (HTLV-III) from patients with AIDS and at risk for AIDS. *Science* 224, 500–503.

Gardner, M.B. (1978) Type C viruses of wild mice: characterization and natural history of amphotropic, ecotropic and xenotropic MuLV. *Curr. Top. Microbiol. Immunol.* 79, 215–259.

Gardner, M.B. and Luciw, P.A. (1988) Simian immunodeficiency viruses and their relationship to the human immunodeficiency viruses. *AIDS* 2, 3–10.

Gartner, S., Markovits, P., Markovits, D.M., Kaplan, M.H., Gallo, R.C. and Popovic, M. (1986) The role of mononuclear phagocytes in HTLV-III/LAV infection. *Science* 233, 215–219.

Gelderblom, H. and Frank, H. (1987) Spumavirinae. In: M.V. Nermut and A.C Steven, (Eds.), *Animal Virus Structure.* Elsevier, Amsterdam, New York, Oxford, pp. 305–311.

Gelderblom, H., Özel, M. and Pauli, G. (1985a) T-Zell-spezifische Retroviren des Menschen: Vergleichende morphologische Klassifizierung und mögliche funktionelle Aspekte. *Bundesgesundh.-Blatt* 28, 161–171.

Gelderblom, H., Reupke, H. and Pauli, G. (1985b) Loss of envelope antigens of HTLV-III/LAV, a factor in AIDS pathogenesis? *Lancet* ii, 1016–1017.

Gelderblom, H., Reupke, H., Winkel, T., Kunze, R. and Pauli, G. (1987a) MHC-antigens: Constituents of the envelopes of human and simian immunodeficiency viruses. *Z. Naturforsch.* 42c, 1328–1334.

Gelderblom, H.R., Hausmann, E., Özel, M., Pauli, G. and Koch, M. (1987b) Fine structure of human immunodeficiency virus (HIV) and immunolocalization of structural proteins. *Virology* 156, 171–176.

Gelderblom, H.R., Özel, M., Hausmann, E.H.S., Winkel, T., Pauli, G. and Koch, M.A. (1988) Fine structure of human immunodeficiency virus (HIV), immunolocalization of structural proteins and virus-cell relation. *Micron Microscopica* 19, 41–60.

Gelderblom, H.R., Özel, M. and Pauli G. (1989) Morphogenesis and morphology of HIV, structure-function relations. *Arch. Virol.* 106, 1–13.

Gendelman, H.E., Narayan, O., Kennedy-Stoskopf, S., Kennedy, P.G.E., Ghotbi, Z., Clements, J.E., Stanley, J. and Pezeshkpour, G. (1986) Tropism of sheep lentiviruses for monocytes: susceptibility to infection and virus gene expression increase during maturation of monocytes to macrophages. *J. Virol.* 58, 67–74.

Gendelman, H.E., Orenstein, J.M., Baca, L.M., Weiser, B., Burger, H., Kalter, D.C. and Meltzer, M.S. (1989) The macrophage in the persistence and pathogenesis of HIV infection. *AIDS* 8, 475–496.

Georgiades, J.A., Billiau, A. and Vanderschueren, B. (1978) Infection of human cell cultures with bovine visna virus. *J. Gen. Virol.* 38, 375–381.

Gheysen, D., Jacobs, E., de Foresta, F., Thiriart, C., Francotte, M., Thines, D. and De Wilde, M. (1989) Assembly and release of HIV-1 precursor $Pr55^{gag}$ virus-like particles from recombinant baculovirus-infected insect cells. *Cell* 59, 103–112.

Gonda, M.A. (1988) Molecular genetics and structure of the human immunodeficiency virus. *J. Electron Microsc. Tech.* 8, 17–40.

Gonda, M.A., Braun, M.J., Carter, S.G., Kost, T.A., Bess Jr., J.W., Arthur, L.O. and Van Der Maaten, M.J. (1987) Characterization and molecular cloning of a bovine lentivirus related to human immundeficiency virus. *Nature* 330, 388–391.

Gonda, M.A., Charman, H.P., Walker, J.L. and Coggins, L. (1978) Scanning and transmission electron microscopic study of equine infectious anemia virus. *Am. J. Vet. Res.* 39, 731–740.

Gonda, M.A., Wong-Stall, F., Gallo, R.C. et al. (1985) Sequence homology and morphologic similarity of HTLV-III and visna virus, a pathogenic lentivirus. *Science* 227, 173–177.

Goto, T., Harada, S., Yamamoto, N. and Nakai, M. (1988) Entry of HIV into MT-2, human T cell leukemia virus carrier cell line. *Arch. Virol.* 102, 29–38.

Grief, C., Hockley, D.J., Fromholc, C.E. and Kitchin, P.A. (1989) The morphology of simian immunodeficiency virus as shown by negative staining electron microscopy. *J. Gen. Virol.* 70, 2215–2219.

Haase, A.T. (1989) Pathogenesis of lentivirus infections. *Nature* 322, 130–136.

Harris, J.R., Kitchen, A.D., Harrison, J.F. and Tovey, G. (1986) Viral release from HIV-1-induced syncytia of CD4+ C8166 cells. *J. Med. Virol.* 28, 81–89.

Harven, E. de (1974) Remarks on the ultrastructure of type A, B, and C virus particles. *Advances Virus Res.* 19, 221–264.

Haseltine, W.A. (1988) Replication and pathogenesis of the AIDS virus. *J. AIDS* 1, 217–240.

Haseltine, W.A. (1989) Development of antiviral drugs for treatment of AIDS, strategies and prospects. *J. AIDS* 2, 311–334.

Hausmann, E.H.S., Gelderblom, H.R., Clapham, P.R., Pauli, G. and Weiss, R.A. (1987) Detection of HIV envelope specific antibodies by immunoelectron microscopy and correlation with antibody titer and virus neutralizing activity. *J. Virol. Meth.* 16, 125–137.

Henderson, L.E., Krutzsch, H.C. and Oroszlan, S. (1983) Myristyl amino-terminal acylation of murine retrovirus proteins: An unusual post-translational protein modification. *Proc. Natl. Acad. Sci.* 80, 339–343.

Henderson, L.E., Sowder, R., Copeland, T.D., Oroszlan, S., Arthur, L.O., Robey, W.G. and Fischinger, P.J. (1987) Direct identification of class II histocompatibility DR proteins in preparations of human T-cell lymphotropic virus type III. *J. Virol.* 61, 629–632.

Henderson, L.E., Sowder, R., Smythers, G.W. and Oroszlan, S. (1987) Chemical and immunological characterization of equine infectious anemia virus *gag*-encoded proteins. *J. Virol.* 61, 1116–1124.

Henderson, L.E., Sowder, R.C., Copeland, T.D., Benveniste, R.E. and Oroszlan, S. (1988) Isolation and characterization of a novel protein (x-orf product) from SIV and HIV-2. *Science* 241, 199–201.

Hockley, D.J., Wood, R.D., Jacobs, J.P. and Garrett, A.J. (1988) Electron microscopy of human immunodeficiency virus. *J. Gen. Virol.* 69, 2455–2469.

Hooks, J.J. and Gibbs Jr., C.J. (1975) The foamy viruses. *Bact. Rev.* 39, 169–185.

Hoxie, J.A., Fitzharris, T.P., Youngbar, P.R., Matthews, D.M., Rackowski, J.L. and Radka, S.F. (1987) Nonrandom association of cellular antigens with HTLV-III virions. *Hum. Immunol.* 18, 39–52.

Jacobs, E., Gheysen, D., Thines, D., Francotte, M. and de Wilde, M. (1989) The HIV-1 *gag* precursor $Pr55^{gag}$ synthesized in yeast is myristoylated and targeted to the plasma membrane. *Gene* 79, 71–81.

Kannagi, M., Kiyotaki, M., King, N.W., Lord, C.I. and Letvin, N.L. (1987) Simian immunodeficiency virus induces expression of class II major histocompatibility complex structures on infected target cells in vitro. *J. Virol.* 61, 1421–1426.

Katsumoto, T., Hattori, N. and Kurimura, T. (1987) Maturation of human immunodeficiency virus, strain LAV, in vitro. *Intervirology* 27, 148–153.

Klatzmann, D., Champagne, E., Chamaret, S., Gruest, J., Guetard, D., Hercend, T., Gluckman, J.-C. and Montagnier, L. (1984) T-lymphocyte T4 molecule behaves as the receptor for human retrovirus LAV. *Nature* 312, 767–768.

Kobayashi, K. (1961) Studies on the cultivation of equine infectious anemia virus in vitro II. Propagation of the virus in horse bone marrow culture. *Virus* 11, 189–201.

Kohl, N.E., Emini, E.A., Schleif, W.A., Davis, L.J., Heimbach, J.C., Dixon, R.A.F., Scolnick, E.M. and Sigal, I.S. (1988) Active human immunodeficiency virus protease is required for viral infectivity. *Proc. Natl. Acad. Sci.* 85, 4686–4690.

Ladhoff, A.-M., Scholz, D., Rosenthal, S. and Rosenthal, H.A. (1986) Zur Struktur des AIDS-Virus—elektronenmikroskopische Untersuchungen. *Z. Klin. Med.* 41, 2209–2214.

Lanzavecchia, A., Roosnek, E., Gregory, T., Berman, P. and Abrignani, S. (1988) T cells can present antigens such as HIV gp120 targeted to their own surface molecules. *Nature* 334, 530–532.

Lasky, L.A., Nakamura, G., Smith, D.H., Fennie, C., Shimasaki, C., Patzer, E., Berman, P., Gregory, T. and Capon, D.J. (1987) Delineation of a region of the human immunodeficiency virus type 1 gp120 glycoprotein critical for interaction with the CD4 receptor. *Cell* 50, 975–985.

Laurent, A.G., Krust, B., Rey, M.A., Montagnier, L. and Hovanessian, A.G. (1989) Cell surface expression of several species of human immunodeficiency virus type 1 major core protein. *J. Virol.* 63, 4074–4078.

Lecatsas, G., Gravell, M. and Sever, J.L. (1984) Morphology of the retroviruses associated with AIDS and SAIDS. *Proc. Soc. Exp. Biol. Med.* 177, 495–498.

Leis, J., Baltimore, D., Bishop, J.M., Coffin, J., Fleissner, E., Goff, S.P., Oroszlan, S., Robinson, H., Skalka, A.M., Temin, H.M. and Vogt, V. (1988) Standardized and simplified nomenclature for proteins common to all retroviruses. *J. Virol.* 62, 1808–1809.

Lever, A., Göttlinger, H., Haseltine, W. and Sodroski, J. (1989) Identification of a sequence required for efficient packaging of human immunodeficiency virus type 1 RNA into virions. *J. Virol.* 63, 4085–4087.

Lifson, J.D., Feinborg, M.B., Reyes, G.R., Rabin, L., Banapour, B., Chakrabarti, S., Moss, B., Wong-Staal, F., Steimer, K.S. and Engleman, E.G. (1986) Induction of CD4-dependent cell fusion by the HTLVIII/LAV envelope glycoprotein. *Nature* 323, 725–728.

Lusso, P., Markham, P.D., Ranki, A., Earl, P., Moss, B., Dorner, F., Gallo, R.C. and Krohn, K.J.E. (1988) Cell-mediated immune response toward viral envelope and core antigens in gibbon apes (*Hylobates lar*) chronically infected with human immunodeficiency virus-1. *J. Immunol.* 141, 2467–2473.

Marsh, M. and Helenius, A. (1989) Virus entry into animal cells. In: K. Maramorosch, F.A. Murphey and A.J. Shatkin (Eds.), *Advances in Virus Research,* Vol. 36. Academic Press, San Diego, pp. 107–158.

Marx, P.A., Munn, R.J. and Joy, K.I. (1988) Computer emulation of thin section electron microscopy predicts an envelope-associated icosadeltahedral capsid for human immunodeficiency virus. *Lab. Invest.* 58, 112–118.

Matthews, R.E.F. (1982) Classification and nomenclature of viruses. *Fourth report of the International Committee on Taxonomy of Viruses.* Karger, Basel, pp. 234–238.

Maurer, B. and Flügel, R.M. (1988) Genomic organization of the human spumaretrovirus and its relatedness to AIDS and other retroviruses. *AIDS Res. Human Retroviruses* 4, 467–473.

McClure, M., Marsh, M. and Weiss, R. (1988) HIV infection of CD4 bearing cells occurs by a pH independent mechanism. *EMBO J.* 7, 513–518.

McCune, J.M., Rabin, L.B., Feinberg, M.B., Liebermann, M., Kosek, J.C., Reyes, G.R. and Weissmann, I.L. (1988) Endoproteolytic cleavage of gp160 is required for the activation of human immunodeficiency virus. *Cell* 53, 55–67.

Modrow, S., Hahn, B.H., Shaw, G.M., Gallo, R.C., Wong-Staal, F. and Wolf, H. (1987) Computer-assisted analysis of envelope protein sequences of seven human immunodeficiency virus isolates: prediction of antigenic epitopes in conserved and variable regions. *J. Virol.* 61, 570–578.

Montagnier, L., Chermann, J.C., Barré-Sinoussi, F., Chamaret, S., Gruest, J., Nugeyre, M.T., Rey, F., Dauguet, C., Axler-Blin, C., Vézinet-Brun, F., Rouzioux, C., Saimot, G.-A., Rozenbaum, W., Gluckman, J.C., Klatzmann, D., Vilmer, E., Griscelli, C., Foyer-Gazengel, C. and Brunet, J.B. (1984) A new human T-lymphotropic retrovirus: characterization and possible role in lymphadenopathy and acquired immune deficiency syndromes. In: R.C. Gallo, M.E. Essex and L. Gross (Eds.), *Human T-cell Leukemia/Lymphoma Virus.* Cold Spring Harbor Laboratory, Cold Spring Harbor, NY, pp. 363–379.

Montelaro, R.C., Robey, W.G., West, M.D., Issel, C.J. and Fischinger, P.J. (1988) Characterization of the serological cross-reactivity between glycoproteins of the human immunodeficiency virus and equine infectious anaemia virus. *J. Gen. Virol.* 69, 1711–1717.

Muesing, M.A., Smith, D.H., Cabradilla, C.D., Benton, C.V., Lasky, L.A. and Capon, D.J. (1985) Nucleic acid structure and expression of the human AIDS/lymphadenopathy retrovirus. *Nature* 313, 450–458.

Munn, R., Marx, P.A., Yamamoto, J.K. and Gardner, M.B. (1985) Ultrastructural comparison of the retroviruses associated with human and simian acquired immunodeficiency syndrome. *Lab. Invest.* 53, 194–199.

Murphey-Corb, M., Martin, L.N., Rangan, S.R.S., Baskin, G.B., Gormus, B.J., Wolf, R.H., Andes, W.A., West, M. and Montelaro, R.C. (1986) Isolation of an HTLV-III-related retrovirus from macaques with simian AIDS and its possible origin in asymptomatic mangabyes. *Nature* 321, 435–437.

Nakai, M., Goto, T. and Imura, S. (1989) Ultrastructural features of the AIDS virus (HIV) and its morphogenesis. *J. Electron Microsc. Tech.* 12, 95–100.

Narayan, O. and Clements J.E. (1989) Biology and pathogenesis of lentiviruses. *J. Gen. Virol.* 70, 1617–1639.

Niedrig, M., Rabanus, J.-P., L'age-Stehr, J., Gelderblom, H.R. and Pauli, G. (1988) Monoclonal antibodies directed against human immunodeficiency virus (HIV) *gag* proteins with specificity for conserved epitopes in HIV-1, HIV-2 and simian immunodeficiency viruses. *J. Gen. Virol.* 69, 2109–2114.

Nixon, D.F., Townsend, A.R.M., Elvin, J.G., Rizza, C.R., Gallwey, J. and McMichael, A.J. (1988) HIV-1 *gag*-specific cytotoxic T lymphocytes defined with recombinant vaccinia virus and synthetic peptides. *Nature* 336, 484–487.

North, T.W., North, G.L.T. and Pedersen, N.C. (1989) Feline immunodeficiency virus, a model for reverse transcriptase-targeted chemotherapy for acquired immune deficiency syndrome. *Antimicrobial Agents Chemother.* 33, 915–919.

Ohta, Y., Masuda, T., Tsujimoto, H., Ishikawa, K., Kodama, T., Morikawa, S., Nakai, M., Honjo, S. and Hayami, M. (1988) Isolation of simian immunodeficiency virus from African green monkeys and seroepidemiologic survey of the virus in various non-human primates. *Int. J. Cancer* 41, 115–122.

Overton, H.A., Fujii, Y., Price, I.R. and Jones, I.M. (1989) The protease and *gag* gene products of the human immunodeficiency virus: authentic cleavage and post-translational modification in an insect cell expression system. *Virology* 170, 107–116.

Özel, M., Pauli, G., and Gelderblom, H.R. (1988) The organization of the envelope projections on the surface of HIV. *Arch. Virol.* 100, 255–266.

Palmer, E. and Goldsmith, C.S. (1988) Ultrastructure of human retroviruses. *J. Electron Microsc. Tech.* 8, 3–15.

Palmer, E., Martin, M.L., Goldsmith, C. and Switzer, W. (1988) Ultrastructure of human immunodeficiency virus type 2. *J. Gen. Virol.* 69, 1425–1429.

Parekh, B., Issel, C.J. and Montelaro, R.C. (1980) Equine infectious anemia virus, a putative lentivirus, contains polypeptides analogous to prototype-C oncornaviruses. *Virology* 107, 520–525.

Patterson, S. and Knight S.C. (1987) Susceptibility of human peripheral blood dendritic cells to infection by human immunodeficiency virus. *J. Gen. Virol.* 68, 1177–1181.

Pauli, G., Rohde, W. and Harms, E. (1978) The structure of the Rous sarcoma virus glycoprotein complex. *Arch. Virol.* 58, 61–64.

Pauza, C.D. and Price, T.M. (1988) HIV infection of T-cells and monocytes proceeds via receptor-mediated endocytosis. *J. Cell Biol.* 107, 959–968.

Pedersen, N.C, Ho, E.M., Brown, M.L. and Yamamoto, J.K. (1987) Isolation of a T-lymphotropic virus from domestic cats with an immunodeficiency-like syndrome. *Science* 235, 790–793.

Perk, K. (1988) Ungulate lentiviruses: pathogenesis and relationship to AIDS. In: K. Perk (Ed.), *Immunodeficiency Disorders and Retroviruses. Advances in Veterinary Science and Comparative Medicine,* Vol. 32. Academic Press, London, pp. 97–124.

Pétursson, G., Pálsson, P.A. and Georgsson, G. (1989) Maedi-visna in sheep: host-virus interactions and utilization as a model. *Intervirology* 30, 36–44.

Pinter, A. and Fleissner, E. (1977) The presence of disulfide-linked gp70-p15E complexes in AKR murine leukemia virus. *Virology* 83, 417–422.

Pinter, A., Honnen, W.J., Tilley, S.A., Bona, C., Zaghouani, H., Gorny, M.K. and Zolla-Pazner, S. (1989) Oligomeric structure of gp41, the transmembrane protein of human immunodeficiency virus type 1. *J. Virol.* 63, 2674–2679.

Popovic, M., Sarngadharan, M.G., Read, E. and Gallo, R.C. (1984) Detection, isolation and continuous production of cytopathic retrovirus (HTLV-III) from patients with AIDS and pre-AIDS. *Science* 224, 497–500.

Putney, S.D. and Montelaro, R.C. (1989) Immunobiology and immunochemistry of lentiviruses. In: A.R. Neurath and M.H.V. van Regenmortel (Eds.), *Immunochemistry of Viruses II.* Elsevier, Amsterdam, 309–346.

Rein, A., McClure, M.R., Rice, N.R., Luftig, R.B. and Schultz, A.M. (1986) Myristylation site in

$Pr65^{gag}$ is essential for virus particle formation by Moloney murine leukemia virus. *Proc. Natl. Acad. Sci.* 83, 7246–7250.

Ribas, T., Hase, E., Hunter, E., Fritz, D., Khan, N. and Burke, D. (1988) HIV enters cells by fusion with cell membrane. *IVth International Conference on AIDS,* Stockholm, Abstract No. 1025.

Riviere, Y., Tanneau-Salvadori, F., Regnault, A., Lopez, O., Sansonetti, P., Guy, B., Kieny, M.-P., Fournel, J.-J. and Montagnier, L. (1989) Human immunodeficiency virus-specific cytotoxic responses of seropositive individuals: distinct types of effector cells mediated killing of targets expressing *gag* and *env* proteins. *J. Virol.* 63, 2270–2277.

Roberts, M.M. and Oroszlan, S. (1989) The preparation and biochemical characterization of intact capsids of equine infectious anemia virus. *Biochem. Biophys. Res. Comm.* 160, 486–494.

Rosenberg, Z.F. and Fauci, A.S. (1989) Immunopathogenic mechanisms of HIV infection. *Clin. Immunol. Immunopathol.* 50, 149–156.

Sarkar, N.H. (1987) Oncovirinae: type B oncovirus. In: M.V. Nermut and A.C. Steven, (Eds.), *Animal Virus Structure.* Elsevier, Amsterdam, New York, Oxford, pp. 257–272.

Schawaller, M., Smith, G.E., Skehel, J.J. and Wiley, D.C. (1989) Studies with crosslinking reagents on the oligomeric structure of the *env* glycoprotein of HIV. *Virology* 172, 367–369.

Schidlovsky, G., Shibley, G.P., Benton, C.V. and Elser, J.E. (1978) Type B and type C RNA tumor virus replication in single cells. Electron microscopy with tannic acid. *J. Natl. Cancer Inst.* 61, 91–95.

Schneider, J. and Hunsmann, G. (1978) Surface expression of murine leukemia structural polypeptides on host cells and the virion. *Int. J. Cancer* 22, 204–213.

Schneider, J. and Hunsmann, G. (1988) Simian lentiviruses—the SIV group. *AIDS* 2, 1–9.

Schneider, J., Jurkiewicz, E., Wendler, I., Jentsch, K.D., Bayer, H., Desrosiers, R.C., Gelderblom, H. and Hunsmann, G. (1987) Structural, biochemical and serological comparison of LAV/HTLV-III and STLV-IIImac, to primate lentiviruses. In: R.C. Gallo, W. Haseltine, G. Klein and H. zur Hausen (Eds.), *Viruses and Human Cancer.* Alan R. Liss, Inc., New York, pp. 319–332.

Schneider, J., Kaaden, O., Copeland, T.D., Oroszlan, S. and Hunsmann, G. (1986) Shedding and interspecies-type seroreactivity of the envelope glycopolypeptide gp120 of the human immunodeficiency virus. *J. Gen. Virol.* 67, 2533–2538.

Schwarz, H., Hunsmann, G., Moenning, V. and Schäfer, W. (1976) Properties of mouse leukemia viruses: XI. Immunoelectron microscopic studies on viral structural antigens on the cell surface. *Virology* 69, 169–178.

Sigurdsson, B. (1954) Observations on three slow infections of sheep. *Br. Vet. J.* 110, 255–270.

Sigurdsson, B., Thormar, H. and Pálsson, P.A. (1960) Cultivation of visna virus in tissue culture. *Arch. Ges. Virusforsch.* 10, 368–381.

Siliciano, R.F., Lawton, T., Knall, C., Karr, R.W., Berman, P., Gregory, T. and Reinherz, E.L. (1988) Analysis of host-virus interactions in AIDS with anti-gp120 T-cell clones: Effect of HIV sequence variation and a mechanism for CD4+ cell depletion. *Cell* 54, 561–575.

Sodroski, J., Goh, W.C., Rosen, C., Campbell, K. and Haseltine, W.A. (1986) Role of the HTLV-III/LAV envelope in syncytium formation and cytopathicity. *Nature* 322, 470–474.

Sölder, B.M., Schulz, T.F., Hengster, P., Löwer, J., Larcher, C., Bitterlich, G., Kurth, R., Wachter, H. and Dierich, M.P. (1989) HIV and HIV-infected cells differentially activate the human complement system independent of antibody. *Immunol. Lett.* 22, 135–146.

Somasundaran, M. and Robinson, H.L. (1988) Unexpectedly high levels of HIV-1 RNA and protein synthesis in a cytocidal infection. *Science* 242, 1554–1557.

Stein, B.S., Gowda, S.D., Lifson, J.D., Penhallow, R.C., Bensch, K.G. and Engleman, E.G. (1987) pH-independent HIV entry into CD4-positive T cells via virus envelope fusion to the plasma membrane. *Cell* 49, 659–668.

Takahashi, I., Takama, M., Ladhoff, A.M. and Scholz, D. (1989) Envelope structure model of human immunodeficiency virus type 1. *J. AIDS* 2, 136–140.

Tsujimoto, H., Cooper, R.W., Kodama, T., Fukasawa, M., Miura, T., Ohta, Y., Ishikawa, K.-J., Nakai, M., Frost, E., Roelants, G.E., Roffi, J. and Hayami, M. (1988) Isolation and characterization of simian immunodeficiency virus from mandrills in Africa and its relationship to other human and simian immunodeficiency viruses. *J. Virol.* 62, 4044–4050.

Vallée, H. and Carré, H. (1904) Sur la nature infectieuse de l'anémie du cheval. *C.R. Acad. Sci.* 139, 331–333.

Van Der Maaten, M.J., Boothe, A.D. and Seger, C.L. (1972) Isolation of a virus from cattle with persistent lymphocytosis. *J. Natl. Cancer Inst.* 49, 1649–1657.

Veronese, F.M., Copeland, T.D., Oroszlan, S., Gallo, R.C. and Sarngadharan, M.G. (1988) Biochemical and immunological analysis of human immunodeficiency virus *gag* gene products p17 and p24. *J. Virol.* 62, 795–801.

Walker, B.D., Flexner, C., Paradis, T.J., Fuller, T.C., Hirsch, M.S., Schooley, R.T. and Moss, B. (1988) HIV-1 reverse transcriptase is a target for cytotoxic T lymphocytes in infected individuals. *Science* 240, 64–66.

Weiland, F. and Bruns, M. (1980) Ultrastructural studies on maedi-visna virus. *Arch. Virol.* 64, 277–285.

Weiland, F., Matheka, H.D., Coggins, L. and Härtner, D. (1977) Electron microscopic studies on equine infectious anemia virus (EIAV). *Arch. Virol.* 55, 335–340.

Weinhold, E. (1974) Visna-Virus-ähnliche Partikel in der Kultur von Plexus choroideus Zellen einer Ziege mit Visna-Symptomen. *Zentralbl. Vet. Med.* B. 21, 32–36.

Weiss, R., Teich, N., Varmus, H. and Coffin, J. (1984) *RNA Tumor Viruses: Molecular Biology of Tumor Viruses,* 2nd edn. Cold Spring Harbor Laboratory, Cold Spring Harbor, NY.

Weiss, R.A. (1988) Foamy retroviruses. A virus in search of a disease. *Nature* 333, 497–498.

Willey, R.L., Ross, E.K., Buckler-White, A.J., Theodore, T.S. and Martin, M.A. (1989) Functional interaction of constant and variable domains of human immunodeficiency virus type 1 gp120. *J. Virol.* 63, 3595–3600.

Yoffe, B., Lewis, D.E., Petrie, B.L., Noonan, C.A., Melnick, J.L. and Hollinger, F.B. (1987) Fusion as a mediator of cytolysis in mixtures of uninfected CD4+ lymphocytes and cells infected by human immunodeficiency virus. *Proc. Natl. Acad. Sci.* 84, 1429–1433.

*Eds. H. Schellekens and M.C. Horzinek*
*Animal Models in AIDS*



# 2

# Human immunodeficiency virus infection: perspectives and challenges

PETER REISS [1] and JOEP M.A. LANGE [1,2]

[1] Department of Medicine, AIDS Unit, and [2] Human Retrovirus Laboratory, Academic Medical Center, Amsterdam, The Netherlands

## Introduction

The acquired immunodeficiency syndrome (AIDS) is caused by a retrovirus known as the human immunodeficiency virus (HIV) (Barre-Sinoussi et al., 1983; Gallo et al., 1984; Levy et al., 1984; Popovic et al., 1984), which is usually classified within the subfamily of lentiviruses (Gonda et al., 1984). However, HIV also has certain characteristics in common with the human oncoviruses HTLV-1 and HTLV-2, such as its T-cell tropism and genomic organization (Reitz and Gallo, 1990).

AIDS represents the extreme of the clinical spectrum of infection with HIV, and is characterized by the occurrence of opportunistic infections, certain malignancies, and neurological disorders.

Primary infection with HIV may be clinically silent, or subjects may show transient signs and symptoms of disease which may vary from a minor flu-like or mononucleosis-like illness to a severe illness accompanied by fever, erythematous rash, enanthema, pneumonitis, oropharyngeal and esophageal ulcers, and less commonly aseptic meningitis or encephalitis (Cooper et al., 1985; Gaines et al., 1988; Reiss et al., 1985). These symptoms occur several weeks after infection with HIV, at which time p24 core antigen can usually be transiently detected in the serum, followed by seroconversion for antibodies to both viral structural and non-structural proteins (Gaines et al., 1987; Lange et al., 1986). A window phase of a few weeks during which no HIV-specific antibodies are detectable may follow the transient detection of serum p24 core antigen (personal observation). Subsequently the HIV-seropositive subject enters an asymptomatic phase, which usually lasts several years, but in exceptional cases only lasts several months.

About half of the subjects develop persistent generalized lymphadenopathy during this asymptomatic phase, the development of which has not been found to be associated with progression to other symptoms of disease, when compared to the course of infection in subjects who remain fully asymptomatic. Following the asymptomatic phase patients may develop AIDS or AIDS-related disorders, as a consequence of the progressive immunodeficiency induced by HIV. The virus preferentially infects CD4 + T-helper lymphocytes, which through several mechanisms leads to a progressive reduction in the number, as well as to functional abnormalities of these cells (Fauci, 1988). Since CD4 + lymphocytes play a central role in the control of most normal immune responses, their depletion and dysfunction lead to severe, both cellular and humoral immunodeficiency. This again results in the wide array of infections (Kovacs and Masur, 1988) and the typical malignancies (Kaposi's sarcoma and malignant lymphomas) (Krigel and Friedman-Kien, 1988; Levine, 1988) associated with AIDS. HIV also has been found to infect both the central and peripheral nervous systems (Rosenblum et al., 1988). Currently, HIV-induced brain damage is thought to result not so much from direct infection of neurons, but rather from infection of microglial cells and astrocytes, resulting in the secretion of "factors" by these cells, which may then subsequently lead to dysfunction and damage of neurons. Clinically neurological symptoms are estimated to occur in 40% of patients with AIDS, and 75% of patients have been found to have nervous system abnormalities at autopsy. The clinical neurological syndromes thought to be the direct result of HIV infection in patients with AIDS are an encephalopathy resulting in the so-called AIDS-dementia complex, vacuolar myelopathy, and various types of peripheral neuropathy (Ho, 1989).

## Epidemiology

Several modes of transmission of HIV have been delineated.

(1) Sexual transmission, by both homosexual (Centers for Disease Control, 1981) and heterosexual (Johnson and Laga, 1988) contact. In the case of heterosexual contact, both male to female and female to male transmission occurs, the latter mode possibly being less frequent. Receptive anal sex (Kingsley et al., 1987; Van Griensven et al., 1987), the presence of genital ulceration (Latif et al., 1989), and sex with uncircumcised men (Bongaarts et al., 1989), have all been reported to increase the likelihood of sexual transmission of HIV.

(2) Exposure to HIV-infected blood, blood components, and tissues, as in the case of intravenous drug users (sharing contaminated needles) (Schoenbaum et al., 1989), hemophiliacs (Goedert et al., 1989), and transfusion recipients (Ward et al., 1989), organ transplant recipients, and people who are accidentally exposed (e.g., needle stick injuries).

(3) Pre- and perinatal transmission of HIV from an HIV-infected mother to her child (Ryder and Hassig, 1988). Transmission is thought to occur before birth through transplacental passage, or at the time of birth, or probably less commonly after birth through breastfeeding.

The distribution of cases of AIDS in adults in the U.S.A., as of July 31, 1989, is shown in Table 1 (Statistics from WHO/CDC, 1989a). In men the majority of

TABLE 1
Distribution of adult cases of AIDS by sex and risk group, in the U.S.A. CDC data as of July 31, 1989

| Risk group | Male (%) | Female (%) |
|---|---|---|
| Homo/bisexual | 67 | |
| IVDU | 17 | 52 |
| Homo/bisexual contact and IVDU | 8 | |
| Hemophilia/coagulation disorder | 1 | |
| Heterosexual contact | 2 | 30 |
| Recipient of transfusion of blood/blood components, or tissues | 2 | 10 |
| Other/undetermined | 3 | 8 |

IVDU, intravenous drug use.

TABLE 2
Cumulative number of cases of AIDS reported by region. WHO/CDC data as of July 31, 1989

| Region | Cumulative number of cases |
|---|---|
| U.S.A. | 98,255 |
| Americas (incl. U.S.A.) | 116,524 |
| Europe | 23,566 |
| Africa | 30,082 |
| S.E. Asia | 59 |
| Western Pacific (incl. Australia) | 1,678 |
| Total | 172,143 |

cases are found in homo- and bisexual men and in intravenous drug users, while in women most cases have been diagnosed in intravenous drug users and in women who have become infected by heterosexual contact with intravenous drug users and bisexual men.

AIDS has become a global problem, with cases having been reported from all areas of the world, as shown in Table 2 (Statistics from WHO/CDC, 1989b). The disease remains incurable, and in the U.S.A. of the 100,000 cases reported by mid-1989 over half had died. Of the cases reported prior to 1986 over 80% have died (Statistics from WHO/CDC, 1989c).

## Management of HIV-infected individuals

The challenges involved in the management of HIV-infected individuals are many, but we will limit our discussion to some of those described in Table 3.

### Treatment of the underlying retroviral infection

No definitive therapy of HIV infection has been developed so far, and therefore prevention of infection by behavioral modification in order to combat

TABLE 3
Challenges in the management of HIV-infected individuals

- Treatment of underlying retroviral infection
- Treatment of the HIV-induced immunodeficiency
- Treatment of opportunistic infections
- Treatment of malignancies
- Treatment of other HIV-related disorders, e.g., HIV-related thrombocytopenia
- Psychosocial management
- Financial issues

the AIDS epidemic remains of the utmost importance. The potential approaches to treatment of established HIV infection can be divided into the following.

(1) Boosting of protective immune responses to the virus (post-exposure vaccination). The prerequisites for such an approach are identification of the nature of the protective immune response in the human host, identification of the epitopes responsible for such a response, and finally development and testing of a vaccine based on these epitopes (Dalgleish, 1988).
(2) Attempts at ameliorating the HIV-induced immunodeficiency.
(3) Development of anti-retroviral drugs. Ideally such drugs should have the following characteristics: (a) high activity against HIV, ultimately leading to eradication of infection; (b) good penetration at all sites of infection, including the central nervous system (CNS); (c) lack of toxicity; (d) lack of induction of resistance; (e) possibility of both oral and parenteral administration; (f) low cost.

At the time of this writing the development within the near future of an effective vaccine seems extremely unlikely, as does the development of anti-retroviral drugs with all of the above characteristics.

When conducting clinical trials of drugs with potential anti-retroviral activity in vivo, one can distinguish trials in subjects with symptoms of HIV-related disease (early symptoms, e.g., oral candidiasis only, or late symptoms characteristic of AIDS), from trials in HIV-infected but still symptom-free subjects. In the former, the ultimate goal of anti-retroviral therapy would be the prevention of further signs and symptoms of HIV-related disease, whereas in the latter the goal would be preventing HIV-related disease manifestations from occurring at all. In this connection one can think of trials involving all such symptom-free individuals, or primarily individuals identified to be at increased risk of (rapid) disease progression. Examples of markers which have been described as being predictive of disease progression are persistence of p24 core antigenemia, low anti-core antibody reactivity, low CD4+ cell numbers, and elevated serum $\beta$-2 microglobulin levels (Lange et al., 1990; Moss and Bacchetti, 1989). However, the set of markers predictive of disease progression may vary over time (De Wolf et al., 1989), and only be identified after the spectrum and time course of HIV-related disease development have fully crystallized. Therefore continuing studies of large cohorts of HIV-infected individuals remain important to identify just such panels

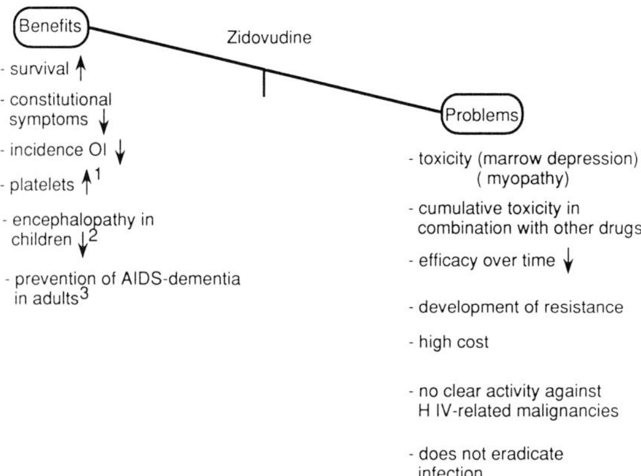


Fig. 1. Benefits and disadvantages of treatment with zidovudine in patients with AIDS and other HIV-related disease manifestations. Numbers refer to references: 1: Hirschel et al., 1988; 2: Pizzo et al., 1988; 3: Portegies et al., 1989.

of markers with optimal predictive power. Here early intervention with anti-retroviral drugs, which may well produce short- or long-term toxicity, could primarily be directed at individuals found to be at highest risk of rapidly developing disease.

The only drug so far shown to have beneficial clinical effects in patients with recently diagnosed AIDS and severe AIDS-related complex (ARC) is the nucleoside analogue zidovudine (AZT or 2′,3′-azidothymidine) (Fischl et al., 1987). Unfortunately, as experience with the use of zidovudine has increased, it has become clear that apart from the beneficial effects, this drug also has very significant drawbacks. Schematically the balance between benefits and drawbacks of zidovudine is depicted in Fig. 1. When put on a scale, the problems encountered when using zidovudine in patients already showing signs of HIV-induced disease seem to outweigh the benefits. Apart from the toxicity of the drug (Richman et al., 1987), which often is accentuated in clinical practice because of the frequent need to use other bone marrow suppressive drugs in these patients, the efficacy of zidovudine in preventing the further occurrence of manifestations of AIDS clearly diminishes over time (Dournon et al., 1988). That this may be due to the recently described in vitro resistance to zidovudine of HIV isolates obtained from patients receiving the drug for prolonged periods (Larder et al., 1989) seems likely but remains to be definitively proven. The lessons learned from the use of zidovudine should obviously be taken into account when judging the benefits and disadvantages of newly developed anti-retroviral agents. Attempts at optimization of anti-retroviral therapy in the near future may well involve the use of combinations or alternating regimens of different drugs, acting at the same or at different levels of the viral life cycle (Yarchoan et al., 1989). The advantages of such an approach may be an increase of the efficacy of therapy both short- and long-term, prevention of the occurrence of resistance, and reduction of toxicities by the possibility of using lower doses of each drug without loss of efficacy. The latter may also lead to a reduction of cumulative toxicity, when combining the anti-retroviral agents with other, e.g., antimicrobial, agents with similar toxicity profiles. Due to its mechanism of action zidovudine may only prevent HIV infection from becoming established in still uninfected cells, but does not prevent or reduce viral replication in already infected cells. Therefore development of therapy maintaining HIV in a latent state in such already infected cells is important as a supplement to therapy preventing HIV infection of uninfected cells. Understanding the viral and host factors which are important in maintaining latency will improve the chances of developing such therapeutic approaches. Since HIV like other retroviruses becomes integrated into the host cell genome, leading to persistent infection, complete eradication of the virus from the host does not seem feasible, and maintenance of latency is all one can hope to achieve in cells that are infected.

### Treatment of HIV-induced immunodeficiency

As has been mentioned, the ultimate mechanism by which HIV produces its devastating effects in man is the induction of a severe state of immunodeficiency. Therefore in treating HIV-infected individuals a possible approach could be to try and reconstitute the damaged immune system. Unfortunately however, the targets of HIV infection are just those cells that play a pivotal role in the immune system, CD4+ helper lymphocytes and blood monocytes as well as tissue macrophages. Activation of these target cells seems important in the switch from latent to productive HIV infection, and therefore one could envision immunomodulating therapies to adversely activate HIV infection, as well as to increase the pool of cells that may be infected by the virus. Consequently, in developing immunomodulating therapies, one seriously has to consider combining such an approach with concomitant anti-retroviral therapy.

### Treatment of opportunistic infections

Although treatment is available for many of the infectious complications of AIDS, substantial problems in managing these infections remain, some of which will be discussed.

#### *Treatment of severe Pneumocystis carinii pneumonia (PCP)*

PCP is the most common opportunistic infection in patients with AIDS and is also the most common primary manifestation of this disease. Mild PCP is easy to treat with drugs such as cotrimoxazole, but severe forms of the infection still carry a high mortality rate. Studies are ongoing to determine whether adjunctive therapy with corticosteroids may reduce mortality in severe PCP (Bozzette et al., 1989; MacFadden et al., 1987; Walmsley et al., 1988). Preliminary results indicate that this may indeed be the case, but investigators are warning that such therapeutic strategies may also increase the risk of other opportunistic infections in the months following treatment of PCP. This could possibly be the result of steroid-induced immunodeficiency, which added to the HIV-induced immunodeficiency may well be imagined to be harmful.

*Primary and secondary prophylaxis of PCP*

The risk of developing PCP in HIV-infected subjects has been found to increase substantially when CD4 + cell numbers drop below 200/mm$^3$ (Masur et al., 1989), raising the issue of primary prophylaxis in such individuals. In addition, in patients who have been successfully treated for PCP there is a high rate of recurrence of this infection, which can be reduced by secondary prophylaxis (maintenance therapy). Cotrimoxazole, which currently remains the first choice for treating PCP, is probably also quite effective as both a primary and a secondary prophylactic agent, but the high incidence of toxicity due to this drug in HIV-infected subjects is an important drawback. Because of this, alternative prophylaxis with nebulized pentamidine which seems to show less systemic toxicity is currently much advocated (Girard et al., 1989; Golden et al., 1989; Murphy et al., 1989). However, though comparative trials still need to be performed, the failure rate of nebulized pentamidine prophylaxis is suspected to be higher than of cotrimoxazole. Also Pneumocystis infections occurring and recurring in patients on nebulized pentamidine prophylaxis may show differences in clinical presentation, with pulmonary upper lobe involvement and extrapulmonary infection being increasingly reported in such patients (Hardy et al., 1989; Poblete et al., 1989; Raviglione et al., 1989).

*Treatment of meningitis due to Cryptococcus neoformans*

The established treatment of cryptococcal meningitis consists of amphotericin B either alone or in combination with fluorocytosine (Bennett et al., 1979). Amphotericin B has to be administered intravenously over a period of at least 4–6 weeks. As is true for most opportunistic infections in patients with AIDS, because of the high recurrence rate of cryptococcal meningitis (Chuck and Sande, 1989), there is a need for lifelong maintenance treatment, involving once or twice weekly infusion of the drug (Zuger et al., 1988). Lifelong parenteral administration of amphotericin B obviously puts a major burden on the patient as well as the health care system, and apart from this the drug may produce severe side effects, most notably nephrotoxicity. Newer antifungal drugs, which are currently being investigated as alternative treatments for cryptococcal meningitis in AIDS, are fluconazole and itraconazole, both belonging to the class of triazoles. Both drugs can be given orally and have favorable toxicity profiles (De Gans et al., 1988; Denning et al., 1989; Stern et al., 1988; Sugar and Saunders, 1988). Preliminary results from clinical trials comparing these agents with amphotericin B indicate that, though active, they may be less effective than amphotericin B. Especially in severe cases of cryptococcal meningitis amphotericin B seems to achieve sterilization of the cerebrospinal fluid (CSF) more frequently and efficiently (Dismukes et al., 1989; Larsen and Leal, 1989). Following effective induction therapy with any regimen, fluconazole and itraconazole both seem able to prevent clinical relapse by chronic suppression of the infection. In the future one may think of designing therapeutic regimens for cryptococcal meningitis involving short courses of amphotericin B to achieve sterilization of the CSF, followed by lifelong maintenance with oral triazoles. Also nephrotoxicity of amphotericin B may possibly be reduced by using liposomal preparations of the drug, which can incorporate higher doses of drug, albeit with reduced nephrotoxicity.

*Treatment of Candida infections*

Oropharyngeal and esophageal candidiasis, which has become clinically refractory to treatment with established as well as newer (fluconazole, itraconazole) antifungal agents, seems to be an emerging clinical problem in patients with AIDS. This may well be due to development of drug resistance, which would not be surprising in view of the *chronic* use of therapy against Candida in many of these patients. Thus there is a clear need for developing reliable sensitivity assays for antifungals, and better drug regimens, possibly involving intermittent rather than continuous administration of single drugs or combinations of drugs.

*Treatment of resistant Herpes virus infections*

Infections with viruses belonging to the Herpes virus family, especially herpes simplex (HSV), cytomegalovirus (CMV) and varicella zoster (VZV), are a frequent cause of morbidity and mortality in patients with AIDS. Mucocutaneous HSV infections and CMV infections in these patients have a strong tendency to recur when therapy is stopped, thereby again producing the need for chronic suppressive treatment with antiviral drugs. This has led to the emerging problem of HSV and CMV infections that have become clinically and virologically less sensitive or even completely resistant to some of the antiviral drugs currently available for the treatment of these infections. So far development of resistance has been noted for HSV infections to aciclovir (Erlich et al., 1989), with potential cross-resistance to ganciclovir ([9-(1,3-dihydroxy-2-propoxymethyl)guanine] or DHPG), and for CMV infections to ganciclovir (Erice et al., 1989). Foscarnet (phosphonophormate) has been found effective in treating HSV and CMV infections that have become resistant to treatment with aciclovir and ganciclovir (Chatis et al., 1989). However, the side effects of foscarnet have not been fully delineated, and once the drug is used more frequently and for longer, the expectation would be that resistance to this drug will also become apparent. Thus a search is needed for alternative regimens, which may be used for prolonged treatment of these infections, without the development of resistance or serious toxicity.

*Infections for which no effective treatment is available*

No truly effective therapy has been established for various opportunistic infections occurring in patients with AIDS. Infections to be mentioned in this category are those caused by Cryptosporidium and Microsporidium, parasites producing diarrhea in these patients, and those caused by "atypical mycobacteria", most notably of the *Mycobacterium avium intracellulare* complex.

These latter pathogens may produce a clinical debilitating syndrome characterized by fever, malaise, wasting, diarrhea, pulmonary and liver involvement.

*Development of alternative treatment for infections, in view of the toxicities of effective "established" treatment*

Examples of drugs used, and their frequently occurring toxicities in patients with HIV infection are:

| Infection | "Established" treatment | Toxicity |
|---|---|---|
| PCP | cotrimoxazole | skin rash, fever, bone marrow suppression |
| Cerebral toxoplasmosis | sulfadiazine + pyrimethamine | skin rash, fever, bone marrow suppression |
| Fungal | amphotericin B, fluorocytosine | nephrotoxicity, bone marrow suppression, hepatotoxicity |
| Tuberculosis | rifampin * | skin rash, fever, hepatotoxicity |
| CMV | ganciclovir | bone marrow suppression |
| CMV | foscarnet | nephrotoxicity |

* Of the anti-tuberculous drugs used, most frequently associated with toxicity in HIV-infected patients.

*Treatment of HIV-associated malignancies*

The types of malignancy which are known to be associated with HIV infection are Kaposi's sarcoma and high grade malignant lymphomas. Both malignancies are also known to occur during other states of cellular immunodeficiency, but their pathogenesis under those circumstances as well as in patients with HIV-induced immunodeficiency remains largely unresolved. Early clinical stages of Kaposi's sarcoma in patients without greatly reduced CD4 + cell numbers seem to have a fair chance of responding to treatment with recombinant $\alpha$-interferon, which may be related to the anti-HIV activity of $\alpha$-interferon in such patients (De Wit et al., 1988; Lane et al., 1988). However, no satisfactory treatment for advanced Kaposi's sarcoma has been reported. Treatment employing various combinations of cytotoxic drugs may induce partial remissions, but usually these are only short-lasting and at the expense of serious side effects, such as bone marrow suppression and occurrence of infections. Similar problems are encountered in treating malignant lymphomas in these patients with multiple drug chemotherapeutic regimens (Bermudez et al., 1989; Kaplan et al., 1989), which have been found reasonably successful in non-HIV-infected individuals with such malignancies. Thus improving our understanding of the pathogenic mechanisms involved in the generation of these malignancies in HIV-infected subjects may lead to more successful and less toxic therapeutic approaches.

*Treatment of HIV-induced thrombocytopenia*

The pathogenesis of this complication of HIV infection, which often occurs when CD4 + cell numbers are still within the normal range, remains unclear, although autoimmune mechanisms have been suggested. Like immune thrombocytopenias in non-HIV-infected individuals the syndrome may respond to treatment with corticosteroids or in steroid-refractory cases to splenectomy. Theoretically however, both these forms of treatment may enhance immune suppression in HIV-infected individuals who, as mentioned, often still have reasonably preserved immunity, and thus possibly induce progression of the HIV infection and increased susceptibility to already pending opportunistic infections and malignancies. HIV-related thrombocytopenia has been reported to be able to respond to treatment with zidovudine (Hirschel et al., 1988; Oksenhendler et al., 1989), but the induced increase in platelet count is often not sustained and has a tendency to wane in a matter of months.

## Conclusion

It is clear that the management of HIV-infected individuals involves many problems, with respect to both the treatment of the underlying retroviral infection and the management of the myriad complications that characterize the disease induced by the retrovirus. Most patients with AIDS will encounter several of these problems in combination or in sequence during the course of their illness, and therefore will often receive treatment directed against HIV as well as several of its disease manifestations at the same time. The necessity to use many drugs in combination in these patients may often result in cumulative toxicity and other types of drug interactions. This should be kept in mind when developing new therapies for AIDS. Animal models of HIV as well as known animal retrovirus infection models may provide important information for the development of vaccines and anti-retroviral drugs. Existing animal models of some of the opportunistic infections found in AIDS may help improve the treatment of these infections. Examples in this respect are the rabbit model of cryptococcal meningitis and the rat model of PCP. In addition there is a need to develop new animal models of other infections, such as those due to *Mycobacterium avium intracellulare.* Animal models could also be helpful in delineating the pathogenesis of HIV-related malignancies and other non-infectious complications, thus providing new approaches to treatment of these HIV-related disease manifestations.

## References

Barre-Sinoussi, F., Nugeyre, M., Dauguet, C., Vilmer, E., Griscelli, C., Brun-Vezinet, F., Rouzioux, C., Gluckman, J., Chermann, J.C. and Montagnier, L. (1983) Isolation of a T-lymphotropic retrovirus from a patient at risk for acquired immune deficiency syndrome. *Science* 220, 868–871.

Bennett, J.E., Dismukes, W.E., Duma, R.J., Medoff, G., Sande, M.A., Gallis, H., Leonard, J., Fields, B.T., Bradshaw, M., Haywood, H., McGee, Z.A., Cate, T.R., Cobbs, C.G., Warner, J.F. and Alling, D.W. (1979) A comparison of amphotericin B alone and combined with flucytosine in the treatment of cryptococcal meningitis. *N. Engl. J. Med.* 301, 126–131.

Bermudez, M.A., Grant, K.M., Rodvien, R. and Mendes, F. (1989) Non-Hodgkin's lymphoma in a population with or at risk for acquired immunodeficiency syndrome: indications for intensive chemotherapy. *Am. J. Med.* 86, 71–76.

Bongaarts, J., Reining, P., Way, P. and Conant, F. (1989) The relationship between male circumcision and HIV infection in African populations. *AIDS* 3, 373–377.

Bozzette, S.A., Wu, A.L., Sattler, F., Chiu, J., Gluckstein, D., Neilson, D., Tilles, J., Leedom, J. and McCutchan, J.A. (1989) A randomized controlled trial of corticosteroids in *Pneumocystis carinii* pneumonia. In: Program and Abstracts of the 29th Interscience Conference on Antimicrobial Agents and Chemotherapy, Houston, TX, Abstract 1068.

Centers for Disease Control (1981) Kaposi's sarcoma and Pneumocystis pneumonia among homosexual men—New York City and California. *MMWR* 30, 305–308.

Chatis, P.A., Miller, C.H., Schrager, L.E. and Crumpacker, C.S. (1989) Successful treatment with foscarnet of an acyclovir-resistant mucocutaneous infection with herpes simplex virus in a patient with acquired immunodeficiency syndrome. *N. Engl. J. Med.* 320, 297–300.

Chuck, S.L. and Sande, M.A. (1989) Infections with *Cryptococcus neoformans* in the acquired immunodeficiency syndrome. *N. Engl. J. Med.* 321, 794–799.

Cooper, D.A., Gold, J., Maclean, P., Donovan, B., Finlayson, R., Barnes, T.G., Michelmore, H.M., Brooke, P. and Penny, R. (1985) Acute AIDS retrovirus infection: definition of a clinical illness associated with seroconversion. *Lancet* i, 537–540.

Dalgleish, A.G. (1988) Human trials of AIDS vaccines: novel means of passive and active immunotherapy. *AIDS* 2 (Suppl. 1), S129–S131.

De Gans, J., Eeftinck Schattenkerk, J.K.M. and Van Ketel, R.J. (1988) Itraconazole as maintenance treatment for cryptococcal meningitis in the acquired immunodeficiency syndrome. *Br. Med. J.* 296, 339.

De Wit, R., Eeftinck Schattenkerk, J.K.M., Boucher, C.A.B., Bakker, P.J.M., Veenhof, K.H.N. and Danner, S.A. (1988) Clinical and virological effects of high-dose recombinant interferon-$\alpha$ in disseminated AIDS-related Kaposi's sarcoma. *Lancet* ii, 1214–1217.

De Wolf, F., Lange, J.M.A., Houweling, J.T.M., Mulder, J.W., Beemster, J., Schellekens, P.T., Coutinho, R.A., Van der Noordaa, J. and Goudsmit, J. (1989) Appearance of predictors of disease progression in relation to the development of AIDS. *AIDS* 3, 563–569.

Denning, D.W., Tucker, R.M., Hanson, L.H., Hamilton, J.R. and Stevens, D.A. (1989) Itraconazole therapy for cryptococcal meningitis and cryptococcosis. *Arch. Intern. Med.* 149, 2301–2308.

Dismukes, W., Cloud, G., Thompson, S., Sugar, A., Tuazon, C., Kaufman, D., Grieco, M., Jacobson, J., Powderly, W. and Robinson, P. (1989) Fluconazole versus amphotericin B therapy of acute cryptococcal meningitis. In: Program and Abstracts of the 29th Interscience Conference on Antimicrobial Agents and Chemotherapy, Houston, TX, Abstract 1065.

Dournon, E., Matheron, S., Rozenbaum, W., Gharakhanian, S., Michon, C., Girard, P.M., Peronne, C., Salmon, D., De Truchis, P., Leport, C., Bouvet, E., Dazza, M.C., Levacher, M. and Regnier, B. (1988) Effects of zidovudine in 365 consecutive patients with AIDS or AIDS-related complex. *Lancet* ii, 1297–1302.

Erice, A., Chou, S., Biron, K.K., Stanat, S.C., Balfour, H.H. Jr and Jordan, M.C. (1989) Progressive disease due to ganciclovir-resistant cytomegalovirus in immunocompromised patients. *N. Engl. J. Med.* 32, 289–293.

Erlich, K.S., Mills, J., Chatis, P., Mertz, G.J., Busch, D.F., Follansbee, S.E., Grant, R.M. and Crumpacker, C.S. (1989) Acyclovir-resistant herpes simplex virus infections in patients with acquired immunodeficiency syndrome. *N. Engl. J. Med.* 320, 293–296.

Fauci, A.S. (1988) The human immunodeficiency virus: infectivity and mechanisms of pathogenesis. *Science* 239, 617–622.

Fischl, M.A., Richman, D.D., Grieco, M.H., Gottlieb, M.S., Volberding, P.A., Laskin, O.L., Leedom, J.O., Groopman, J.E., Mildvan, D., Schooley, R.T., Jackson, G.G., Durack, D.T., King, D. and the

AZT Collaborative Working Group (1987) The efficacy of azidothymidine (AZT) in the treatment of patients with AIDS and AIDS-related complex. A double-blind placebo-controlled trial. *N. Engl. J. Med.* 317, 185–191.

Gaines, H., Von Sydow, M., Pehrson, P.O. and Lundbergh, P. (1988) Clinical picture of primary HIV infection presenting as a glandular-fever-like illness. *Br. Med. J.* 297, 1363–1368.

Gaines, H., Von Sydow, M., Sönnerborg, A., Albert, J., Czajkowski, J., Pehrson, P.O., Chiodi, F., Moberg, L., Fenyö, E.M., Åsjö, B. and Forsgren, M. (1987) Antibody response in primary human immunodeficiency virus infection. *Lancet* i, 1249–1253.

Gallo, R.C., Salahuddin, S.Z., Popovic, M., Shearer, G.M., Kaplan, M., Haynes, B.F., Palker, T.J., Redfield, R., Oleske, J., Safai, B., White, G., Foster, P. and Markham, P.D. (1984) Frequent detection and isolation of cytopathic retroviruses (HTLV-III) from patients with AIDS and at risk of AIDS. *Science* 224, 500–503.

Girard, P.-M., Landman, R., Gaudebout, C., Lepretre, A., Lottin, P., Michon, C., De Truchis, P., Matheron, S., Camus, F., Farinotti, R., Marche, C., Coulaud, J.-P. and Saimot, A.G. (1989) Prevention of *Pneumocystis carinii* pneumonia relapse by pentamidine aerosol in zidovudine-treated AIDS patients. *Lancet* i, 1348–1353.

Goedert, J.J., Kessler, G.M., Aledort, L.M., Biggar, R.J., Andes, W.A., White, G.C. II, Drummond, J.E., Vaidya, K., Mann, D.L., Eyster, M.E., Ragni, M.V., Lederman, M.M., Cohen, A.R., Bray, G.L., Rosenberg, P.S., Friedman, R.M., Hilgartner, M.W., Blattner, W.A., Kroner, B. and Gail, M.H. (1989) A prospective study of human immunodeficiency virus type 1 infection and the development of AIDS in subjects with hemophilia. *N. Engl. J. Med.* 321, 1141–1148.

Golden, J.A., Chernoff, D., Hollander, H., Feigal, D. and Conte, J.E. (1989) Prevention of *Pneumocystis carinii* pneumonia by inhaled pentamidine. *Lancet* i, 654–657.

Gonda, M.A., Wong-Staal, F., Gallo, R.C., Clements, J.E., Narayan, O. and Gilden, R.V. (1984) Sequence homology and morphologic similarity of HTLV-III and visna, a pathogenic lentivirus. *Science* 227, 173–177.

Hardy, W.D., Northfelt, D.W. and Drake, T.A. (1989) Fatal, disseminated pneumocystosis in a patient with acquired immunodeficiency syndrome receiving prophylactic aerosolized pentamidine. *Am. J. Med.* 87, 329–331.

Hirschel, B. and the Swiss Group for Clinical Studies on AIDS (1988) Zidovudine for the treatment of thrombocytopenia associated with human immunodeficiency virus (HIV). *Ann. Intern. Med.* 109, 718–721.

Ho, D.D. (Moderator) (1989) The acquired immunodeficiency syndrome (AIDS) dementia complex. *Ann. Intern. Med.* 111, 400–410.

Johnson, A.M. and Laga, M. (1988) Heterosexual transmission of HIV. *AIDS* 2 (Suppl. 1), S49–S56.

Kaplan, L.D., Abrams, D.I., Feigal, E., McGrath, M., Kahn, J., Neville, P., Ziegler, J. and Volberding, P.A. (1989) AIDS-associated non-Hodgkin's lymphoma in San Francisco. *JAMA* 261, 719–724.

Kingsley, L.A., Detels, R., Kaslow, R., Polk, B.F., Rinaldo, C.R., Chmiel, J., Detre, K., Kelsey, S.F., Odaka, N., Ostrow, D., VanRaden, M. and Visscher, B. (1987) Risk factors for seroconversion to human immunodeficiency virus among male homosexuals. *Lancet* i, 345–349.

Kovacs, J.A. and Masur, H. (1988) Opportunistic infections. In: V.T. DeVita Jr., S. Hellman and S.A. Rosenberg (Eds.), *AIDS, Etiology, Diagnosis, Treatment and Prevention.* J.B. Lippincott Company, Philadelphia, PA, pp. 199–225.

Krigel, R.L. and Friedman-Kien, A.E. (1988) Kaposi's sarcoma in AIDS: diagnosis and treatment. In: V.T. DeVita Jr., S. Hellman and S.A. Rosenberg (Eds.), *AIDS, Etiology, Diagnosis, Treatment and Prevention.* J.B. Lippincott Company, Philadelphia, PA, pp. 245–261.

Lane, H.C., Kovacs, J.A., Feinberg, J., Herpin, B., Davey, V., Walker, R., Deyton, L., Metcalf, J.A., Baseler, M., Salzman, N., Manischewitz, J., Quinnan, G., Masur, H. and Fauci, A.S. (1988) Anti-retroviral effects of interferon-$\alpha$ in AIDS-associated Kaposi's sarcoma. *Lancet* ii, 1218–1222.

Lange, J.M.A., de Wolf, F. and Goudsmit, J. (1990) Markers for progression in HIV infection. *AIDS* 3 (Suppl. 1), S153–S160.

Lange, J.M.A., Paul, D.A., Huisman, H.G., de Wolf, F., van den Berg, H., Coutinho, R.A., Danner,

S.A., van der Noordaa, J. and Goudsmit, J. (1986) Persistent HIV-antigenaemia and decline of HIV core antibodies associated with transition to AIDS. *Br. Med. J.* 293, 1459–1462.

Larder, B.A., Darby, G. and Richman, D.D. (1989) HIV with reduced sensitivity to zidovudine (AZT) isolated during prolonged therapy. *Science* 243, 1731–1734.

Larsen, R.A. and Leal, M.E. (1989) Fluconazole compared to amphotericin B as treatment of cryptococcal meningitis. In: Program and Abstracts of the 29th Interscience Conference on Antimicrobial Agents and Chemotherapy, Houston, TX, *Abstract* 1062.

Latif, A.S., Katzenstein, D.A., Bassett, M.T., Houston, S., Emmanuel, J.C. and Marowa, E. (1989) Genital ulcers and transmission of HIV among couples in Zimbabwe. *AIDS* 3, 519–523.

Levine, A.M. (1988) Reactive and neoplastic lymphoproliferative disorders and other miscellaneous cancers associated with HIV infection. In: V.T. DeVita Jr., S. Hellman and S.A. Rosenberg (Eds.), *AIDS, Etiology, Diagnosis, Treatment and Prevention.* J.B. Lippincott Company, Philadelphia, PA, pp. 265–271.

Levy, J.A., Hoffman, A.D., Kramer, S.M., Landis, J., Shimabukuro, J. and Oshiro, L. (1984) Isolation of lymphadenopathic retroviruses from San Francisco patients with AIDS. *Science* 225, 840–842.

MacFadden, D.K., Edelson, J.D., Hyland, R.H., Rodriguez, C.H. and Rebuck, A.S. (1987) Corticosteroids as adjunctive therapy in treatment of *Pneumocystis carinii* pneumonia in patients with acquired immunodeficiency syndrome. *Lancet* i, 1477–1479.

Masur, H., Ognibene, F.P., Yarchoan, R., Shelhamer, J.H., Baird, B.F., Travis, W., Suffredini, A.F., Deyton, L., Kovacs, J.A., Falloon, J., Davey, R., Polis, M., Metcalf, J., Baseler, M., Wesley, R., Gill, V.J., Fauci, A.S. and Lane, H.C. (1989) CD4 counts as predictors of opportunistic pneumonias in human immunodeficiency virus (HIV) infection. *Ann. Intern. Med.* 111, 223–231.

Moss, A.R. and Bacchetti, P. (1989) Natural history of HIV infection. *AIDS* 3, 55–61.

Murphy, R., MacDonell, K., Newquist, S., Skoutelis, T. and Phair, J. (1989) Aerosolized pentamidine prophylaxis following *Pneumocystis carinii* pneumonia in AIDS patients. In: Program and Abstracts of the 29th Interscience Conference on Antimicrobial Agents and Chemotherapy, Houston, TX, Abstract 1072.

Oksenhendler, E., Bierling, P., Ferchal, F., Clauvel, J.-P. and Seligmann, M. (1989) Zidovudine for thrombocytopenic purpura related to human immunodeficiency virus (HIV) infection. *Ann. Intern. Med.* 110, 365–368.

Pizzo, P.A. Eddy, J., Falloon, J. et al. (1989) *N. Engl. J. Med.* 319, 889–896.

Poblete, R.B., Rodriguez, K., Foust, R.T., Reddy, R. and Saldana, M.J. (1989) *Pneumocystis carinii* hepatitis in the acquired immunodeficiency syndrome (AIDS). *Ann. Intern. Med.* 110, 737–738.

Popovic, M., Sarngadharan, M.G., Read, E. and Gallo, R.C. (1984) Detection, isolation and continuous production of cytopathic retroviruses (HTLV-III) from patients with AIDS and pre-AIDS. *Science* 224, 497–500.

Portegies, P., de Gans, J., Lange, J.M.A. et al. (1989) *Br. Med. J.* 299, 819–821.

Raviglione, M.C., Mariuz, P., Sugar, J. and Mullen, M.P. (1989) Extrapulmonary Pneumocystis infection. *Ann. Intern. Med.* 111, 339.

Reiss, P., Lange, J.M.A. and Goudsmit, J. (1985) LAV/HTLV-III infectie na eenmalig sexueel contact met een AIDS-patient. *Ned. Tijdschr. Geneesk.* 129, 1933–1934.

Reitz, M.S. Jr. and Gallo, R.C. (1990) Human immunodeficiency virus. In: G.L. Mandell, R.G. Douglas and J.E. Bennett (Eds.), *Principles and Practice of Infectious Diseases.* Churchill Livingstone, New York, NY, pp. 1344–1352.

Richman, D.D., Fischl, M.A., Grieco, M.H., Gottlieb, M.S., Volberding, P.A., Laskin, O.L., Leedom, J.M., Groopman, J.E., Mildvan, D., Hirsch, M.S., Jackson, G.G., Durack, D.T., Nusinoff-Lehrman, S. and the AZT Collaborative Working Group (1987) The toxicity of azidothymidine (AZT) in the treatment of patients with AIDS and AIDS-related complex. *N. Engl. J. Med.* 317, 192–197.

Rosenblum, M.L., Levy. R.M. and Bredesen, D.E. (1988) *AIDS and the Nervous System.* Raven Press, New York, NY.

Ryder, R.W. and Hassig, S.E. (1988) The epidemiology of perinatal transmission of HIV. *AIDS* 2 (Suppl. 1), S83–S89.

Schoenbaum, E.E., Hartel, D., Selwyn, P.A., Klein, R.S., Davenny, K., Rogers, M., Feiner, C. and

Friedland, G. (1989) Risk factors for human immunodeficiency virus infection in intravenous drug users. *N. Engl. J. Med.* 321, 874–878.

Statistics from the World Health Organization and the Centers for Disease Control (1989a) *AIDS* 3, 621.

Statistics from the World Health Organization and the Centers for Disease Control (1989b) *AIDS* 3, 619–620.

Statistics from the World Health Organization and the Centers for Disease Control (1989c) *AIDS* 3, 623.

Stern, J.J., Hartman, B.J., Sharkey, P., Rowland, V., Squires, K.E., Murray, H.W. and Graybill, R. (1988) Oral fluconazole therapy for patients with acquired immunodeficiency syndrome and cryptococcosis: experience with 22 patients. *Am. J. Med.* 85, 477–480.

Sugar, A.M. and Saunders, C. (1988) Oral fluconazole as suppressive therapy of disseminated cryptococcosis in patients with acquired immunodeficiency syndrome. *Am. J. Med.* 85, 481–489.

Van Griensven, G.J.P., Tielman, R.A.P., Goudsmit, J., van der Noordaa, J., de Wolf, F., de Vroome, E.M.M. and Coutinho, R.A. (1987) Risk factors and prevalence of HIV antibodies in homosexual men in The Netherlands. *Am. J. Epidemiol.* 125, 1048–1057.

Walmsley, S., Salit, I.E. and Brunton, J. (1988) The possible role of corticosteroid therapy for pneumocystis pneumonia in the acquired immunodeficiency syndrome (AIDS). *J. AIDS* 1, 354–360.

Ward, J.W., Bush, T.J., Perkins, H.A., Lieb, L.E., Allen, J.R., Goldfinger, D., Samson, S.M., Pepkowitz, S.H., Fernando, L.P., Holland, P.V., Kleinman, S.H., Grindon, A.J., Garner, J.L., Rutherford, G.W. and Holmberg, S.D. (1989) The natural history of transfusion-associated infection with human immunodeficiency virus. *N. Engl. J. Med.* 321, 947–952.

Yarchoan, R., Mitsuya, H. and Broder, S. (1989) Clinical and basic advances in the antiretroviral therapy of human immunodeficiency virus infection. *Am. J. Med.* 87, 191–200.

Zuger, A., Schuster, M., Simberkoff, M.S., Rahal, J.J. and Holzman, R.S. (1988) Maintenance amphotericin B for cryptococcal meningitis in the acquired immunodeficiency syndrome (AIDS). *Ann. Intern. Med.* 109, 592–593.

*Eds. H. Schellekens and M.C. Horzinek*
*Animal Models in AIDS*



3

# Safety in the use of animal models for AIDS

J.R. KEDDIE

Health and Safety Executive, Technology Division, Stanley Precinct, Bootle, Merseyside, U.K.

## Introduction

Research into the causal agent of acquired immunodeficiency syndrome (AIDS) has increased significantly in recent years in response to the growing incidence of infection in the community. The causal agent of AIDS, human immunodeficiency virus (HIV), has been isolated and extensive research into anti-HIV pharmaceuticals and anti-HIV vaccines is under way. As new products and candidate vaccines appear on the scene, effective models for the screening and evaluation of these products are required. The use of animal models for product screening and research poses additional risks to those encountered when handling HIV in the laboratory. This paper discusses the hazards associated with the use of animal models for work with HIV/SIV and describes the standards currently adopted in the U.K.

## Animal models

A wide range of animal models have been suggested as suitable for work with HIV and associated viruses including chimpanzees (Saxinger et al., 1987), cynomolgus monkeys (Daniel et al., 1985), rabbits (Filice et al., 1988), mice (Mosier et al., 1988) and cats (Pedersen et al., 1987). Clearly, not all models are appropriate for every purpose and the most reliable models to date remain the higher order non-human primates such as the chimpanzee. The problems inherent in the use of this type of model have prompted the development of other non-primate systems.

## HIV and associated viruses

In the U.K., pathogens are categorised by the Advisory Committee on Dangerous Pathogens (ACDP, 1984, 1989) into one of four hazard groups based on the inherent hazard of the organism, the transmissibility of the organisms and the effectiveness of prophylaxis/treatment following infection. HIV is categorised as a hazard group 3 organism. Laboratory propagation/concentration of the virus should therefore be undertaken at ACDP containment level 3, although routine diagnostic work with HIV may be undertaken at ACDP containment level 2 with certain additional caveats. Certain viruses such as feline immunodeficiency virus (FIV) are not recognised as being pathogenic to man and hence are not categorised by ACDP. Others such as simian immunodeficiency virus (SIV) are closely analogous to HIV and the possibility of human infection cannot be excluded. SIV is therefore also categorised as a group 3 pathogen along with HIV, requiring a similar standard of containment.

The routes of transmission of HIV are by now well characterised (Friedland and Klein, 1987) and the standard of laboratory containment necessary is well established. The use of animal models for work with HIV and associated viruses, however, poses additional concerns in terms of worker protection and potential contamination of the working environment. Whilst the aerosol route of transmission has not been conclusively established in any documented case of infection with HIV, the possibility of infectious aerosols must be considered with work with animals in addition to bites, scratches and parenteral inoculation. This is of particular significance when handling concentrated virus.

## Animal containment standards

ACDP in their 1984 categorisation report specify the physical containment standards necessary for work in both laboratories and animal containment facilities. Animal containment level 3 is required for work with vertebrates deliberately infected with both HIV and SIV. This standard of containment is higher than the equivalent standard proposed by CDC for the prevention of SIV infection in animal handlers (CDC, 1988).

The main requirements of ACDP containment level 3 include the following.

(i) All surfaces within the animal suite should be impervious to spillages and be easy to clean. Floor drain traps must be kept filled and regularly disinfected.

(ii) The suite should be entered via a separate ante-room with two doors and should contain suitable hand washing and shower facilities.

(iii) The suite should be sealable for fumigation purposes.

(iv) A continuous airflow into the suite should be maintained with exhaust air ducted direct to atmosphere via a HEPA filter. Where a powered air supply system is provided, the extract and supply systems should be interlocked to prevent positive pressurisation of the suite in the event of extract from failure.

(v) An autoclave and incinerator should be available on site with the autoclave within the same building. All waste should be made safe prior to disposal and all animal carcases should be incinerated.

(vi) A microbiological safety cabinet (BS 5726, 1979) should be provided for all procedures likely to create significant aerosols such as inoculation, necropsy, tissue harvesting etc. Alternatively, high performance respiratory protective equipment may be used.

(vii) Animals should be housed in safety cabinets or isolators, or in ventilated enclosures fitted with HEPA filtered exhaust ventilation. Alternatively, high performance respiratory protective equipment may be used.

(viii) All accidents, bites, scratches, etc. should be reported and recorded.

(ix) Protective clothing including footwear, gloves, gowns and additional heavy duty clothing should be provided. Protective clothing should be disinfected or autoclaved after use.

(x) All animal house workers and research staff should be fully experienced in handling animals infected with group 3 pathogens.

(xi) A detailed code of practice should be prepared for all work within the animal containment facility.

The risks of infection to research and animal house technicians are clearly very different when handling small animals such as infected mice from those encountered when handling non-human primates. The U.K. philosophy towards the handling of dangerous pathogens is that of containment at source. This is relatively straight-forward with animals such as mice, rabbits and cats which can be housed in microbiological safety cabinets or isolators fitted with HEPA filtered ventilation. Access to the animals is by means of glove ports and all activities likely to generate aerosols can be undertaken within the isolator or cabinet.

Containment at source involving the use of safety cabinets or isolators is clearly not practicable, however, for the handling of non-human primates in animal houses. In these cases, animals are held in crush back cages within a room fitted with a HEPA filtered ventilation system and the use of respiratory protective equipment (RPE) is recommended for all employees involved in handling monkeys. The RPE recommended for this type of work comprises a 'blouse' covering the head and upper body which is positively supplied with air by means of a small motorised fan back pack carried by the worker. This type of RPE must be used with high efficiency (99.997%) disposable filters. Positive pressure RPE of this type is more efficient than other types of respirator and provides additional protection from splashes, scratches, etc. Respirators which cover the face and rely on the use of a cannister under negative pressure will provide a high standard of protection but are crucially dependent on the correct fitting and maintenance of the equipment. The breathing resistance of negative pressure respirators also increases the discomfort of the wearer during physical work.

It is important that attention is also paid to other protective clothing such as gowns, overalls and gloves. Heavy duty gloves should be worn whenever there is a risk of scratching or biting by animals. Non-human primates should only be handled when anaesthetised. When handling infected primates, it is important suitable systems of work and procedures are available for the recapture of animals which may escape from their enclosures.

When working with non-human primates consideration should also be given to the risk of infection with simian herpes B virus (Wansburgh-Jones et al., 1988; Anon., 1989). The precautions mentioned for work with HIV/SIV will be adequate to prevent exposure to B virus, but primates known to be free from the virus should be used where possible. Guidance on the prevention of B virus infection are given by MRC (1985) and CDC (1987), and Appendix C of the ACDP report (1984).

## HIV and animals in the U.K.

All premises in the U.K. which propagate/concentrate HIV are required to notify the U.K. Health and Safety Executive. These premises are inspected by specialist inspectors from the headquarters of the Health and Safety Executive to assess compliance with the U.K. Health and Safety legislation. Standards and systems of work are assessed in the light of the ACDP guidelines, and comprehensive advice given based on the nature of the work proposed. Where the use of non-human primates is proposed, inspectors are involved at an initial stage to ensure good standards and best practice are incorporated at an early stage of design.

## Conclusions

High standards have been established in premises in the U.K. where animal models are used for HIV/SIV research. A flexible approach has been implemented for the establishment of these premises involving extensive dialogue with research staff, based on a detailed framework provided by the Advisory Committee on Dangerous Pathogens. The risks inherent in the use of animals infected with HIV/SIV are higher than those commonly encountered in laboratories, but safe working can be achieved if accepted guidelines are followed.

## References

Advisory Committee on Dangerous Pathogens (1984) Categorisation of Pathogens According to Hazard and Categories of Containment. *HMSO*, London.

Anon. (1989) Fourth lab worker hospitalised for monkey virus symptoms: state investigates. *Occup. Safety Health Rep.* 9 June, 623.

BS 5726 (1979) Microbiological Safety Cabinets. *BSI*, London.

CDC (1987) Guidelines for the prevention of Herpesvirus simiae (B virus) infection in monkey handlers. *MMWR* 36, 680–682, 687–689.

CDC (1988) Guidance to prevent Simian Immunodeficiency Virus infection in laboratory workers and animal handlers. *MMWR* 37, 693–704.

Daniel, M.D., Letvin, N.L., King, N.W. et al. (1985) Isolation of T-cell tropic HTLV-III-like retrovirus from macaques. *Science* 228, 1201–1204.

Filice, G., Cereda, P.M. and Varnier, O.E. (1988) Infection of rabbits with human immunodeficiency virus. *Nature* 335, 366–368.

Friedland, G.H. and Klein, R.S. (1987) Transmission of the Human Immunodeficiency Virus. *N. Engl. J. Med.* 317, 1125–1135.

Mosier, D.E., Gulizia, R.J., Baird, S.M. and Wilson, D.B. (1988) Transfer of a functional human immune system to mice with severe combined immunodeficiency. *Nature* 335, 256–259.

Medical Research Council (1985) The Management of Simians in Relation to Infectious Hazards to Man. *MRC,* London.

Pedersen, N.C., Ho, E.W., Brown, M.L. and Yamamoto, J.K. (1987) Isolation of a T-lymphotropic virus from domestic cats with an immunodeficiency-like syndrome. *Science* 235, 790–793.

Saxinger, C., Alter, H.I., Eichberg, J.W. et al. (1987) Stages in the progression of HIV infection in chimpanzees. *AIDS Res. Hum. Retrovir.* 3, 375–385.

Wansburgh-Jones, M.H., Cooper, B. and Sarantis, N. (1988) Prophylaxis against B virus infection. *Br. Med. J.* 297, 909.

# *HIV-1 and HIV-2 in animal models*

*Eds. H. Schellekens and M.C. Horzinek*
*Animal Models in AIDS*



4

# The chimpanzee, rhesus monkey, and baboon as models for HIV infection, disease, and vaccine development

JORG W. EICHBERG

Department of Virology and Immunology, Southwest Foundation for Biomedical Research, San Antonio, TX 78284, U.S.A.

## Animal models

Since 1983 our laboratory has been involved in the comparative immunopathogenesis of human and simian immunodeficiency viruses (HIV and SIV) in the chimpanzee and other non-human primates (Table 1). Inoculation of HIV-1 resulted in infection only in the chimpanzee, whereas rhesus monkeys and baboons were not susceptible (Alter et al., 1984; Morrow et al., 1989). However, at present, 6.5 years post infection, only two chimpanzees receiving presumably high doses of HIV have demonstrated a temporary lymphadenopathy (Alter et al., 1984; Hu et al., 1987). The exquisite sensitivity of the chimpanzee to infection with HIV-1 has now been demonstrated in approximately 120 animals worldwide.

In contrast, rhesus monkeys and baboons, but not chimpanzees, were susceptible to SIV infection (Kanki et al., 1990). However, only rhesus monkeys developed disease symptoms and died of typical simian immunodeficiency syndrome (SAIDS). Most notable was the fact that these rhesus monkeys displayed severe immune dysfunctions long before developing SAIDS. Both lymphocyte subset

TABLE 1
Inoculation of primates with HIV or SIV

| | HIV | | SIV | |
|---|---|---|---|---|
| | Infection | Disease | Infection | Disease |
| Chimpanzee | + | − | − | − |
| Rhesus | − | − | + | + |
| Baboon | − | − | + | − |

TABLE 2
$SIV_{mac}$ in rhesus monkeys

| Monkeys | T-cell subsets | | | | | | Mitogen | | |
|---|---|---|---|---|---|---|---|---|---|
| | $L_5$ | $L_3$ | 3/2 | $L_2$ | $L_8$ | $L_{12}$ | PHA | PWM | ConA |
| 1 | | | | | | | | | |
| Control | 69.2 | 27.9 | 1.92 | 14.5 | 28.0 | 4.3 | 265.8 | 193.6 | 246.6 |
| 6 mo p.i. | 79.9 | 8.7 | 0.22 | 39.2 | 17.5 | 0.7 | 5.6 | 51.2 | 16.0 |
| 2 | | | | | | | | | |
| Control | 72.3 | 30.6 | 1.34 | 22.9 | 40.0 | 9.3 | 322.2 | 99.7 | 250.0 |
| 6 mo p.i. | 83.1 | 7.1 | 0.17 | 40.8 | 15.3 | 1.4 | 46.3 | 24.5 | 49.5 |
| 3 | | | | | | | | | |
| Control | 62.6 | 21.9 | 1.02 | 21.5 | 31.1 | 7.0 | 137.6 | 178.4 | 312.3 |
| 6 mo p.i. | 89.2 | 10.3 | 0.27 | 38.5 | 25.9 | 1.5 | 66.4 | 42.4 | 107.3 |

Control: prior to infection.
6 mo p.i.: 6 months post infection.

populations and mitogen responsiveness were severely compromised 6 months post infection (p.i.), long before death at approximately 1.5 years p.i. (Table 2). The ease with which rhesus monkeys can be infected with $SIV_{mac}$ and the following period of immunodeficiency with and without disease make the rhesus monkey an excellent model for vaccine development and antiviral therapy.

Our laboratory has been involved in several efforts to induce disease with HIV-1 in chimpanzees through the use of co-factors. Neither HIV-1 infection of hepatitis B or hepatitis C carrier animals nor experimental infection with cytomegalovirus and HIV-1 resulted in disease development (Eichberg et al., 1989). In addition, neither the use of immunosuppression nor immunoenhancement resulted in disease (Table 3). This lack of disease development in the chimpanzee, with the exception of the two cases of lymphadenopathy mentioned above, could be due simply to a time factor; the recently described average incubation period

TABLE 3
Experimental co-factors to induce disease in chimpanzees

| Co-factor | Effect | Disease |
|---|---|---|
| HIV dose ↑ | T4 ↓ | Temporary LAD |
| NANB, HBV | – | – |
| CMV | HIV ↑ | – |
| Prednisone | – | – |
| ATG | WBC ↓, subsets ↓ mitogens ↓ | – |
| Anti-Leu2a | T8 ↓ HIV ↑ | – |
| Factor VIII | HIV ↑ | – |
| Allogeneic lymphocytes | HIV ↑ | – |

TABLE 4
HIV vaccine trials in chimpanzees: active and passive immunization

| | Animals (n) | ELISA | | | | Challenge virus | Virus dose ($TCID_{50}$) |
|---|---|---|---|---|---|---|---|
| | | CMI | WB | NB | Protection | | |
| Synthetic peptide (735–752) | 3 | – | + | – | no | NY5 | $10^3$ |
| Vaccinia-*env* | 9 | + | + | – | no | LAV | $10^2$–$10^5$ |
| rgp120 | 4 | + | + | ± | no | IIIB | $10^{2.4}$ |
| HIVIG | 5/1 | NA | + | + | no/yes | IIIB | $10^{1-2.4}$ |

CMI: cell-mediated immunity.
WB: Western blot.
NB: neutralizing antibodies.
HIVIG: HIV immunoglobulin.

is 9.8 years in humans (Bacchetti and Moss, 1989) and has not yet been reached in the chimpanzee experiments. However, even if chimpanzees should develop disease, they still would not be a good disease model. It would simply be too much time in an experimental system.

## Vaccine development

As discussed above, their 100% sensitivity to infection with HIV-1 makes chimpanzees an ideal model for vaccine development. This is particularly true if the objective of an AIDS vaccine is to prevent infection. In view of the fact that most people infected with HIV-1 develop disease and die, this objective is obviously desirable. While the rhesus monkey SIV model system is a good model to study the efficacy of SIV vaccines, it has one major problem: HIV-1 and $SIV_{mac}$ are only approximately 45% similar. Therefore, we have been involved in extensive HIV-1 vaccine development in the chimpanzee.

Table 4 summarizes our findings to date with three active and two passive immunization protocols. Synthetic peptide 735–752 linked to KLH and administered with Freund's complete adjuvant did not induce measurable cell-mediated immunity (CMI) but did induce a definite anti-gp41 response in a Western blot assay (WB). Neutralizing antibodies were not detected and two experimentally immunized and one control animal were not protected when challenged with $10^3$ $TCID_{50}$ of HIV-1 (NY5). Vaccinia-*env* recombinant virus (Hu et al., 1987) induced strong CMI, ELISA, and WB responses (Zarling et al., 1987) but no neutralizing antibodies nor protection from infection was achieved whether $10^2$ or $10^5$ $TCID_{50}$ of LAV was used as challenge dose. In the low challenge dose (100 $TCID_{50}$) group of animals, earlier seroconversion was noted in the immunized chimpanzees versus the control animal. Both strong CMI and WB responses were detected in the recombinant gp120 (expressed in Chinese hamster ovary cells) immunized chimpanzee (Berman et al., 1988). However, it was interesting to note that, although this response was always transient, there was a strong response to

TABLE 5
Immune status of chimpanzees passively immunized with HIVIG prior to challenge with 258 or 34 $TCID_{50}$ of HIV IIIB

| Sample | Dose of HIVIG | ELISA | ADCC | NA | HIV challenge ($TCID_{50}$) | HIV isolation p.i. (weeks) |
|---|---|---|---|---|---|---|
| HIVIG | – | 1,024,000 | 1:200,000 | 1:944 | 258 | – |
| Chimp 212 | 1 ml/kg | 6,400 | 1:1800 | <1:20 | 258 | 3 |
| Chimp 233 | 1 ml/kg | 6,400 | 1:1900 | <1:20 | 258 | 13 |
| Chimp 130 | 10 ml/kg | 204,800 | >1:20,000 | 1:354 | 258 | 3 |
| Chimp 310 | 10 ml/kg | 204,800 | >1:20,000 | 1:178 | 258 | 9 |
| Chimp 304 | Control | < 400 | 0 | <1:20 | 258 | 7 |
| Chimp 106 | 10 ml/kg | 409,800 | ND | 1:640 | 34 | – |

NA: Neutralizing antibodies.
p.i.: post infection.

booster immunizations. In spite of low and cross-neutralizing antibodies, the immunized animals were not protected when challenged with HIV-1 (IIIB).

The low or absent levels of neutralizing antibodies prompted us to attempt to passively immunize chimpanzees with HIV immunoglobulin (HIVIG) prepared from a human donor pool with high HIV neutralizing antibody titer (Prince et al., 1988). One day following infusion of either a low or a high dose of HIVIG, the animals were challenged intravenously (i.v.) with approximately 258 $TCID_{50}$ of HIV IIIB. Their immune status 1 day post infusion prior to challenge is depicted in Table 5. In spite of the fact that the high dose animals had significantly higher neutralizing antibody titers, HIV could be isolated from all animals as early as 3 weeks p.i. In a subsequent experiment, one animal was also infused with high dose HIVIG but was challenged with a 10-fold higher diluted HIV stock virus, i.e., 34 $TCID_{50}$. The outcome of this study was much more favorable than in the previous five animals. Only on one occasion, one week 15, one lymphocyte co-culture revealed borderline p24 antigen. Most interesting, when lymphocytes were analyzed by DNA-PCR they were positive only until week 23 and subsequently became negative. This suggested that the animal became infected but cleared the infection or positive PCR was introduced through the inoculum. Whatever the answer might be, this experiment represents a successful outcome following passive immunization with HIVIG and transfer of high neutralizing antibodies.

## Conclusion

Based on published work from our laboratory and others, a summary of possible prerequisites for a successful HIV vaccine is given in Table 6. It is apparent that the immune response to the neutralizing loop determinants is

TABLE 6
Requisites for HIV vaccine success

- Immune response to loop and other epitopes
- Immunogenicity: peptides, glycoproteins, virus
- Conformation: hidden epitopes
- Induction of NeAb (cell-free): titer
- Induction of CTL (cell-associated): circulating, clones
- Adjuvants: alum, MDP, MTP, iscom
- Interval, dose
- Relevance of animal models

important but might require the participation of additional epitopes. It is probable that a successful vaccine might be developed first with more crude preparations such as a whole virus preparation, and some successes have been reported in the SIV-rhesus monkey model. Our experiments demonstrate the prerequisite of high neutralizing antibodies for potential success with a cell-free HIV challenge. The importance of cytotoxic T cells in a cell-associated virus challenge has not yet been addressed. It is quite clear how important adjuvants are in enhancing immune responsiveness. However, only alum is approved for human use at this point. In addition, from a recently completed immunogenicity study with rgp120 in baboons, it is quite apparent that the interval of immunization is more important than the dose of the immunogen (Anderson et al., 1990). Finally, in an ideal sense, many questions related to HIV vaccinology should be addressed in the SIV model system where there is no shortage of animals. Once the lessons learned in this model system are sufficiently positive, equivalent HIV constructs should be tested for efficacy in the HIV-chimpanzee model before being administered to humans.

## Acknowledgements

This work was supported in part by Contracts NO1-HB-7-7029 of the National Heart, Lung, and Blood Institute and NO1-CL-6-2101 of the Research Contracts Branch, NIH.

## References

Alter, H.J., Eichberg, J.W., Masur, H., Saxinger, W.C., Gallo, R.C., Macher, A.M., Lane, H.C. and Fauci, A.S. (1984) Transmission of HTLV-III from human plasma to chimpanzees: an animal model for the acquired immunodeficiency syndrome. *Science* 226, 549–552.

Anderson, K.P., Lucas, C., Hansen, C.V., Izu, A., Gregory, T., Berman, P.W., Lie, Y., Ammann, A. and Eichberg, J.W. (1990) Effect of dose and immunization schedule on immune response of baboons to recombinant gp120 of HIV-1. *J. Infect. Dis.* (in press).

Bacchetti, P. and Moss, A.R. (1989) Incubation period of AIDS in San Francisco. *Nature* 338, 251–253.

Berman, P.W., Groopman, J.E., Gregory, T., Clapham, P.R., Weiss, R.A., Ferriani, R., Riddle, L., Shimasaki, C., Lucas, C., Lasky, L.A. and Eichberg, J.W. (1988) Human immunodeficiency virus type 1 challenge of chimpanzees immunized with recombinant envelope glycoprotein gp120. *Proc. Natl. Acad. Sci. U.S.A.* 85, 5200–5204.

Dreseman, G.R., Kennedy, R.C., Kanda, P., Chanh, T.C., Eichberg, J.W., Sparrow, J.T., Ho, D.D., Allan, J.S., Lee, T.H. and Essex, M. (1986) Synthetic HIV peptide vaccine candidates and protection studies in chimpanzees. In: M. Girard, G. DeThe and L. Valette (Eds.), *Retroviruses of Human AIDS and Related Animal Diseases.* Pasteur Vaccins, Paris, pp. 175–178.

Eichberg, J.W., Levy, J.A. and Alter, H.J. (1989) Primates as models to understand cofactors in AIDS. In: R.R. Watson (Ed.), *Cofactors in HIV-1 Infection and AIDS.* CRC Press, Boca Raton, FL, pp. 223–229.

Hu, S.-L., Fultz, P.N., McClure, H.M., Eichberg, J.W., Kinney-Thomas, E., Zarling, J.M., Shinghal, M.C., Kosowski, S., Swenson, R.B., Anderson, D.C. and Todaro, G. (1987) Effect of immunization with vaccinia-HIV *env* on HIV infection of chimpanzees. *Nature* 328, 721–723.

Kanki, P.J., Eichberg, J.W. and Essex, M. (1990) Relevant aspects of HIV related viruses to vaccine development. In: S.D. Putney and D. Bolognesi (Eds.), *AIDS Vaccine: Basic Research and Clinical Trials.* Marcel Dekker, New York, NY (in press).

Morrow, W.J.W., Homsy, J., Eichberg, J.W., Krowka, J., Pan, L.-Z., Gaston, I., Legg, H., Lerche, N., Thomas, J. and Levy, J.A. (1989) Long-term observation of baboons, rhesus monkeys, and chimpanzees inoculated with HIV and given periodic immunosuppressive treatment. *AIDS Res. Human Retroviruses* 5, 233–246.

Prince, A.M., Horowitz, B., Baker, L., Shulman, R.W., Ralph, H., Valinsky, J., Cundell, A., Brotman, B., Boehle, W., Rey, F., Piet, M., Reesink, H., Lelie, N., Tersmette, M., Miedema, F., Barbosa, L.H., Nemo, G.J., Nastula, C.L., Allan, J.S., Lee, D.R. and Eichberg, J.W. (1988) Failure of an HIV immunoglobulin to protect chimpanzees against experimental challenge with HIV. *Proc. Natl. Acad. Sci. U.S.A.* 85, 6944–6948.

Zarling, J.M., Eichberg, J.W., Moran, P.A., McClure, J., Sridhar, P. and Hu, S.-L. (1987) Proliferative and cytotoxic T cells to AIDS virus glycoproteins in chimpanzees immunized with a recombinant vaccinia virus expressing AIDS virus envelope glycoproteins. *J. Immunol.* 139, 988–990.

*Eds. H. Schellekens and M.C. Horzinek*
*Animal Models in AIDS*



# 5

# Infectivity and pathogenicity of HIV-2ben in macaques

C. STAHL-HENNIG, O. HERCHENRÖDER, S. NICK, M. EVERS, K.-D. JENTSCH, F. KIRCHHOFF, T. TOLLE, T.J. GATESMAN, W. LÜKE and G. HUNSMANN

Deutsches Primatenzentrum, Abteilung Virologie und Immunologie, 3400 Göttingen, F.R.G.

**Summary**

Infectivity and pathogenicity of a new HIV-2 isolate (HIV-2ben) was examined in macaques. Ten rhesus (Mm) and six cynomolgus (Mf) monkeys received different virus preparations by varying routes of application. Seroconversion occurred in 13 of the 16 inoculated monkeys 2–6 weeks after infection (p.i.). Three Mm remained seronegative. In the seropositive animals ELISA antibody titers of 80–40,000 were measured. All seroconverted monkeys developed antibodies against gp160 and gp130, as well as in varying degrees against gp32 and core proteins. Virus isolation succeeded in 11 of the 13 seropositive macaques. Mm showed a transient viremia 6–14 weeks p.i. whereas all Mf have been persistently viremic from 2–7 weeks p.i. until now. During 6–18 months of follow-up one Mm lost 20% of its body weight. Two Mf showed transient lymphadenopathy and splenomegaly; the other monkeys remained clinically healthy. By Southern blot analysis a re-isolated virus was indistinguishable from the parental HIV-2ben used for infection.

Our data show that two readily available macaque species are infectable with cell-free HIV-2ben by a single intravenous injection. Furthermore, persistent viremia and early seroconversion in Mf are valuable and reliable criteria of infection required for studies on antivirals and vaccines.

## Introduction

An adequate animal model for the human acquired immunodeficiency syndrome (AIDS) with human immunodeficiency virus (HIV) as its causative agent (Barre-Sinoussi et al., 1983; Gallo et al., 1984; Levy et al., 1984) is still lacking. Such a model is most important for studies on pathogenicity, antiviral drugs and vaccines. Ideally, the two types of HIV, HIV-1 and HIV-2, should reproducibly infect and cause AIDS in an animal species which is closely related to humans. This kind of model should closely mimic the situation in HIV-infected man and should also be readily available.

To date, only chimpanzees (Alter et al., 1984; Fultz et al., 1986; Morrow et al., 1989) and gibbons (Lusso et al., 1988) are infectable with HIV-1, whereas infection of these two species with HIV-2 has not been reported so far. However, these models are of limited value since both species are endangered. Chimpanzees are expensive and difficult to keep, and apart from transient lymphadenopathy in one chimpanzee no other AIDS-related disorders were observed.

At present, experimental infection of macaques with several simian immunodeficiency viruses (SIV) seems to represent the only animal model in which an AIDS-like disease can be induced (Letvin et al., 1985; Daniel et al., 1987; Benveniste et al., 1988; Baskin et al., 1988; McClure et al., 1989; Fultz et al., 1989). However, with some SIV isolates also persistent infection for more than 3 years with no signs of illness has been observed (Daniel et al., 1987; Baskin et al., 1989; McClure et al., 1989).

HIV-2 is more closely related to SIV from macaques and sooty mangabeys than is HIV-1 (Guyader et al., 1987; Chakrabarti et al., 1987). Therefore HIV-2 might also be suited for developing a macaque model for AIDS. Initial experiments on the infectivity and pathogenicity of HIV-2 in macaques, baboons and mangabeys (Letvin et al., 1987; Dormont et al., 1988; Nicol et al., 1989) have generated contradictory data.

This prompted us to investigate the infectivity and pathogenicity of a novel HIV-2 isolate (HIV-2ben). The influence of different virus preparations and routes of inoculation was examined in two different macaque species. HIV-2ben was isolated from a patient with mainly neurological symptoms (Klemm et al., 1988) and seems to have evolved early from the main stem of HIV-2 (Kirchhoff et al., 1990).

## Material and methods

### Animals

Ten rhesus (*Macaca mulatta,* Mm) and six cynomolgus monkeys (*Macaca fascicularis,* Mf), all juvenile, of either sex and seronegative for simian T-cell leukemia virus type I, SIV, type D virus, foamy virus, HIV-1 and HIV-2 were used for infection. The rhesus monkeys were either born in the colony of the German Primate Center (DPZ), originating from an Indian breeding stock or imported from China. The cynomolgus monkeys were imported from the Philippines or Mauritius. During the study all animals were kept in single cages in an isolation facility with P3 level. The animals were examined daily for their clinical status and bled before and at regular intervals after infection for serology, virus isolation, immunology, hematology and blood chemistry. Physical examination was done at the time of blood collection.

### Inoculation protocol

An early passage of HIV-2ben which had been isolated at the DPZ (Schneider et al., 1990) was propagated in Molt-4 cells and used either for in vitro infection of rhesus peripheral mononuclear blood cells (PBMC) or directly for inoculation into monkeys. In detail (see also Table 1), two Mm received intravenously (i.v.) $10^7$ Molt-4 cells permanently infected with HIV-2ben. Two Mm were administered $10^7$ HIV-ben infected, autologous monkey PBMC. Two Mm were intrathecally (i.t.) inoculated with cell-free HIV-2ben corresponding to a reverse transcriptase (RT) incorporation rate of $8 \times 10^5$ counts per minute (cpm). Finally, six Mf and four Mm received i.v. cell-free HIV-2ben with a dose of $2 \times 10^6$ cpm RT activity.

### Virus isolation

Virus isolation was performed by cocultivation of PBMC from the HIV-2ben inoculated monkeys with phytohemagglutinin (PHA) stimulated human PBMC from normal blood donors. Cultures were fed once a week with prestimulated fresh human PBMC. Culture supernatants were examined for magnesium-dependent RT activity every 7 days (Hoffman et al., 1985; Jentsch et al., 1987) with slight modifications to optimize conditions using poly(rC):oligo dG as exogenous template primer. Cultures were discarded when no RT activity was observed during 6 weeks of cultivation.

### Serology

Seroconversion of the monkeys against HIV-2ben was determined by ELISA using whole, detergent treated HIV-2ben as antigen (Hunsmann et al., 1984). The humoral immune response was also specified with the more sensitive methods of radioimmunoprecipitation assay (RIPA) (Schneider et al., 1984) using lysates of $^{35}$S-cysteine labeled HIV-2ben infected Molt-4 clone 8 cells (Kikukawa et al., 1986) and Western blotting (WB) using alkaline phosphatase for the enzymatic reaction (Harlow and Lane, 1988).

### Immunology

For unspecific mitogenic stimulation monkey PBMC were stimulated in vitro with PHA and concanavalin A in optimal concentrations for 3 days. DNA synthesis of these cultures was assessed by $^3$H-thymidine incorporation (Ochs et al., 1980). Proliferative responses to viral HIV-2ben antigens were performed using soluble whole antigen which was added to cultures at a concentration of 5 $\mu$g antigen per $10^5$ cells. After 9 days of cultivation DNA synthesis was measured as described before. Stimulation indices were calculated as reported recently (Morrow et al., 1989).

Lymphocyte subpopulations were analyzed by flow cytometry (Schroff et al., 1983) in an EPICS Profile (Coulter Electronics, Krefeld, F.R.G.) after labeling the cells with the monoclonal antibodies Leu5b, Leu-2a (Becton Dickinson, Heidelberg, F.R.G.) and OKT4 (Ortho Diagnostic System, Neckargemünd, F.R.G.).

SOUTHERN BLOT ANALYSIS

Total genomic DNA was extracted by standard techniques from Molt-4 clone 8 cells infected with the parental HIV-2ben or a re-isolate obtained from an infected monkey 3 weeks after infection. The DNA was digested with *Kpn*I, *Eco*RI, *Pst*I, *Bam*HI and *Xho*I. These restriction endonucleases are known to yield DNA fragments specific only for HIV-2ben (Schneider et al., 1990). After electrophoretic separation DNA fragments were transferred to nitrocellulose (Southern, 1975). Hybridization was carried out according to published methods using the *gag* fragment pROD4.8 and the *env*-LTR region pSBE2 of HIV-2rod (Clavel et al., 1986). Finally, the filters were washed and exposed overnight to X-ray films.

## Results

Independent of the route of inoculation seroconversion was observed within 2–6 weeks p.i. in 13 of the 16 inoculated monkeys (seven Mm and six Mf). Two Mm from DPZ which received cell-bound virus and one Chinese Mm inoculated i.v. with cell-free virus remained seronegative for 6–18 months (Table 1). Generally, in all animals 2–6 weeks p.i. antibodies against the envelope proteins gp160 and gp130 were detected by RIPA, followed by antibodies against the *gag* gene products and gp32 determined by RIPA and WB with a delay of 2 weeks (data not shown). ELISA antibody titers either rose rapidly within 10–20 weeks p.i. to peak levels or increased constantly to values of 80–40,000 (Fig. 1). The weakest immune response to HIV-2ben was observed in the one Mm inoculated with permanently infected Molt-4 cells with an ELISA titer of 80 and a faint reactivity with gp160 in RIPA (data not shown). In contrast, highest antibody titers were found in three of the Mf infected with HIV-2ben with values of $1–4 \times 10^4$ (Fig. 1).

Virus was transiently re-isolated from five of the seven seroconverted Mm during 2–14 weeks p.i. From one Mm inoculated i.v. with cell-bound virus and the two Mm which received HIV-2ben i.t. virus isolation was successful only once 6 weeks p.i., whereas two Mm were repeatedly viremic. In contrast to Mm, all inoculated Mf developed a persistent viremia from 2–7 weeks p.i. onwards (Table 1). In these animals virus was recovered at almost every attempt.

As clinical alterations only two Mf showed transient lymphadenopathy and splenomegaly 2–3 months p.i., but these alterations disappeared completely 8–10 weeks later. One Mm inoculated i.v. with cell-free virus lost 20% of its body weight.

The immunologic studies on cellular immune response indicated no change in all seropositive monkeys during follow-up when compared to preimmune data and the negative controls. The helper-suppressor ratio and the absolute CD4 + lymphocytes remained within the normal range. Blastogenic responses to PHA and concanavalin A showed no considerable changes. So far, 10 of the 16

TABLE 1
Inoculation scheme, virus isolation, immune response and clinical alterations in HIV-2ben infected macaques

| Species [a] | Origin [b] | Inoculum [c] | Route [d] | Viremia [e] | Seroconversion [f] | Lymphocyte proliferation [g] | Clinical signs [h] |
|---|---|---|---|---|---|---|---|
| Mm | DPZ | aPBMC | i.v. | – | – | < 2.0 | – |
| Mm | DPZ | aPBMC | i.v. | – | 4 | < 2.0 | – |
| Mm | DPZ | Molt-4 | i.v. | tr(6) | 6 | < 2.0 | – |
| Mm | DPZ | Molt-4 | i.v. | – | – | < 2.0 | – |
| Mm | DPZ | c-f | i.t. | tr (6) | 4 | < 2.0 | – |
| Mm | DPZ | c-f | i.t. | tr (6) | 4 | < 2.0 | – |
| Mm | DPZ | c-f | i.v. | tr (2–14) | 4 | < 2.0 | – |
| Mm | DPZ | c-f | i.v. | tr (2–8) | 2 | 26.8 | 20% WL |
| Mm | CN | c-f | i.v. | – | 4 | nd | – |
| Mm | CN | c-f | i.v. | – | – | nd | – |
| Mf | PH | c-f | i.v. | per ( > 7) | 4 | 10.3 | trL, trS |
| Mf | PH | c-f | i.v. | per ( > 7) | 2 | 10.0 | trL, trS |
| Mf | PH | c-f | i.v. | per ( > 4) | 4 | nd | – |
| Mf | PH | c-f | i.v. | per ( > 4) | 4 | nd | – |
| Mf | MU | c-f | i.v. | per ( > 2) | 4 | nd | – |
| Mf | MU | c-f | i.v. | per ( > 4) | 4 | nd | – |

[a] Mm, *Macaca mulatta;* Mf, *Macaca fascicularis.*
[b] DPZ, German Primate Center; CN, China; PH, Philippines; MU, Mauritius.
[c] aPBMC, autologous infected PBMC; Molt-4, Molt-4 cells permanently infected; c-f, cell-free virus.
[d] i.v., intravenous; i.t., intrathecal.
[e] tr, transient; per, persistent; (weeks after inoculation).
[f] Weeks after inoculation.
[g] Proliferation of monkey lymphocytes to HIV-2ben antigen expressed as stimulation index (Morrow et al., 1989); nd, not done.
[h] WL, weight loss; trL, transient lymphadenopathy; trS, transient splenomegaly.

inoculated monkeys have been tested for proliferative responses of their PBMC to whole HIV-2ben antigen. Lymphocytes of one Mm receiving i.v. cell-free virus and of the two tested Mf proliferated significantly in response to HIV-2ben compared to the other infected and the uninfected control animals (data not shown). Stimulation indices of 10–27 were measured (Table 1).

The original infecting HIV-2ben and one re-isolate from an experimentally infected rhesus monkey were indistinguishable by Southern blotting. Digestion of proviral DNA from the original HIV-2ben and the re-isolated HIV-2ben provirus with the restriction enzymes indicated generated fragments of the same size (Fig. 2).

## Discussion

We could demonstrate that HIV-2ben isolated at the DPZ in 1987 (Schneider et al., 1990) from an AIDS patient who suffered from mainly neurological

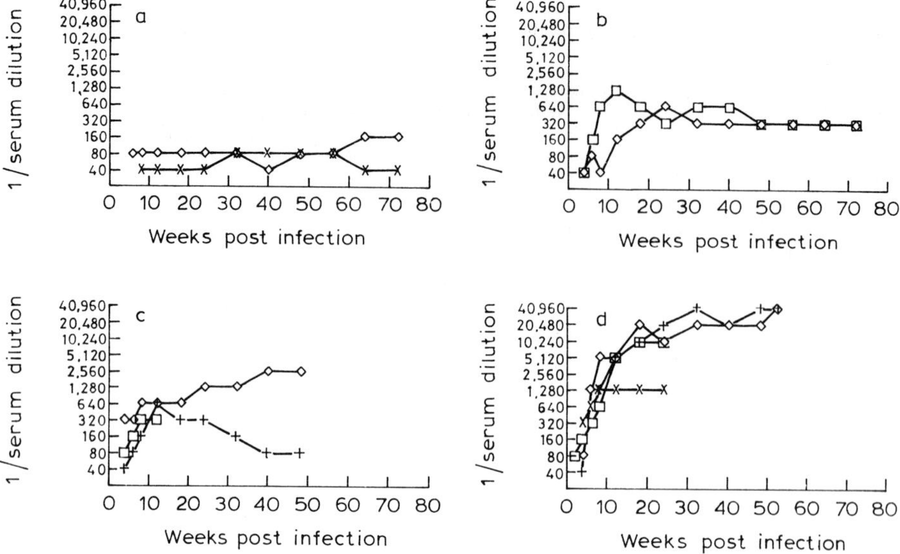


Fig. 1. Kinetics of serum antibody titers in macaques following inoculation of HIV-2ben. The influence of different virus preparations and routes of inoculation is demonstrated in panels a–d. Antibody titers were measured by ELISA. (a) Mm inoculated i.v. with cell-bound virus; (b) Mm receiving cell-free virus intrathecally; (c) Mm inoculated i.v. with cell-free virus; (d) Mf administered i.v. cell-free virus.

disorders (Klemm et al., 1988) was infectious for two macaque species (*Macaca mulatta* and *Macaca fascicularis*).

Only little has been reported on the experimental infection of non-human primates with HIV-2 or infectious molecular clones. In the first experiment described (Letvin et al., 1987) baboons and Mm had been inoculated with HIV-2 MIR. Only the baboons seroconverted and showed a transient viremia, whereas the Mm remained seronegative suggesting no susceptibility of the latter species to HIV-2, as has also been reported for HIV-1 (Morrow et al., 1989). More recently, another study described the successful infection of Mm with HIV-2rod and HIV-2 EHO (Dormont et al., 1989). However, the inoculation protocol was rather complicated including in vitro adaptation of the viruses and combination of different routes of inoculation and different virus preparations. In this experiment 90% of the inoculated animals seroconverted. Virus was recovered at variable frequencies. The molecular clone of HIV-2rod failed to infect Mm and baboons (Naidu et al., 1988). Most recently, data on the infectivity of HIV-2 NIH-DZ in three monkey species (mangabey, rhesus macaque and baboon) were published (Nicol et al., 1989). According to this report, two different virus preparations, the use of varying routes of inculation and in two cases repeated injection of virus led to seroconversion in all animals. The strongest immune response was observed in the four mangabeys, the weakest in the one Mm. Virus isolation was successful in all monkeys to a varying extent.

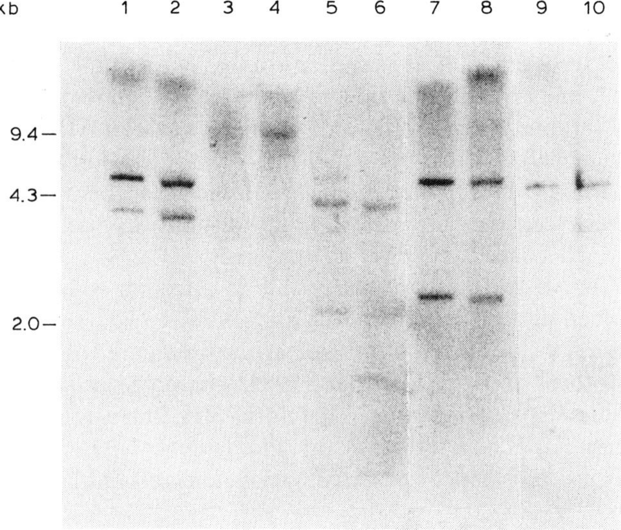


Fig. 2. Southern blot analysis of total genomic DNA from Molt-4 clone 8 cells infected with HIV-2ben. The original HIV-2ben from the AIDS patient and an HIV-2ben re-isolate from an experimentally infected monkey (same as in Fig. 1) obtained 3 weeks after infection were examined. Molecular size markers are indicated on the left (in kilobases, kb). Lanes with odd numbers represent DNA from cells infected with parental HIV-2ben, lanes with even numbers DNA from cells infected with the re-isolate from the monkey. Numbers above the lanes indicate digest with *Kpn*I (1, 2), *Eco*RI (3, 4), *Pst*I (5, 6), *Bam*HI (7, 8) and *Xho*I (9, 10).

To shed more light on the issue of infectivity and possible pathogenicity of HIV-2 in macaques we investigated HIV-2ben for these properties in two easily available macaque species. HIV-2ben is distinct from all known HIV-2 isolates (Schneider et al., 1990) and is thought to have branched off early from the main HIV-2 stem (Kirchhoff et al., 1990).

In 81% of our inoculated monkeys seroconversion was observed 2–6 weeks p.i. Virus was sporadically recovered from five Mm early after infection whilst the Mf became persistently viremic. Evaluation of different virus preparations and routes of application showed that i.v. or i.t. inoculation of cell-free virus reliably led to infection of the macaques. Application of cell-bound virus seemed to be less efficient because only two of four monkeys showed signs of infection.

Moreover, infectability of Mm seemed to depend on the origin of the macaques, most likely reflecting differences in their genetic background. Chinese Mm seemed to be less susceptible to HIV-2ben infection since only one of these two Mm seroconverted and virus isolation failed. In contrast, the two Mm with an Indian background and bred at the DPZ both became infected with the same virus dose.

Most interesting was the interspecies variation of HIV-2ben susceptibility. All Mf receiving cell-free virus i.v. seroconverted rapidly, developed a persistent viremia and lymphocytes of the two Mf tested so far for proliferative response to HIV-2ben antigen exhibited stimulation indices of 10.

Southern blot analysis of parental and re-isolated HIV-2ben from an infected Mm clearly showed that the two viruses were indistinguishable.

Whether the transient clinical alterations in two Mf and the weight loss in one Mm were due to the experimental infection with HIV-2ben remains uncertain. So far, only one Mm infected with HIV-2rod seemed to exhibit AIDS-like symptoms (Dormont et al., 1989), whereas other monkeys did not develop any AIDS-specific disease (Letvin et al., 1987; Nicol et al., 1989). However, because the HIV-2ben infected monkeys have only been followed up for up to 18 months, pathogenicity of this virus in macaques cannot yet be excluded.

In conclusion, Mf and Mm are susceptible to infection with HIV-2ben. Early markers of infection such as seroconversion and viremia were observed in Mf after one single i.v. injection of cell-free virus. Compared to the complicated inoculation protocol of Dormont et al. (1989) our protocol is easy to perform inducing reliable signs of infection. Therefore, HIV-2ben infection of Mf may serve as an animal model at least for the latent phase of HIV infection. Moreover, this model is suited for vaccine trials and certain therapy studies.

## Acknowledgements

Subclones of HIV-2rod were kindly provided by Dr. M. Alizon, Institut Pasteur, Paris, France. Molt-4 clone 8 cells were a gift of Dr. M. Hayami, Kyoto, Japan. We thank Dr. J. Schneider, Hoffmann-La Roche, Basel, Switzerland for helpful suggestions, Claudia Oeffner and Marion Stäger for excellent technical assistance. Part of the study was supported by a grant from the EC.

## References

Alter, H.J., Eichberg, J.W., Masur, H., Saxinger, W.C., Gallo, R.C., Macher, A.M., Lane, H.C. and Fauci, A.S. (1984) Transmission of HTLV-III infection from human plasma to chimpanzees: an animal model for AIDS. *Science* 226, 549–552.

Barre-Sinoussi, F., Chermann, J.C., Rey, F., Nugeyre, M.T., Chamaret, S., Gruest, J., Dauguet, C., Axler-Blin, C., Brun-Vezinet, F., Rouzioux, C., Rozenbaum, W. and Montagnier, L. (1983) Isolation of a T-lymphotropic retrovirus from a patient at risk for acquired immunodeficiency syndrome (AIDS). *Science* 220, 868–871.

Baskin, G.B., Murphey-Corb, M., Watson, E.A. and Martin, L.N. (1988) Necropsy findings in rhesus monkeys experimentally infected with cultured simian immunodeficiency virus (SIV)/delta. *Vet. Pathol.* 25, 456–467.

Benveniste, R.E., Morton, W.R., Clark, E.A., Tsai, C.-C., Ochs, H.D., Ward, J.M., Kuller, L., Knott, W.B., Hill, R.W., Gale, M.J. and Thouless, M.E. (1988) Inoculation of baboons and macaques with simian immunodeficiency virus/Mne, a primate lentivirus closely related to human immunodeficiency virus type 2. *J. Virol.* 62, 2091–2101.

Chakrabarti, L., Guyader, M., Alizon, M., Daniel, M.D., Desrosiers, R.C., Tiollais, P. and Sonigo, P. (1987) Sequence of simian immunodeficiency virus from macaque and its relationship to other human and simian retroviruses. *Nature* 328, 543–547.

Clavel, F., Guyader, M., Guetard, D., Salle, M., Montagnier, L. and Alizon, M. (1986) Molecular cloning and polymorphism of the human immunodeficiency virus type 2. *Nature* 324, 691–695.

Daniel, M.D., Letvin, N.L., Sehgal, P.K., Hunsmann, G., Schmidt, D.K., King, N.W. and Desrosiers, R.C. (1987) Long-term persistent infection of macaque monkeys with the simian immunodeficiency virus. *J. Gen. Virol.* 68, 3183–3189.

Dormont, D., Livartowski, J., Chamaret, S., Guetard, D., Henin, D., Levagueresse, R., van der Moortelle, P.F., Larke, B., Gourmelon, P., Vazeux, R., Metivier, H., Flageat, J., Court, L., Hauw, J.J. and Montagnier, L. (1989) HIV-2 in rhesus monkeys: serological, virological and clinical results. *Intervirology* 30 (Suppl.), 59–65.

Fultz, P.N., McClure, H.M., Swenson, R.B., McGrath, C.R., Brodie, A., Getchell, J.P., Jensen, F.C., Anderson, L.D.C., Broderson, J.R. and Francis, D.P. (1986) Persistent infection of chimpanzees by human T-lymphotropic virus type III/lymphadenopathy-associated virus: a potential model for acquired immunodeficiency syndrome. *J. Virol.* 58, 116–124.

Fultz, P.N., McClure, H.M., Anderson, D.C. and Switzer, W.M. (1989) Identification and biologic characterization of an acutely lethal variant of simian immunodeficiency virus from sooty mangabeys (SIV/SMM). *AIDS Res. Hum. Retrovir.* 5, 397–409.

Gallo, R.C., Salahuddin, S.Z., Popovic, M., Shearer, G.M., Kaplan, M., Haynes, B.F., Palker, T.J., Redfield, R., Oleske, J., Safai, B., White, G., Foster, P. and Markham, P.D. (1984) Frequent detection and isolation of cytopathic retrovirus (HTLV-III) from patients with AIDS. *Science* 224, 500–503.

Guyader, M., Emerman, M., Sonigo, P., Clavel, F., Montagnier, L. and Alizon, M. (1987) Genome organization and transactivation of the human immunodeficiency virus type 2. *Nature* 326, 662–664.

Harlow, E. and Lane, D. (1989) *Antibodies: A Laboratory Manual.* Cold Spring Harbor Laboratory Press, Cold Spring Harbor, NY.

Hoffmann, A.D., Banapour, B. and Levy, J.A. (1985) Characterization of the AIDS-associated retrovirus reverse transcriptase and optimal conditions for its detection in virions. *Virology* 147, 326–335.

Hunsmann, G., Schneider, J., Bayer, H., Berthold, H., Schimpf, K., Kabisch, H., Bienzle, U., Ritter, K., Schmitz, H., Kern, P. and Dietrich, M. (1984) Antibodies to adult T-cell leukemia virus (ATLV/HTLV-I) in AIDS patients and people at risk of AIDS in Germany. *Med. Microbiol. Immunol.* 173, 241–250.

Jentsch, K.-D., Hunsmann, G., Hartmann, H. and Nickel, P. (1987) Inhibition of human immunodeficiency virus type I reverse transcriptase by suramin-related compounds. *J. Gen. Virol.* 68, 2183–2192.

Kikukawa, R., Koyanagi, S., Harada, N., Kobayashi, N., Hatanaka, M. and Yamamoto, N. (1986) Differential susceptibility to the acquired immunodeficiency syndrome retrovirus in cloned cells of human leukemic T-cell line MOLT-4. *J. Virol.* 57, 1159–1162.

Kirchhoff, F., Jentsch, K.-D., Stuke, A., Bachmann, B., Laloux, C., Lüke, W., Stahl-Hennig, C., Schneider, J., Nieselt, K., Eigen, M. and Hunsmann, G. (1990) A novel proviral clone of HIV-2: biological and phylogenetic relationship to other primate immunodeficiency viruses. *Virology* (in press).

Klemm, E., Schneeweis, K.E, Horn, R., Tackmann, W., Schulze, G. and Schneider, J. (1988) HIV-2 infection with initial neurologic manifestation. *J. Neurol.* 235, 304–307.

Letvin, N.L., Daniel, M.D., Sehgal, P.K., Desrosiers, R.C., Hunt, R.D., Waldron, L.M., MacKey, J.J., Schmidt, D.K., Chalifoux, L.V. and King, N.W. (1985) Induction of AIDS-like disease in macaque monkeys with T-cell tropic retrovirus STLV-III. *Science* 230, 71–73.

Letvin, N.L., Daniel, M.D., Prabhat, K.S., Yetz, J.M., Solomon, K.R., Kannagi, M., Schmidt, D.K., Silva, D.P., Montagnier, L. and Desrosiers, R.C. (1987) Infection of baboons with human immunodeficiency virus-2 (HIV-2). *J. Infect. Dis.* 156, 406–407.

Levy, J.A., Hoffmann, A.D., Kramer, S.M., Landis, J.A., Shimabukuro, J.M. and Oshiro, L.S. (1984) Isolation of lymphocytopathic retroviruses from San Francisco patients with AIDS. *Science* 225, 840–842.

Lusso, P., Markham, P.D., Ranki, A., Earl, P., Moss, B., Dorner, F., Gallo, R.C. and Krohn, K.J.E. (1988) Cell-mediated immune response toward viral envelope and core antigens in gibbon apes (*Hylobates lar*) chronically infected with human immunodeficiency virus-1. *J. Immunol.* 141, 2467–2473.

McClure, H.M., Anderson, D.C., Fultz, P.N., Ansari, A.A., Lockwood, E. and Brodie, A. (1989) Spectrum of disease in macaque monkeys chronically infected with SIV/SMM. *Vet. Immunol. Immunopathol.* 21, 13–24.

Morrow, W.J.W., Homsey, J., Eichberg, J.W., Krowka, J., Li-Zhen, P., Gaston, I., Legg, H., Lerche, N., Thomas, J. and Levy, J.A. (1989) Long-term observation of baboons, rhesus monkeys, and chimpanzees inoculated with HIV and given periodic immunosuppressive treatment. *AIDS Res. Hum. Retrovir.* 5, 233–245.

Naidu, Y.M., Kestler, H.W. III, Li, Y., Butler, C.V., Silva, D.P., Schmidt, D.K., Troup, C.D., Sehgal, P.K., Sonigo, P., Daniel, M.D. and Desrosiers, R.C. (1988) Characterization of infectious molecular clones of simian immunodeficiency virus (SIVmac) and human immunodeficiency virus type 2: persistent infection of rhesus monkeys with molecularly cloned SIVmac. *J. Virol.* 62, 4691–4696.

Nicol, E., Flamminio-Zola, G., Dubouch, P., Bernard, J., Snart, R., Jouffre, R., Reveil, B., Fouchard, M., Seportes, I., Nara, P., Gallo, R. and Zagury, D. (1989) Persistent HIV-2 infection of rhesus macaque, baboon, and mangabeys. *Intervirology* 30, 258–267.

Ochs, H.D., Slichter, S.J., Harker, L.A., von Behrens, W.E., Clark, R.A. and Wedgwood, R.J. (1980) The Wiskott-Aldrich syndrome: studies of lymphocytes, granulocytes, and platelets. *Blood* 55, 243–252.

Schneider, J., Yamamoto, N., Hinuma, Y. and Hunsmann, G. (1984) Sera from adult T-cell leukemia patients react with envelope and core polypeptides of adult T-cell leukemia virus. *Virology* 132, 1–11.

Schneider, J., Lüke, W., Jentsch, K.D., Kirchhoff, F., Jung, R., Jurkiewicz, E., Stahl-Hennig, C., Klemm, E. and Hunsmann, G. (1990) Isolation and characterization of HIV-2ben, a new HIV-2 from a patient with predominantly neurological defects. *AIDS* (in press).

Schroff, R.W., Gottlieb, M.S., Prince, H.E., Chai, L.L. and Fahey, J.L. (1983) Immunological studies of homosexual men with immunodeficiency and Kaposi's sarcoma. *Clin. Immunol. Immunopathol.* 27, 300–314.

Southern, E. (1975) Detection of specific sequences among DNA fragments separated by gel electrophoresis. *J. Mol. Biol.* 98, 503–519.

*Eds. H. Schellekens and M.C. Horzinek*
*Animal Models in AIDS*



# 6

# Second in vivo passage of HIV-2 in rhesus monkeys

D. DORMONT [1,2], J. LIVARTOWSKI [1], G. VOGT [1], S. CHAMARET [2], I. NICOL [1], D. DWYER [2], P. LEBON [3], D. GUETARD [2] and L. MONTAGNIER [2]

[1] Centre de Recherches du Service de Santé des Armées, Commissariat à l'Energie Atomique, DPS/SPE, 92265 Fontenay aux Roses Cedex, France, [2] Unité d'Oncologie Virale, Institut Pasteur, Paris, France and [3] Hôpital Saint Vincent de Paul, Paris, France

**Summary**

HIV-2 has been inoculated into rhesus monkeys after being in vitro adapted to monkey lymphocytes. First in vivo passage of these viruses in 10 animals induced six seroconversions (days 13–180) and reproducible detection of HIV-2 in PBL and CSF cell cultures; two animals exhibited clinical symptoms which might be related to HIV infection: one animal showed generalized actinomycete infection, with a dramatic decrease in CD4+ cells (monkey 1), and the other is pancytopenic (monkey 2). Therefore we performed a second passage of the virus isolated from monkey 1, and we inoculated the eight monkeys without clinical symptoms 15 months after the first inoculation (both seropositive and seronegative animals), and one animal as positive control of this HIV-2 strain. The inoculation protocol consisted in double inoculation by the intracerebral (i.c.) and intravenous (i.v.) routes of a great amount of virus ($10^6$ cpm of reverse transcriptase equivalent). We report here the virologic, clinical, and immunologic follow up of these nine monkeys during 8 months after inoculation. Four animals lost more than 15% of their weight within 3 months following the second infection, and in seven of nine animals we observed a decrease in CD4+ cells. A transient enhancement of anti-HIV-2 antibody reaction was observed in previously seropositive animals. PCR was positive in all animals' PBL DNA for at least two primers. As preliminary conclusions, these results might suggest that (1) all animals are infected with HIV-2; (2) there are differences in in vivo susceptibility to lentiviruses; and (3) the second passage of HIV-2-ROD may be more pathogenic than the first.

## Introduction

Human immunodeficiency virus type 1 (HIV-1) has been identified as the etiologic agent of AIDS, by F.C. Barre-Sinoussi et al. (1983), and since that time other lentiviruses have been described in both humans and primates: HIV-2 in humans (Clavel et al., 1986), and SIVs in African green monkeys ($SIV_{AGM}$) (Kanki et al., 1985), in mandrills ($SIV_{MND}$), in mangabeys ($SIV_{SMN}$) (Fultz et al.,

1986), and in macaques ($SIV_{MAC}$) (Daniel et al., 1985; Benveniste et al., 1986). Several of these lentiviruses are not pathogenic in their natural hosts, and therefore may constitute only infection models for HIV infections in humans ($SIV_{AGM}$, $SIV_{MND}$, $SIV_{SMN}$). Others may induce diseases in recipients, and these diseases resemble human AIDS and AIDS-related complexes (Desrosiers, 1988). These experimental infections of macaques with $SIV_{MAC}$ are good models for human AIDS and may be used for pathogenesis and therapeutic studies, and in testing vaccine strategies.

Chimpanzees inoculated with HIV-1 seroconverted but did not develop any clinical symptom which might be related to HIV infection; nevertheless, HIV is identifiable in peripheral blood cell (PBL) culture supernatants (Gajdusek et al., 1985; Fultz et al., 1986, 1989). Therefore, HIV-1 inoculated chimpanzees could not be considered today as a good model for human HIV infection, possibly the last animal test of vaccines before human trials.

The molecular sequence of $SIV_{MAC}$ appears to be closer to HIV-2 (Chakrabarti et al., 1987; Guyader et al., 1987) than to HIV-1. Therefore, from a theoretical point of view, HIV-2 might be a better candidate than HIV-1, for establishing a human HIV infection animal model. Several experimental infections of macaques or other species of monkeys (baboons, mangabeys, etc.) with HIV-2 have been performed, using massive inoculations of several strains of HIV-2. Seroconversion occurred in all published experiments (Dormont et al., 1987; Fultz et al., 1988; Nicol et al., 1989), and, in our laboratory, biological and clinical symptoms of HIV infection have been described in two out of 10 inoculated macaques (Dormont et al., 1989). We report here the biological and/or clinical pattern of two successive in vivo passsages of one HIV-2 isolate (HIV-2-ROD), the second passage being performed with the viral isolate which was pathogenic in macaques at the first passage.

## Material and methods

### In vitro adaptation of HIV-2 strains before the first passage

Two HIV-2 strains (HIV-2-ROD, and HIV-2-EHO) were in vitro adapted to monkey cells (baboon, cynomolgus, or rhesus monkey). Five different viruses were obtained: HIV-2-ROD (wild type); HIV-2-ROD adapted to baboon cells (HIV-2-ROD/BAB); HIV-2-ROD/BAB adapted to rhesus cells (HIV-2-ROD/BAB/MAC); HIV-2-ROD adapted to cynomolgus cells (HIV-2-ROD/CYN); HIV-2-EHO adapted to baboon cells (HIV-2-EHO/BAB).

### Inoculation protocols

#### *First passage*

Each virus was inoculated in two rhesus monkeys, which were caged in special high security facilities (P4), in accordance with official animal experimentation rules and recommendations.

The inoculation protocol was as follows. Day −3: intravenous (i.v.) injection of $10^7$ normal human PBL. Day 0: (1) i.v. injection of $10^6$ cpm of reverse transcriptase (RT) viral equivalent; (2) i.v. injection of $10^7$ human PBL (same donor as at day −3) infected with correspondent HIV-2 at the time of the RT peak; (3) Intracerebral (i.c.) injection (right hippocampus) of $10^6$ cpm of RT viral equivalent.

*Second passage*

Animals were inoculated with both $10^6$ cpm of viral equivalent by the i.v. route and $10^6$ cpm of viral equivalent by the i.c. route into the right hippocampus.

### Biological and clinical survey

*Clinical survey*

Animals were anesthetized every 2 weeks. They were clinically examined: lymphadenopathies, splenomegaly, hepatomegaly, cutaneous symptoms, temperatures, and weights were recorded.

Non-anesthetized animals were examined by experimenters and videotaped in order to detect any neurologic or psychophysiologic symptoms.

*Biological survey*

Every 2 weeks, blood was drawn from animals for biological survey.

*General biological parameters.* Blood cell counts, platelet counts and routine blood chemistry, including γ-globulin dosage were performed every month.

*Serologic tests.* HIV-2 radioimmunoprecipitation assay and HIV-2 Western blot analysis (New LAV-BLOT) were performed every 2 weeks until seroconversion, and every 2 months thereafter.

*CD4+ and CD8+ peripheral blood lymphocyte determination (absolute numbers).* Peripheral blood mononuclear cells (PMC) were isolated as usually described by Ficoll gradient. After cell washing, cell suspensions were adjusted to $10^7$ cells/ml. Samples of 50 μl were then incubated for 30 min with either anti-leu 3a + b, anti-leu 2a, or anti-leu 5b (Becton Dickinson). Cells were washed and incubated for 30 min with FITC anti-mouse immunoglobulin antibodies. Labeled cell numbers were counted by epifluorescence.

*Jacaline T cell proliferation.* Jacaline is an extract from *Artocarpus heterophyllus.* It has been reported to be a specific mitogen of the CD4+ lymphocytes in humans. Previous results have demonstrated that, in humans, a good correlation may exist between jacaline proliferation and both clinical staging of the patients and the absolute number of CD4+ lymphocytes (N. Pineau et al., in preparation).

Proliferation assays of PMC were performed in the presence of 50, 100, and 200 pg/ml of this specific mitogen, by measuring 24 h tritiated thymidine incorporation after 3 days of culture.

*Retrovirus isolation.* PMC were isolated as described above. Cocultures with phytohemagglutinin-p (PHA-p) stimulated human cord lymphocytes (three human lymphocytes for one monkey PMC) were performed in RPMI 1640 supplemented with 10% recombinant human interleukin 2 (IL-2), 10% fetal calf serum, antibiotics, 20 mM glutamine, hexadimethrine bromide (2 mg/ml), and anti-$\alpha$-recombinant interferon antibodies.

Reverse transcriptase assays were performed at each passage on cell culture supernatants, as previously described (poly(rA)-oligo($dT_{12-18}$)) (Barre-Sinoussi et al., 1983).

*Antigenemia.* Commercial kits allow the detection of HIV-1 major core protein (P25) in serum, CSF, and biological fluids. Because antibodies cross-react with HIV-2 major core protein (P26), these kits may be used to detect HIV-2 P26 in infected individuals. Nevertheless one must take into consideration a constant loss of sensitivity of 1 log (G. Vogt, unpublished data).

The P26 seric level was determined sequentially during the experimental infection (Abbott Kit).

*Polymerase chain reaction (PCR).* DNA was extracted from PMC as previously described (Loche et al., 1988). Three different primers were used: LTR(7410,01.3) (NP 39–49, CP 192–215), *gag* 1,3 (NP 303–320, CP 637–656), and *env* (7367–7368) (NP 8265–8267, CP 8412–8434). The reaction mixture included 10 $\mu$l of reaction buffer (50 mM Tris–HCl, pH 8.3, 1.5 mM $MgCl_2$, and 0.1% gelatin), 16 $\mu$l of dNTP, 10 pM of normal primer, 10 pM of complementary primer, 1 $\mu$g DNA, 0.5 $\mu$l of Taq polymerase (5 U/ml), and distilled water (q.s.p. 100 $\mu$l). Thirty cycles were performed. Amplification products were run on an agarose 1% gel, stained with ethidium bromide, and transferred onto a nitrocellulose membrane. Hybridization was performed with a total $^{32}$P-labeled oligoprobe corresponding to the viral genome included between the primers.

*Interferon dosage.* $\alpha$-Interferon was measured on MDBK cells, and total interferon levels in serum were determined using the Vero cell assay.

*Complementary investigations.* When clinical or biological symptoms of infection were suspected in our animals, specific investigations were performed: hemoculture in the case of fever, electroencephalogram (EEG) in the case of neurologic symptoms, and tomodensitometry if EEG abnormalities were noticed.

## Results

### Results of the first passage

Results of the first passage (24 months of experiment) have been previously published (Dormont et al., 1989). Briefly, seven monkeys seroconverted between week 2 and week 20: antibodies were directed against *env* and *gag* proteins and/or *nef* protein. One monkey exhibited antibodies only against *nef* protein (33219). HIV-2 was detectable in PMC cocultures in seven monkeys (five

TABLE 1
Jacaline T cell proliferation

| Animal | Jacaline concentration (pg/ml) | | |
|---|---|---|---|
| | 50 | 100 | 200 |
| 33209 | 8555 | 5421 | 4956 |
| 33210 | 9258 | 14945 | 13545 |
| 33219 | 37437 | 40399 | 30289 |
| 34435 | 50125 | 37736 | 26959 |
| 34771 | 12740 | 9540 | 17841 |
| 34782 | 62313 | 38679 | 20217 |
| 37202 | 85948 | 62896 | 21954 |
| Negative control | 47357 | 26919 | 13055 |

seropositive and two seronegative animals); no viral replication could be identified in the PMC culture of monkey 33219 (only anti-*nef* antibodies).

CD4 + and CD8 + PMC were modified significantly in eight animals (> 40% decrease in CD4 cell number) 22 months after inoculation (see Table 1). T cell proliferation was identical to or greater than controls in five out of the eight tested animals; no correlation could be made between this proliferation index and the clinical or immunological status of the animal. No major interferon level abnormality was recorded. PCR results are summarized in Table 2. Four of the eight tested animals were positive for the three primers; one (33219) was positive for both *gag* and LTR primers, and one was positive only for the *gag* primer. Antigenemia was detectable in four animals between week 71 and week 100. Clinical records showed no specific symptoms of primary infection. Two monkeys exhibited clinical symptoms, which started 5 and 7 months after inoculation, and which might be related to lentivirus infection: one animal showed generalized actinomycete infection, with a dramatic decrease in CD4 + cells (monkey 33215) and was euthanized 6 months after inoculation, and the other remained very

TABLE 2
Polymerase chain reaction

| Animal | First passage | | | Second passage | | |
|---|---|---|---|---|---|---|
| | *Gag* | LTR | *Env* | *Gag* | LTR | *Env* |
| 33209 | + + + | + + + | + | + + + | + | + + + |
| 33210 | – | – | – | + + | – | + + + |
| 33219 | + + | + + | – | + + | – | + + + |
| 34433 | nd | nd | nd | – | + + | + + + |
| 34435 | nd | nd | nd | + + + | + + | + + + |
| 34771 | – | – | – | – | + | + + + |
| 34773 | + + + | + + | + | nd | nd | nd |
| 34782 | + | – | – | + | – | + + |
| 37202 | Negative control of the first passage | | | + + | + | + + + |

pancytopenic with severe non specific bone marrow abnormalities between 8 and 22 months after inoculation (monkey 33216); this monkey lost 20% of its body weight and died at month 22; the causes of death are under investigation.

## RESULTS OF THE SECOND PASSAGE

Because one of the monkeys died from generalized opportunistic infection (33215), we propagated its virus isolate in human PMC, and with this virus re-inoculated all the monkeys without clinical symptoms, seropositive (five animals) or not (three animals). A previously not inoculated monkey was also infected as positive control of the experiment.

### *Serologic results*

After the second inoculation, an increase in antibody titer was observed in monkeys 34435 and 34433. One animal seroconverted 2 weeks after the second inoculation (33209), and two sera were slightly positive for GP in RIPA at week 7 (34771, 34782). Monkey 33219, in whose serum only anti-*nef* antibodies were detectable after the first infection, did not develop any other antibody after the second experimental infection.

The positive control (monkey 37202) seroconverted in week 5.

### *Evolution of CD4 + and CD8 + absolute cell numbers*

Absolute numbers of CD4 + cells and CD4 + /CD8 + ratios are summarized in Table 3.

All eight re-inoculated animals showed a significant decrease in CD4 + cells 180 days after the second inoculation. Today CD4/CD8 ratios are < 1 except in one animal (33219), which has only anti-*nef* antibodies.

TABLE 3
Evolution of CD4+ cell numbers and CD4/CD8 ratios

| Animal | Before inoculation | | Last determination | | |
|---|---|---|---|---|---|
| | CD4+/CD8+ | CD4+ cells/ml | CD4+/CD8+ | CD4+ cells/ml | Day |
| 33209 | 1.99 | 1705 | 0.45 | 717 | 580 |
| 33210 | 1 | 1179 | 0.54 | 624 | 620 |
| 33215 | 2.3 | 2033 | 0.7 [a] | 269 [a] | 190 [a] |
| 33216 | 1.07 | 1391 | 0.5 [a] | 512 [a] | 620 [a] |
| 33219 | 1.89 | 1572 | 1.57 | 974 | 580 |
| 34433 | 1.7 | 1595 | 0.96 | 577 | 620 |
| 34435 | 2.4 | 1441 | 0.68 | 691 | 650 |
| 34771 | 2.61 | 2005 | 0.6 | 644 | 620 |
| 34773 | 2.93 | 2043 | 0.47 | 268 | 580 |
| 34782 | 1.6 | 2121 | 0.62 | 612 | 620 |

[a] First passage only.

*PCR results*

Results are summarized in Table 3.

All the animals are positive in PCR for primer *env* including the positive control (37202). All monkey PMN DNAs are positive for at least two primers, suggesting that all animals may be infected.

*Clinical results*

Lymphadenopathies were observed in three monkeys 5 weeks after inoculation, and 7 months after the second inoculation they are persistent.

Four animals lost more than 15% of their weight. One of them exhibited generalized chronic dermatosis, which resembles that described in HIV infected humans.

## Discussion

After the first passage, one may conclude that rhesus monkeys can be infected with HIV-2. Seroconversion occurred in seven of 10 animals 13–150 days after infection, which agrees with previously published data, and it is of interest to note that monkeys may develop only anti-*nef* protein antibodies. Reproducible viral isolation of HIV-2 in cell culture supernatants was possible in inoculated animals, suggesting that rhesus monkeys can be infected with HIV-2. The virus can be isolated in seronegative monkeys, as has also been described for humans. Antigenemia is sometimes detectable, but this in vivo HIV replication parameter does not seem to be as efficient as it is in HIV-1 infected humans. Two monkeys developed clinical symptoms which can be related to lentivirus infection: pancytopenic syndrome, wasting syndrome, and opportunistic infection are clinical symptoms of AIDS. Moreover, the association of these clinical AIDS-like symptoms with biological symptoms of HIV infection (decrease in CD4+ cell numbers, decrease in CD4+/CD8+ ratios, and hypergammaglobulinemia) may support a diagnosis of full-blown AIDS in our two monkeys. No effect of the previous virus in vitro adaptation to monkey cells has been detected, either in seroconversion delay or in in vivo pathogenicity. Therefore, infection of rhesus monkeys may depend on individual susceptibility, including animal genetic background, and immune status at the time of infection.

Because in other fields of virology successive in vivo passages of human viruses in primates or rodents are required to obtain a reproducible disease model, we decided to inoculate all our monkeys with the most clinically pathogenic HIV-2 isolated in our animals. This second passage was performed with a lower amount of virus than for the first infection. The main results are: all our animals were infected, because PCR results were positive for at least two primers. None of the inoculated animals remained seronegative; anti-GP antibodies were identifiable 50 days after infection (RIPA) in eight of the nine macaques, and the last monkey, which had no anti-structural protein antibodies, exhibited anti-*nef* protein antibodies. In seven of eight doubly inoculated animals, CD4+ absolute cell numbers and CD4 + /CD8 + ratios decreased significantly; it is interesting to note that the only animal that had no modified CD4/CD8 ratio (33219) exhibits only anti-*nef* antibodies, suggesting that, in vivo, *nef* protein might slow down viral replication. Clinical follow-up made it possible to record symptoms of lentivirus infection: weight loss (four animals), lymphadenopathies, and chronic dermatosis; these clinical parameters were not identifiable at the corresponding time after the first infection. Therefore, one might suspect an increase of HIV-2 pathogenicity in rhesus monkeys during this second in vivo passage.

These encouraging data suggest that it might be useful (1) to carry out a third passage of this HIV-2 strain, in both asymptomatic seropositive monkeys and in not previously inoculated animals, (2) to analyze, at the molecular level, the potential differences which may have occurred during these two in vivo passages of HIV-2-ROD and (3) to focus our attention on the immune system of monkey 33219, in whose blood only anti-*nef* antibodies are identifiable.

If these preliminary results are confirmed, HIV-2 inoculation of rhesus monkeys may be both an infection model and a disease model, and this model may be involved in testing vaccine efficiency, determining pathogenesis mechanisms, and in therapeutic monitoring trials. Because of the low number of chimpanzees nowadays, available for HIV vaccine trials, HIV-2 inoculation of monkeys might be an alternative for the HIV-1-inoculated chimpanzee model, and may constitute the last experimental step before testing a vaccine in humans.

## Acknowledgements

This work has been made possible by a generous donation of the 'Fondation Mérieux'. The authors wish to thank Dr. R. Masse, Dr. H. Metivier, Dr. J.C. Mestries, Dr. N. Pineau and Dr. F. Barre-Sinoussi for their scientific contribution.

## References

Barre-Sinoussi, F.C., Chermann, J.C., Rey, F. et al. (1983) Isolation of a T lymphotropic retrovirus from a patient at risk for AIDS. *Science* 220, 868–870.

Benveniste, R.E., Lo, A., Tsai, C.C. et al. (1986) Isolation of a lentivirus from macaque with lymphoma: comparison with HTLVIII/LAV and other lentiviruses. *J. Virol.* 60, 483–490.

Chakrabarti, L., Guyader, M., Alizon, M. et al., (1987) Sequence of simian immunodeficiency virus from macaque and its relationship to other human and simian retroviruses. *Nature* 328, 543–547.

Clavel, F., Guetard, D., Brun-Vezinet, F. et al. (1986) Isolation of a new retrovirus from West African patients with AIDS. *Science* 233, 343–346.

Daniel, M.D., Letvin, N.I., King, N.W., et al. (1985) Isolation of a T-cell tropic HTLVIII-like retrovirus from macaques. *Science* 228, 1201–1204.

Desrosiers, R.C. (1988) Simian immunodeficiency viruses. *Annu. Rev. Microbiol.* 42, 607–625.

Dormont, D., Van De Moortelle, P.F., Guetard, D. et al. (1988) HIV-2 in rhesus monkey. In: Retroviruses of Human AIDS and Related Animal Diseases; Colloque des Cent Gardes, 1987, Paris, O. Robert, Paris, pp. 171–173.

Dormont, D., Livartowski, J., Chamaret, S. et al. (1989) HIV-2 in rhesus monkeys; serological, virological and clinical results. *Intervirology* 30 (Suppl. 1), 59–65.

Fultz, P.N., McClure, H.M., Swenson, R.B. et al. (1986) Persistent infection of chimpanzees with HTLVIII/LAV: a potential model for acquired immunodeficiency syndrome. *J. Virol.* 58, 116–124.

Fultz, P.N., McClure H.M., Anderson, D.C. et al. (1986) Isolation of a T-lymphotropic retrovirus from naturally infected sooty mangabey monkeys *(Cercocebus atys). Proc. Natl. Acad. Sci. U.S.A.* 83, 5286–5290.

Fultz, P.N., McClure, H.M., Switzer, W.M., et al. (1988) Responses of macaques to infection by SIV/SMM and HIV-2. In: *Retroviruses of Human AIDS and Related Animal Diseases;* Colloque des Cent Gardes, 1987, Paris. O. Robert, Paris, pp. 166–170.

Fultz, P.N., McClure, H.M., Swenson, R.B. et al. (1989) HIV infection of chimpanzees as a model for testing chemotherapeutics. *Intervirology* 30 (Suppl. 1), 51–58.

Gajdusek, D.C., Amyx, H.L., Gibbs, C.J. et al. (1985) Infection of chimpanzees by human T lymphotropic retroviruses in brain and other tissues from AIDS patients. *Lancet* i, 55–56.

Guyader, M., Emerman, M., Sonigo. P. et al. (1987) Genome organization and transactivation of the human immunodeficiency virus type 2. *Nature* 326, 662–669.

Kanki, P.J., Alroy, J. and Essex, M. (1985) Isolation of a T-lymphotropic retrovirus related to HTLVIII/LAV from wild caught African green monkeys. *Science* 230, 951–954.

Loche, M. and Mach, B. (1988) Identification of HIV infected seronegative individuals by a direct diagnostic test based on hybridization to amplified viral DNA. *Lancet* i, 418–421.

Nicol, I., Flamminio-Zola, G., Dubouch, P. et al. (1989) Persistent HIV-2 infection of rhesus macaque, baboon, and mangabeys. *Intervirology* 30, 258–267.

*Eds. H. Schellekens and M.C. Horzinek*
*Animal Models in AIDS*



# 7

# Infection of non-human primates with $SIV_{agm}$ and HIV-2

S. HARTUNG [1], S. NORLEY [1], G. KRAUS [1], A. WERNER [1], M. VOGEL [1], L. BERGMANN [2], M. BAIER [1] and R. KURTH [1]

[1] Paul Ehrlich Institute, 6070 Langen, F.R.G. and [2] J.W. Goethe University, 6000 Frankfurt, F.R.G.

## Introduction

For economic, ecological and ethical reasons it is no longer acceptable to use the HIV-1/chimpanzee animal model for anything but the most crucial of vaccine trials and the development of alternative models has been a high priority research goal in many laboratories, including our own, for some time (Desrosiers and Letvin, 1987). Consequently, a number of lentiviruses have been isolated from different primate species which are closely related in terms of their genomic organization to HIV-1 and HIV-2, the simian immunodeficiency viruses (SIV) (Kurth et al., 1988). The most thoroughly examined virus of this group, because of its property of inducing an AIDS-like disease in rhesus macaques, is $SIV_{mac}$. However, members of another family of SIV which have recently been isolated from African green monkeys (AGM) by a number of groups, including our own, are of particular interest because judging from the seroprevalence (20–40%) amongst wild AGMs (Kanki et al., 1985), this monkey represents the natural host of the virus. Despite the close relationship between $SIV_{agm}$ and HIV, $SIV_{agm}$ infected AGMs do not appear to succumb to an immunodeficiency disease and the question of why the animals remain healthy despite an active infection urgently requires an answer. As part of our efforts to provide such an answer, we have inoculated different primate species with our $SIV_{agm}$ isolate, both wild type and a biologically active molecular clone, and have characterized the ensuing infection.

## Materials and methods

Three adult pig-tailed macaques (*Macaca nemestrina*), three adult rhesus macaques (*M. mulatta*) and one juvenile cynomolgus monkey (*M. fascicularis*) were infected intravenously with wild type $SIV_{agm3}$ (Kraus et al., 1989), produced by permanently infected Molt 4/8 cells. Each animal received an inoculation of culture supernatant containing $4 \times 10^5$ $TCID_{50}$ virus. Additionally one adult pig-tailed macaque, two juvenile African green monkeys and one juvenile cynomolgus monkey were infected with molecularly cloned $SIV_{agm3}$ (Baier et al., 1989) also propagated in permanently infected Molt 4/8 cells. In these cases each animal received $5 \times 10^6$ $TCID_{50}$ of the cloned virus. Animals were bled before infection and at monthly intervals thereafter for serology, blood chemistry and hematology studies. In addition, virus isolation was attempted by cocultivation of the monkeys' peripheral blood cells (PBL) with Molt 4/8 cells and culture supernatants were examined at weekly intervals for reverse transcriptase activity. Seroconversion was monitored by immunoblotting (Werner et al., 1989) using purified $SIV_{agm}$ as antigen. The levels of antibody specific for $SIV_{agm}$ were determined by ELISA (Kurth et al., 1984). Plates were coated either with whole purified $SIV_{agm}$ or with highly purified $SIV_{agm}$ p28*gag*. Goat anti-human IgG peroxidase conjugate was used as second antibody.

For Southern blot analysis of sequential isolates from one pig-tailed macaque genomic DNAs were digested with *Eco*RI, *Kpn*I and *Hinc*II. Genomic DNA from molecularly cloned $SIV_{agm}$ infected Molt 4/8 cells digested with the same enzymes served as a positive control. The filter was hybridized with the *Eco*RI fragment of the cloned $SIV_{agm}$.

Variations in the different T-cell subpopulations were measured by flow cytometry after labeling of cells with the monoclonal antibodies Leu-2a, Leu-3a and OKT11.

For indicating functional immunity, the ability of sera from infected animals to neutralize virus infectivity or to elicit antibody dependent cellular cytotoxicity (ADCC) of infected cells in the sera was measured. The neutralization assays, performed in microtiter plates, involved incubating dilutions of heat inactivated sera with a very low challenge dose (7 $TCID_{50}$) of $SIV_{agm}$ before addition of the highly sensitive indicator cell subclone Molt 4/8-79. After 7 days incubation, wells were scored for the presence of replicating virus as indicated by syncytia formation. For target cells in the ADCC assays, chromium labeled Molt 4/8-SAM cells (persistently infected with $SIV_{agm}$) were used. The ability of sera to initiate lysis of these cells in the presence of healthy human effector PBLs was measured in a standard 4-h chromium release assay.

## Results

### Infection with wild type $SIV_{agm}$

*Serological and clinical data*

Fig. 1 shows the Western blot results with sera obtained at various times after inoculation. The pig-tailed macaques had developed antibodies to gp45 and

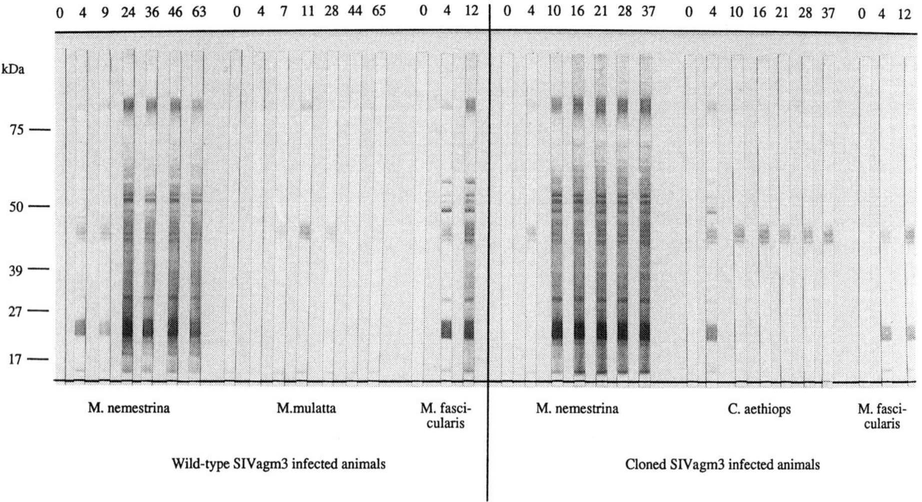


Fig. 1. Western blot analysis of sera from $SIV_{agm}$ infected AGMs and macaques using purified $SIV_{agm}$ as antigen. The animals were infected artificially by an intravenous injection of $SIV_{agm}$ (wild type or cloned).

gp140 envelope (*env*) and to p28/p18 core (*gag*) proteins by 4–9 weeks after infection while antibodies to other viral proteins, including antibodies to *pol* gene products, (p64/p48) were delayed by a few weeks. The cynomolgus monkey developed antibodies to *env, gag* and *pol* gene products at approximately the same time, 4 weeks after infection. The Rhesus monkeys seroconverted approximately 7 weeks post infection (p.i.). They only showed a weak response against the envelope proteins and the core protein p17. Virus could be readily isolated from the PBL of the two species which showed a strong serological response, the pig-tailed macaques and the cynomolgus monkey, beginning at 4 weeks after inoculation and continuously thereafter. In contrast, it was not possible to rescue virus from the rhesus at any time.

By ELISA the antibody response in the rhesus monkeys to whole virus antigen was shown to peak at 11 weeks and then to decline (Fig. 2). In contrast, the level of specific antibody in *M. nemestrina* was high and remained so over a period of 16 months after infection.

Monitoring of the T-cell numbers, including CD4+ and CD8+ subsets, showed that the inoculated pig-tailed macaques and the cynomolgus monkey did not experience significant changes in their lymphocyte subset levels. The rhesus macaques experienced large fluctuations in their CD4+/CD8+ ratios, although there was no clear tendency.

Measurement of conventional hematological and blood chemistry parameters failed to reveal any significant changes. In addition, all infected animals regularly underwent a clinical examination. However, up to the present time (17 months

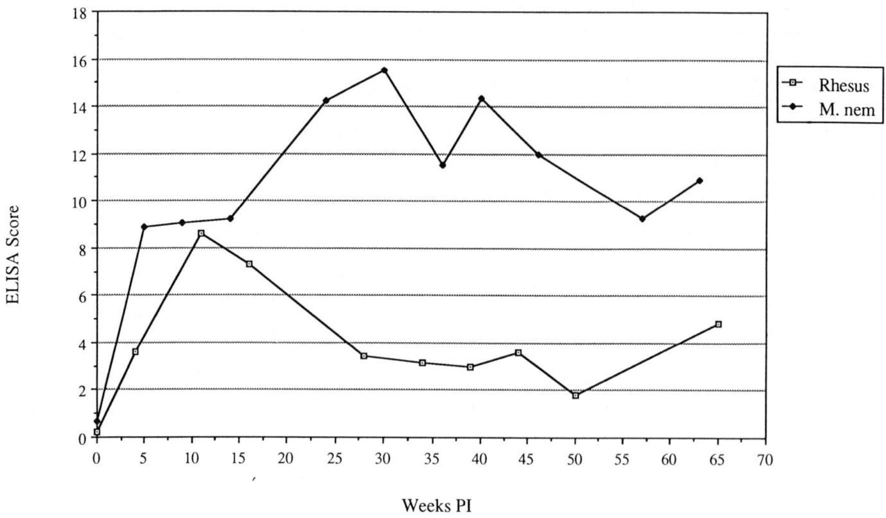


Fig. 2. ELISA reactivity of antisera from $SIV_{agm}$ infected macaques against whole virus. Sera were titrated from 1/50 to 1/819,200 in fourfold dilution steps. Results are expressed as ELISA score, defined as the area under the dilution curve for each serum.

p.i. for the pig-tailed macaques and the rhesus and 5 months p.i. for the cynomolgus) no indications of disease have been observed.

Southern blot analysis of sequential isolates from an infected *M. nemestrina* (Fig. 3) showed differences in banding patterns between the viruses isolated 2

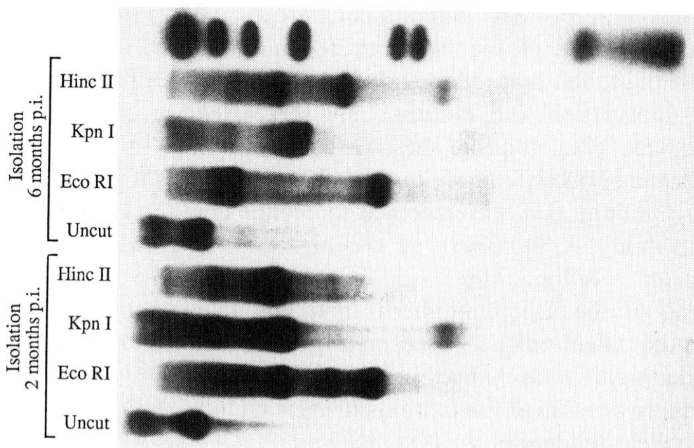


Fig. 3. Southern blot analysis of two sequential isolates from one *Macaca nemestrina* infected with $SIV_{agm}$. Genomic DNAs were digested with different restriction enzymes and hybridized with the *Eco*RI fragment of the cloned $SIV_{agm}$.

and 6 months p.i. Digestion with *Eco*RI revealed the loss of one *Eco*RI site in the isolate obtained 6 months p.i.

## Infection with molecularly cloned $SIV_{agm}$

To enable a more precise evaluation of the immunological and genetic situation in vivo, including studies of in vivo variability, animals were infected with a biologically active molecular clone of $SIV_{agm}$. Two African green monkeys, one cynomolgus and one pig-tailed macaque were infected with $5 \times 10^6$ $TCID_{50}$ of cloned virus. Following inoculation all animals seroconverted within 4 weeks (Fig. 1). The pig-tailed macaque showed an antibody response that corresponded to the serological response of the wild type infected *M. nemestrina* with a strong and persistent expression of antibodies to virtually all viral proteins. The cynomolgus monkey had only a weak expression of antibodies to *env* and *gag* proteins, compared with the wild type infected animal. Virus could be readily isolated from the PBL of all three species beginning approximately 3 weeks after inoculation and continuously thereafter. All animals remained healthy up to the present time (8 months p.i.).

AGMs infected with $SIV_{agm}$, although having a strong anti-*env* response, showed only a weak transient anti-*gag* response (Fig. 1). This reflects the serological response of naturally infected AGMs which rarely have a significant reaction to the core protein p28. This response was confirmed in ELISA studies using either whole virus or highly purified p28*gag* as antigen. All infected animals had high antibody titers against the whole virus, but whereas sera from the pig-tailed macaque also contained high titer anti-p28 antibodies, few or no such antibodies could be detected in the AGM sera (Fig. 4).

## Functional immune response of $SIV_{agm}$ infected primates

The neutralizing activity and antibody dependent cellular cytotoxicity capacity of sera from $SIV_{agm}$ infected animals were measured to provide information about the hosts' ability to eliminate virus or virus infected cells. Nearly all naturally infected animals possessed high titers of antibodies able to initiate lysis of $SIV_{agm}$ infected cells in the presence of human effector PBLs. However, the level of neutralizing antibody in the sera of naturally infected animals was low or completely absent, even when an absolutely minimum challenge dose (7 $TCID_{50}$/well) was used. Interestingly, the highest levels of neutralizing antibody were found either in the sera of animals which had recently seroconverted as a result of natural infection or in the experimentally infected primates, in particular the *M. nemestrina*.

## Infection of cynomolgus monkeys with HIV-2

Two cynomolgus monkeys recently infected with HIV-2 showed a serological response to the virus, as shown by Western blot, in particular against the

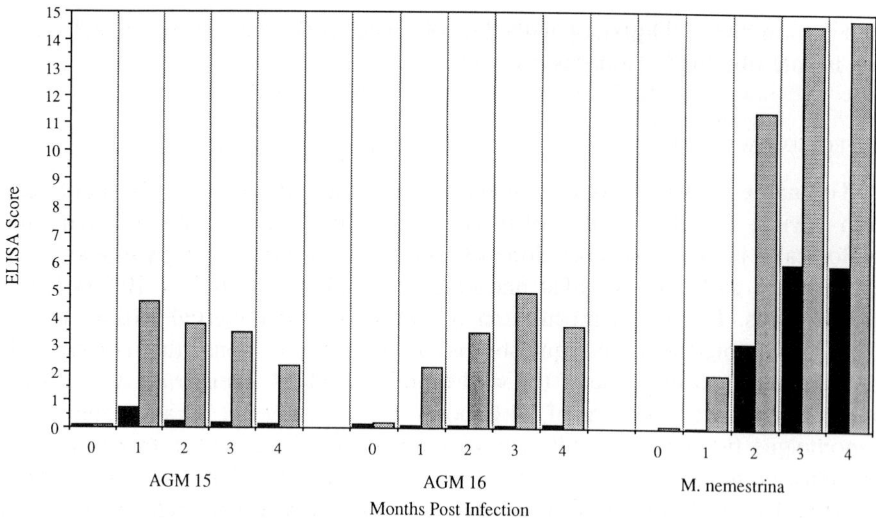


Fig. 4. ELISA reactivity of antisera from artificially $SIV_{agm}$ infected AGMs and *M. nemestrina* against whole virus (▨) and against purified *gag* (■). Sera were titrated from 1/50 to 1/819,200 in fourfold dilution steps. Results are expressed as ELISA score, defined as the area under the dilution curve for each serum.

envelope glycoproteins. Furthermore, sera from these animals reacted well in an ELISA using as antigen a synthetic peptide corresponding to a major immunogenic epitope in the transmembrane gp36 (kindly provided by Prof. B. Wahren, Stockholm). Virus was readily isolated from the infected animals at different times after infection, confirming the potential of this animal model for the study of HIV infection.

## Discussion

Judging from the relatively weak serological response and the failure to reisolate virus, $SIV_{agm}$ appears to replicate rather poorly in rhesus macaques. The *M. nemestrina* species, in comparison, is readily infectable, exhibiting a rapid, strong and persistent antibody response and permitting reisolation of the virus at every attempt. However, at 17 months after infection, even the *M. nemestrina* shows no sign of illness. Whether this simply reflects a long period of latency (like HIV-1 in humans) or confirms the inherent apathogenicity of this SIV remains to be seen. We are presently carrying out in vivo passage of the virus in susceptible, heterologous species in an attempt to produce a pathogenic strain. The genomic changes revealed by the Southern blot analysis of sequential isolates from an infected pig-tailed macaque either suggest a rapid mutation of the dominant viral species in vivo or may reflect the outgrowth of variants from a mixed inoculum.

Naturally infected African green monkeys do not succumb to an immunodeficiency disease and one possible reason for this might be that this species reacts to SIV $_{agm}$ infection with a particularly vigorous immune response which is able to control the virus. However, examination of the functional immune response revealed that infected animals have, if anything, a weaker immune status than HIV infected humans. The levels of neutralizing antibody were low or non-existent and the ADCC response was similar in strength to that in HIV seropositive humans. One striking difference was that $SIV_{agm}$ infected African green monkeys show a weak or absent anti-*gag* response. In comparison, *M. nemestrina* infected with the same virus have a very strong reaction to the core proteins, indicating that this is a property of the host rather than of the virus. Whether this failure to react to *gag* has any significance in terms of pathogenesis (perhaps through an auto-immune mechanism) remains to be seen.

Cynomolgus monkeys were infected with our own isolate of HIV-2 (PEI-2), and reacted with a specific serological response. Furthermore, virus was readily recoverable from these animals and as HIV-2 is a human virus, the potential for this model is clear. To allow more precise studies to be performed, we are in the process of molecularly cloning the virus for sequencing and subsequently for in vivo studies of variability and immune response.

## References

Baier, M., Garber, C., Müller, C., Werner, A., Kraus, G., Ferdinand, F.J., Cichutek, K., Papas, T.S., Hartung, S. and Kurth, R. (1989) Molecularly cloned $SIV_{agm3}$ is highly divergent from other $SIV_{agm}$ isolates and is biologically active in vitro and in vivo. *J. Virol.* 63, 5119–5123.

Desrosiers, R.C. and Letvin, N.L. (1987) Animal models for acquired immunodeficiency syndrome. *Rev. Infect. Dis.* 9, 438–446.

Kanki, P.J., Kurth, R., Becker, W., Dreesman, G., McLane, M.F. and Essex, M. (1985) Antibodies to simian T-lymphotropic retrovirus type III in African green monkeys and recognition of STLV-III viral proteins by AIDS and related sera. *Lancet* i, 1330–1332.

Kraus, G., Werner, A., Baier, M., Binninger, D., Ferdinand, F.J., Norley, S. and Kurth, R. (1989) Isolation of human immunodeficiency virus-related simian immunodeficiency viruses from African green monkeys. *Proc. Natl. Acad. Sci. U.S.A.* 86, 2892–2896.

Kurth, R., Mikschy, U., Tondera, C., Lizonova, A., Brede, H.D., Helm, E.B., Bergmann, L., Frank, H., Popovic, M. and Gallo, R.C. (1984) HTLV-III Infektionen bei Patienten mit AIDS und Lymphadenopathie-Syndrom. *Münch. Med. Wschr.* 46, 1363–1368.

Kurth, R., Kraus, G., Werner, A., Hartung, S., Centner, P., Baier, M., Norley, S. and Löwer, J. (1988) AIDS: animal retroviruses and vaccines. *J. AIDS* 1, 284–294.

Werner, A., Baier, M., Löwer, J., Norley, S. and Kurth, R. (1989) Human sera from healthy blood donors and multiple sclerosis patients recognize human and animal retrovirus antigens. *AIFO* 2, 70–71.

in SIV$_{agm}$ infection with a particularly vigorous immune response which is able to control the virus. However, examination of the functional immune response revealed that infected animals have, if anything, a weaker immune status than HIV infected humans. The levels of neutralizing antibodies were low or absent, [illegible] and the ADCC response was similar in strength to that in HIV-seropositive humans. One striking difference was that SIV$_{agm}$ infected African green monkeys show [illegible] response. In [illegible], AGMs were [illegible] with the same virus [illegible] reaction to the core proteins. This means that this is a property of the host rather than of the virus. Whether this [illegible] [illegible]

[illegible]

References

[illegible]

*Eds. H. Schellekens and M.C. Horzinek*
*Animal Models in AIDS*



# 8

# Animal models for HIV infection and AIDS: HIV-2 and $SIV_{sm}$ infections of cynomolgus monkeys

PER PUTKONEN [1], RIGMOR THORSTENSSON [1],
REINHOLD BENTHIN [2], KARL-GÖRAN HEDSTRÖM [2],
BO ÖBERG [3], ERLING NORRBY [3] and GUNNEL BIBERFELD [1]

[1] Department of Immunology, National Bacteriological Laboratory, [2] SBL Primate Research Center and [3] Department of Virology, Karolinska Institute, Stockholm, Sweden

**Summary**

Twenty-two healthy cynomolgus monkeys (*Macaca fascicularis*) were inoculated with two different isolates of human immunodeficiency virus type 2 (HIV-2), namely HIV-$2_{SBL-6669}$ (n = 10) or HIV-$2_{SBL-K135}$ (n = 12), to establish an animal model for HIV infection and AIDS. These animals were compared with 13 cynomolgus monkeys inoculated with $SIV_{sm}$. All HIV-2 infected animals seroconverted and virus was recovered from blood mononuclear cells of most of the animals, but they have remained clinically healthy and have shown no CD4 cell decrease after 4–18 months of follow-up. In contrast, all SIV infected monkeys have shown a decrease in CD4 cells and six of 13 animals died or had to be killed because of an AIDS-like disease within a year after infection.

Comparison of HIV-2 inocula grown on fresh PBMC and in continuous cell lines indicates that extensive passage of HIV-2 in continuous cell lines decreases the in vivo replicative capacity of HIV-2.

HIV-2 infection and SIV infection of cynomolgus monkeys represent useful experimental models for HIV vaccine studies.

## Introduction

Substantial advances have already been made in the understanding of the human immunodeficiency virus (HIV) and the acquired immunodeficiency syndrome (AIDS). Progress has, however, been seriously hampered by the lack of a suitable and inexpensive animal model which can be employed to help solve the two most urgent problems: the lack of a vaccine to prevent HIV infection and an effective drug to combat the clinical syndrome. Chimpanzees (Alter et al., 1984; Fultz et al., 1986; Gajdusek et al., 1985) and gibbon apes (Lusso et al., 1988) are the only animals known to be susceptible to HIV-1 infection. However, these primates are too rare and too expensive to serve as animal models on a large scale. We (Putkonen et al., 1989b) and others (Fultz et al., 1989; Dormont et al., 1989; Nicol et al., 1989) have previously shown that it is possible to infect macaques with HIV-2.

The best model at present is to infect Asian macaques with simian immunodeficiency virus ($SIV_{mac}$, $SIV_{sm}$, $SIV_{mne}$) (Scheider and Hunsmann, 1989) as these monkeys develop an AIDS-like disease following infection. SIV is the closest relative to HIV types 1 and 2 identified today. $SIV_{sm}$ and HIV-2 are closely related viruses (Hirsch et al., 1989a) and show a clear serological relationship (Gardner and Luciw, 1988).

In this report, we describe the experimental infection of cynomolgus macaques with $SIV_{sm}$ and with two strains of HIV-2. The aim of this work was to establish an animal model for the development of a vaccine for HIV and AIDS. A second objective was to determine if passage of HIV-2 in continuous cell lines causes lower in vivo replicative capacity.

## Material and methods

Thirty-five cynomolgus macaques (*Macaca fascicularis*) were inoculated intravenously with cell-free, undiluted supernatants of two different isolates of HIV-2, $HIV\text{-}2_{SBL\text{-}6669}$ (n = 10) or $HIV\text{-}2_{SBL\text{-}K135}$ (n = 12) or with $SIV_{sm}$ (n = 13) (SIV/SMM-3, the Yerke strain). The two strains of HIV-2 had been grown in fresh human and monkey lymphocyte cultures or in continuous cell lines. Six of 10 monkeys received $HIV\text{-}2_{SBL\text{-}6669}$ which had been propagated for a long time in continuous cell lines (Table 2). Virus isolation was done by coculture of peripheral blood mononuclear cells (PBMC) from each animal with phytohemagglutinin-stimulated human PBMC and monitoring of culture supernatants for reverse transcriptase activity. Serum or plasma antigenemia was determined using a commercial HIV-1 antigen capture ELISA (Abbott). HIV-2 or SIV antibodies were determined by ELISA, Western blot and radioimmunoprecipitation assay (RIPA) using $HIV\text{-}2_{SBL\text{-}6669}$ as antigen (for details see Putkonen et al., 1989a,b). The observation time was up to 18 months.

## Results

All 35 cynomolgus monkeys experimentally infected with cell-free supernatants of SIV or HIV-2 became infected as shown by seroconversion. Table 1 shows a comparison of cynomolgus monkeys infected with $SIV_{sm}$ or $HIV\text{-}2_{SBL\text{-}K135}$. $SIV_{sm}$ is pathogenic for this macaque species, since six of 13 animals died or had to be killed because of an AIDS-like disease within a year after infection. In contrast, all HIV-2 inoculated monkeys have remained clinically healthy. SIV has been recovered repeatedly over the course of infection. $HIV\text{-}2_{SBL\text{-}K135}$ could be

TABLE 1
Cynomolgus monkeys infected with $SIV_{sm}$ or HIV-$2_{SBL-K135}$

| Monkeys infected with | Antibody response | Virus isolation | Antigenemia in serum | Lymphadenopathy | CD4 cell decrease | Dead (follow-up >12 months) |
|---|---|---|---|---|---|---|
| SIV | 13/13 | 13/13 | 13/13 | 13/13 (persistent) | 13/13 | 6/13 |
| HIV-2 | 12/12 | 11/12 | 7/12 | 6/12 (fluctuating) | 0/12 | 0/12 |

isolated from PBMC from 11 of 12 animals, but only for about a month after inoculation. Antigenemia was demonstrated in all SIV infected but only in seven of 12 HIV-2 infected monkeys. All 13 SIV inoculated animals developed persistent substantial lymphadenopathy (which regressed terminally), while the monkeys inoculated with HIV-2 developed intermittent fluctuating swollen lymph nodes. All 13 SIV-infected monkeys showed a pronounced decrease in CD4 + lymphocytes, whereas none of the HIV-2 infected monkeys developed a CD4 cell decrease.

Cynomolgus monkeys inoculated with HIV-$2_{SBL-K135}$ or HIV-$2_{SBL-6669}$ cultured only in fresh PBMC developed antibodies to envelope and core proteins and virus recovery was successful (Table 2). In contrast six monkeys, which had received virus passaged in continuous cell lines, developed antibodies to envelope but not to core proteins and all virus isolation attempts have been negative in these animals.

## Discussion

SIV and HIV-2 infections of cynomolgus macaques represent useful experimental models for testing whether immunization protects against infection and in the SIV-macaque system whether vaccination will prevent development of disease. The SIV-macaque system has the advantage that an AIDS-like disease can be induced in a relatively short time, and promising vaccine candidates can thus be tested for the ability to protect against development of disease, even if they do not protect against infection.

TABLE 2
Cynomolgus monkeys infected with HIV-2. Study comparing in vivo replicative capacity of the SBL-6669 and SBL-K135 viruses grown in fresh PBMC or in continuous cell lines

| Virus | Antibody against | | Virus isolation | Antigenemia |
|---|---|---|---|---|
| | *env* | core p26 | | |
| SBL-K135 cultured in fresh PBMC | 12/12 | 12/12 | 11/12 | 7/12 |
| SBL-6669 cultured in fresh PBMC | 4/4 | 4/4 | 4/4 | 0/4 |
| SBL-6669 passaged in continuous cell lines | 6/6 | 0/6 | 0/6 | 0/6 |

Passage of HIV-2 in continuous cell lines seems to decrease the in vivo replicative capacity of HIV-2. All six monkeys that had received virus passaged in continuous cell lines developed only antibodies to envelope proteins and all attempts to recover virus from these animals were unsuccessful. The mechanism of the low in vivo replicative capacity is unknown. The amount of virus inoculated into these six animals was equivalent to or greater than the inoculum injected into the other groups of animals, as determined by measurement of reverse transcriptase activity in the supernatants. The lower in vivo replicative capacity may have occurred by selection by extensive passage in U937-2 cells (continuous monocytoid human cell line). It has recently been shown that SIV adapted to human cells expresses a transmembrane glycoprotein with the size of 32 kDa rather than 41 kDa (Hirsch et al., 1989b). The possibility of adaptation and attenuation is a matter of concern in developing reliable inocula for use in animal studies.

In this context it should be noted that African green monkeys naturally infected with $SIV_{agm}$ develop an antibody response against envelope antigens but not against core antigens (Kraus et al., 1989), like our monkeys infected with HIV-2 passaged in human cell lines.

In conclusion, HIV-2 infection and SIV infection of cynomolgus monkeys represent useful experimental models for HIV vaccine trials. Furthermore, these experimental models can be used for testing whether preinfection of cynomolgus monkeys with a non-pathogenic HIV-2 protects animals against challenge with virulent SIV.

## Acknowledgements

This work was supported by the Swedish National Board for Technical Development (Project 87-03356) and by the Swedish Medical Research Council (Project 16H-2380). We thank K. Warstedt and H. Linder for the skilled technical assistance.

## References

Alter, H.J., Eichberg, J.W., Masur, H., Saxinger, W.C., Gallo, R., Macher, A.M., Lane, H.C., and Fauci, A.S. (1984) Transmission of HTLV-III infection from human plasma to chimpanzees. An animal model for AIDS. *Science* 226, 549–552.

Dormont, D., Livartovski, J., Chamaret, S., Guetard, D., Henin, R., Levagueresse, R., Moortelle, P.F., Larke, B., Gourmelon, P., Vazeaux, R., Metivier, H., Flageat, J. Court, L., Hauw, J.J. and Montagnier, L. (1989) HIV-2 in rhesus monkeys: serological, virological and clinical results. *Intervirology* 30 (Suppl. 1), 59–65.

Fultz, P.N., McClure, H.M., Swenson, R.B., McGrath, C.R., Brodie, A., Getchell, J.P., Jensen, F.C., Andersson, D.C., Broderson, J.R. and Francis, D.P. (1986) Persistent infection of chimpanzees with human T lymphotropic virus type III/LAV: a potential model for acquired immunodeficiency syndrome. *J. Virol.* 58, 116–124.

Fultz, P.N., Switzer, W., McClure, H.M., Anderson, D. and Montagnier, L. (1988) Simian models for AIDS: SIV/SMM and HIV-2 infection of macaques. In: Chancock, Lerner, Brown and Ginsberg (Eds.) *Vaccines 88.* Cold Spring Harbor Laboratory Press, Cold Spring Harbor, NY, pp. 167–170.

Gajdusek, D.C., Gibbs, C.J., Rogers-Johnson, P., Amyx, H.L., Asher, D.M., Epstein, L.G., Sarin, P.S., Gallo, R.C., Malluish, A., Arthur, L.O., Montagnier, L. and Mildvan, D. (1985) Infection of chimpanzees by human T-lymphotropic retroviruses in brain and other tissues from AIDS patients. *Lancet* i, 55–56.

Gardner, M.B. and Luciw, P.A. (1988) Simian immunodeficiency viruses and their relationship to human immunodeficiency viruses. *AIDS* 2 (Suppl. 1), 3–10.

Hirsch, V.M., Omlsted, R.A., Murphey-Corb, M., Purcell, R.H. and Johnson, P.R. (1989) An African primate lentivirus ($SIV_{sm}$) closely related to HIV-2. *Nature* 339, 389–392.

Hirsch, V.M., Edmonsson, P., Murphey-Corb, M., Arbeille, B., Johnsson, P.R. and Mullins, J.I. (1989) SIV adaption to human cells. *Nature* 341, 573–574.

Kraus, G., Werner, M., Baier, M., Binniger, D., Ferdinand, F.J., Norley, S. and Kurth, R. (1989) Isolation of human immunodeficiency virus-related simian immunodeficiency viruses from African green monkeys. *Proc. Natl. Acad. Sci. U.S.A.* 86, 2892–2896.

Lusso, P., Markham, P.D., Ranki, A., Earl, P., Moss, B., Dorner, F., Gallo, R.C. and Krohn, K.J.E. (1988) Cell-mediated immune response toward viral envelope and core antigens in gibbon apes (*Hylobates tar*) chronically infected with human immunodeficiency virus-1. *J. Immunol.* 7, 2467–2473.

Nicol, I., Flamminio-Zola, G., Dubouch, P., Bernard, J., Snart, R., Jouffre, R., Reveil, B., Fouchard, M., Desportes, I., Nara, P., Gallo, R.C. and Zagury, D. (1989) Persistent infection of rhesus macaque, baboon and mangabeys. *Intervirology* 30, 258–267.

Putkonen, P., Warstedt, K., Thorstensson, R., Benthin, R., Albert, J., Lundgren, B., Öberg, B., Norrby, E. and Biberfeld, G. (1989a) Experimental infection of cynomolgus monkeys (*Macaca fascicularis*) with simian immunodeficiency virus (SIVsm). *J. AIDS* 2, 359–365.

Putkonen, P., Böttiger, B., Warstedt, K., Thorstensson, R., Albert, J. and Biberfeld, G. (1989b) Experimental infection of cynomolgus monkeys (*Macaca fascicularis*) with HIV-2. *J. AIDS* 2, 366–373.

Schneider, J. and Hunsmann, G. (1988) Simian lentiviruses – the SIV group. *AIDS* 2, 1–9.

*Eds. H. Schellekens and M.C. Horzinek*
*Animal Models in AIDS*



9

# Characterization of simian foamy virus proviral DNA

MATTHIAS SCHWEIZER, ROLF RENNE and
DIETER NEUMANN-HAEFELIN

Abteilung Virologie, Institut für Medizinische Mikrobiologie und Hygiene, Universität Freiburg, D-7800 Freiburg, F.R.G.

## Introduction

Foamy viruses or Spumavirinae constitute the third subfamily of Retroviridae in addition to Oncovirinae and Lentivirinae. They cause persistent infections in different mammalian species, mainly in primates and possibly also in man.

Our work with the simian foamy virus (SFV) LK-3 may be of special interest because of its T-cell lymphotropic properties and because it was derived from an African green monkey living in a colony where two infections have occurred in animal house personnel. We have characterized proviral LK-3 DNA, which is present in infected cells as a non-integrated, linear duplex DNA molecule of about 13 kb containing a single-stranded "gap" near the center.

## Materials and methods

### Cells and viruses

Molt-4 (human T-cell leukemia) cells were kept in RPMI 1640 medium, HeLa, BHK-21 cells, and human diploid fibroblasts in Eagle's minimal essential medium, supplemented with fetal calf serum (10% and 5%, respectively), penicillin, and streptomycin (100 U/ml each).

Simian foamy virus LK-3 was isolated (zur Hausen and Gissmann, 1979) and characterized (Neumann-Haefelin et al., 1983, 1986; Schweizer et al., 1988, 1989) in this laboratory. Prototype strains of simian foamy virus types 1, 2, 3, 5, 6, 7 and 8 were obtained from the American Type Culture Collection, and human spumaretrovirus was kindly provided by Dr. M.A. Epstein, Bristol.

Molecular cloning, extraction of DNA, Southern blotting and hybridization, and sequencing of DNA were carried out as described elsewhere (Maniatis et al., 1982).

## Results and discussion

### Molecular cloning

DNA from LK-3-infected Molt-4 cells was digested with nuclease S1 to cleave unintegrated LK-3 DNA into a pair of 6 and 6.5 kb fragments (Neumann-Haefelin et al., 1986). These fragments were molecularly cloned in phage and plasmid vectors using *Sal*I linkers (Schweizer et al., 1988, 1989). The clones obtained were designated pMS02 and pMS03. To prove complete cloning of LK-3 DNA, proviral DNA from uninfected cells was investigated on Southern blots with or without previous nuclease S1 digestion in parallel to cloned DNA (Fig. 1). Since every restriction fragment of nuclease S1-digested proviral DNA was found in either pMS02 or pMS03, these clones appear to represent the entire viral genome left hand and right hand of the site sensitive to nuclease S1. For cloning the nuclease S1-sensitive portion of DNA in the center of the genome, the central *BamH*I fragment containing this "gap" was cloned after completing the double strand with Klenow polymerase and T4 DNA ligase. The DNA clone obtained by this procedure was designated pMS04 and further investigated.

### Structure of proviral LK-3 DNA

The restriction map of the LK-3 DNA (Fig. 2) was derived from double digests of cloned and proviral DNA (not shown). Mutual cross-hybridization of

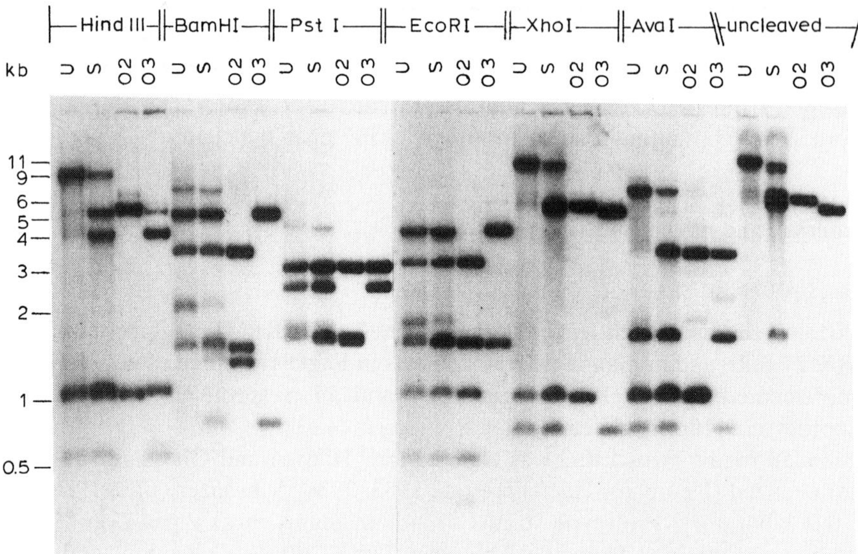


Fig. 1. Southern blot comparing cloned and native proviral LK-3 DNA. Native proviral DNA was digested with nuclease S1 as indicated. For hybridization, pMS02 and pMS03 were used. U: 5 μg DNA from infected Molt-4 cells. S: 5 μg DNA from infected Molt-4 cells, cleaved with nuclease S1. 02: 500 pg pMS02 insert. 03: 500 pg pMS03 insert.

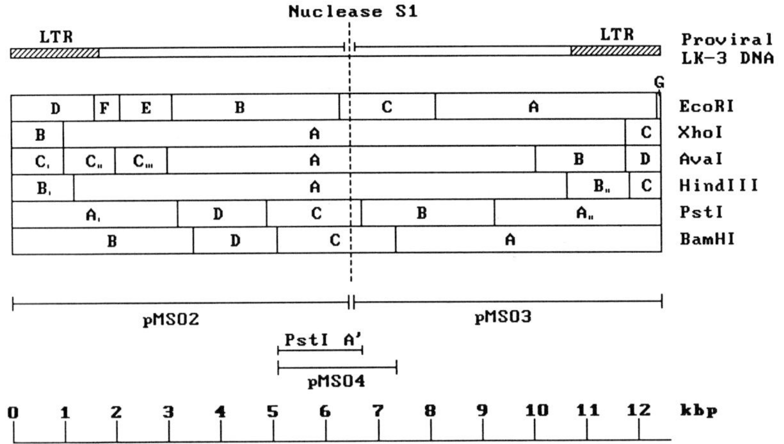


Fig. 2. Restriction maps of cloned and native proviral LK-3 DNA.

pMS02 and pMS03 revealed homologous regions of 1.7 kb at the termini of the LK-3 DNA, which appear to be the long terminal repeats (LTRs) of this retroviral genome. The unusual length of the LTRs was confirmed by identifying a binding site for a primer tRNA, which is typical of the 5′ end of the unique sequence of retroviral genomes (Coffin, 1982). In LK-3 DNA, the binding site for $tRNA^{lys}$ (TGGCGCCCAACGTGGGG) (Wain-Hobson et al., 1985) was found 1.7 kb from the 5′ end.

The nuclease S1-sensitive site was investigated on the molecular level. Since the ends of pMS02 and pMS03 define the limits of the single-stranded DNA, the nucleotide sequence of this gap could be localized on pMS04 (Fig. 3). At the 3′ end of the obtained 109 nucleotide gap sequence, a polypurine tract (PPT, AGGAGAGGGTA) was found, which is similar to the putative initiation site of plus strand DNA synthesis in various other retroviruses (Coffin, 1982; Varmus and Swanstrom, 1982). As was speculated for HIV-1 and visna virus (Sonigo et al., 1985; Wain-Hobson et al., 1985), which possess a central PPT besides the common PPT close to the 3′ LTR, this may point to a discontinuous synthesis of plus strand DNA in the replication cycle of LK-3.

After digestion of DNA from infected cells with nuclease S1, a 1.7 kb fragment in addition to the 6.5 and 6 kb fragments was detected (Fig. 1, "uncleaved S"), which hybridized exclusively to LTR fragments (not shown). As

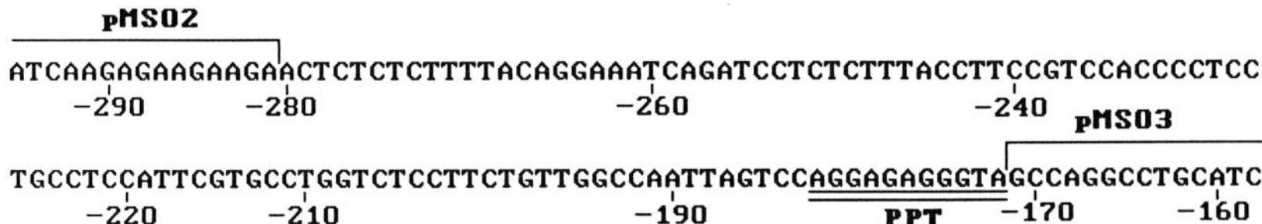


Fig. 3. Nucleotide sequence of the gap region. The positions, relative to the sequenced pMS04 *Pst*I A′ fragment (Fig. 2), of the 3′ end of pMS02 and the 5′ end of pMS03 are indicated. PPT: polypurine tract. Numbers of nucleotides refer to the 3′ end of the pMS04 *Pst*I A′ fragment.

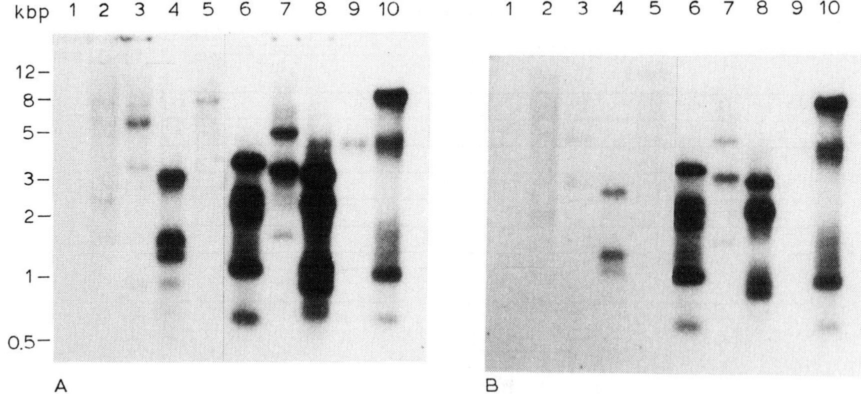


Fig. 4. Southern blots of *Hind*III-cleaved DNAs from cells infected with different SFV prototypes. (A) Hybridization under conditions of low stringency (20% formamide, 5×SSC, 42°C). (B) Hybridization under conditions of higher stringency (50% formamide, 5×SSC, 42°C). DNAs originated from: uninfected BHK-21 cells (1), SFV-8-infected human diploid fibroblasts (2), SFV-7-infected BHK-21 (3), SFV-6-infected BHK-21 (4), SFV-5-infected HeLa cells (5), SFV-3-infected BHK-21 (6), SFV-2-infected BHK-21 (7), SFV-1-infected BHK-21 (8), human spumaretrovirus-infected BHK-21 (9), and LK-3-infected BHK-21 (10). The viral inserts of pMS02 and pMS03 were used as hybridization probes.

no further nuclease S1-sensitive site besides the gap region was found in the complete proviral DNA by double cleavage with nuclease S1 and restriction enzymes (Fig. 1), the 1.7 kb fragment seems to be generated from a particular form of replicating viral DNA. This may be plus strand "strong-stop" DNA accumulated during reverse transcription of retroviral genomes (Varmus and Swanstrom, 1982), which consists of an LTR plus strand and the homologous minus strand being transcribed from the RNA template. Only after hydrolysis of the variably sized minus strand by nuclease S1 do double-stranded LTR fragments become detectable.

### Relationship of LK-3 to other retroviruses

Using cloned LK-3 DNA as hybridization probes, no DNA of onco- or lentiviruses could be detected on Southern blots, whereas DNA of all investigated foamy viruses was recognized (Fig. 4). Thus, in spite of several common features in the biology and genomic architecture, spuma- and lentiviruses form clearly distinct divisions of the retrovirus family. Therefore, LK-3 specific probes can be used to exclude the presence of foamy viruses as contaminants in HIV culture experiments.

## Acknowledgement

This work was supported by the Deutsche Forschungsgemeinschaft, Grant Ne 213/4-3.

## References

Coffin, J.M. (1982) Structure of the retroviral genome. In: R. Weiss, N. Teich, H. Varmus and J.M. Coffin (Eds.), *RNA Tumor Viruses.* Cold Spring Harbor Laboratory Press, Cold Spring Harbor, NY, pp. 261–368.

Maniatis, T., Fritsch, E.F. and Sambrook, J. (1982) *Molecular Cloning: A Laboratory Manual.* Cold Spring Harbor Laboratory Press, Cold Spring Harbor, NY.

Neumann-Haefelin, D., Rethwilm, A., Bauer, G., Gudat, F. and zur Hausen, H. (1983) Characterization of a foamy virus isolated from *Cercopithecus aethiops* lymphoblastoid cells. *Med. Microbiol. Immunol.* 172, 75–86.

Neumann-Haefelin, D., Schweizer, M., Corsten,, B. ,and Matz, B. (1986) Detection and characterization of infectious DNA intermediates of a primate foamy virus. *J. Gen. Virol.* 67, 1993–1999.

Schweizer, M., Corsten, B. and Neumann-Haefelin, D. (1988) Heterogeneity of primate foamy virus genomes. *Arch. Virol.* 99, 125–134.

Schweizer, M., Renne, R. and Neumann-Haefelin, D. (1989) Structural analysis of proviral DNA in simian foamy virus (LK-3)-infected cells. *Arch. Virol.* 109, 103–114.

Sonigo, P., Alizon, M., Staskus, K., Klatzmann, D., Cole, S., Danos, O., Retzel, E., Tiollais, P., Haase, A. and Wain-Hobson, S. (1985) Nucleotide sequence of the Visna lentivirus: relationship to the AIDS virus. *Cell* 42, 369–382.

Varmus, H. and Swanstrom, R. (1982) Replication of retroviruses. In: R. Weiss, N. Teich, H. Varmus and J.M. Coffin (Eds.), *RNA Tumor Viruses.* Cold Spring Harbor Laboratory Press, Cold Spring Harbor, NY, pp. 369–512.

Wain-Hobson, S., Sonigo, P., Danos, O., Cole, S. and Alizon, M. (1985) Nucleotide sequence of the AIDS virus, LAV. *Cell* 40, 9–17.

zur Hausen, H. and Gissmann, L. (1979) Lymphotropic papovaviruses isolated from African green monkey and human cells. *Med. Microbiol. Immunol.* 167, 137–153.

*Eds. H. Schellekens and M.C. Horzinek*
*Animal Models in AIDS*



# 10

# Utility of the rabbit in HIV-1 and HTLV-1 infection

H. KULAGA[1], M.E. TRUCKENMILLER[2], T.M. FOLKS[3] and T.J. KINDT[2]

[1] Neuropsychiatry Branch, NIMH Neurosciences Center at St. Elizabeths, Washington, DC 20032, U.S.A., [2] Laboratory of Immunogenetics, NIAID, Bethesda, MD, U.S.A. and [3] Retroviral Research Branch, CDC, Atlanta, GA, U.S.A.

Recent investigations on human retroviral infections and their consequences in the laboratory rabbit indicate that the rabbit may provide a much needed model for studying at least two infectious agents, human T-cell lymphoma virus (HTLV-1) and human immunodeficiency virus (HIV-1). Miyoshi, Seto and their colleagues have shown that the rabbit is an excellent host for HTLV-1 (Miyoshi et al., 1983; Akagi et al., 1985; Seto et al., 1987, 1988). Their reports indicate that certain strains of inbred rabbits can acquire a fatal leukemia-like disease when injected with cell lines that are HTLV-1 producers, and that modes of HTLV-1 transmission in rabbits may be similar to those in humans (Uemura et al., 1986).

Recently, rabbit cells, including an HTLV-1 transformant, have been infected in vitro with HIV-1 (Kulaga et al., 1988). More important, however, are studies from our laboratory and others (Filice et al., 1988; Kulaga et al., 1989) showing that in vivo HIV-1 infection is possible. In Filice et al.'s in vivo protocol, HIV-1 is administered intraperitoneally (i.p.) following macrophage activation by administration of thioglycollate. In our own studies in vivo infection was established by intravenous inoculation of HIV-1-infected human T-cells. Although no overt disease was reported following HIV-1 infection of rabbits, certain gross and microscopic pathological findings not unlike human AIDS were observed. It has further been demonstrated that infection with HIV-1 in rabbits previously infected with HTLV-1 leads to more pronounced signs of infection in these animals.

In human populations, HIV-1 may remain latent for as long as 6 years (Anderson et al., 1988). The mechanism(s) which stimulate HIV-1 from a latent to the productive phase are unknown, although human viral agents, including HTLV-1, have been implicated (Quinn et al., 1987; Gendelman et al., 1987; Mosca et al., 1987). It has been reported that individuals doubly infected with

HTLV-1 and HIV-1 may develop AIDS more aggressively than those infected only with HIV-1 (Bartholomew et al., 1987; Hattori et al., 1989). Several mechanistic possibilities that suggest synergism between HTLV-1 and HIV-1 have been reported. Molecular studies demonstrated direct transactivation of HIV-1 by the HTLV-1 *rex* protein (Rinsky et al., 1988). HTLV-1 has been shown to be mitogenic for T-cells (Gazzolo and Dodon, 1987) and can stimulate HIV-1 production in infected T-cells in vitro (Zack et al., 1988). Therefore it is of great value to have an animal model system in which both viruses may be studied alone or in combination.

Recently, studies from our laboratory described infection with HTLV-1 and subsequently with HIV-1. Infection was shown by the presence of antibodies specific for both viruses in doubly infected animals and by the presence of proviral sequences in PCR-amplified samples. Initially the HIV-1 *gag* sequence (Kulaga et al., 1989) and *env* sequence (Truckenmiller et al., 1989) were detected after virus was amplified by growing rabbit peripheral mononuclear blood cells (PMBC) in culture with recombinant interleukin-2 (rIL-2) and/or growing A3.01 cells (a human indicator T-cell line) in the presence of supernatants from cultured infected rabbit PMBC. In a subsequent report (Truckenmiller et al., 1989), PMBC taken directly from doubly infected rabbits contained sufficient HIV-1 DNA to be detected by PCR analysis. In all the preceding cases, amplified fragments were proven to be specific by hybridization with probes derived from viral sequences. It is notable that some animals retain HTLV-1 and/or HIV-1 proviral DNA that could be detected in PMBC for at least 12 months post HIV-1 infection and 14 months post HTLV-1 infection. These findings clearly indicate persistent infection in the rabbit over an extended period of time.

## References


Akagi, T., Takeda, I., Oka, T., Ohtsuki, Y., Yano, S. and Miyoshi, I. (1985) *Gann* 76, 86–94.

Anderson, R.M. and May, R.M. (1988) *Nature* 333, 514–519.

Bartholomew, C., Blattner, W. and Cleghorn, F. (1987) *Lancet* ii, 1469.

Filice, G., Cereda, P.M. and Varnier, O.E. (1988) *Nature* 335, 366–369.

Gazzolo, L. and Dodon, M.D. (1987) *Nature* 236, 714–717.

Gendelman, H.E., Phelps, W., Feigenbaum, L., Ostrove, J.M., Adachi, A., Howley, P.M., Khoury, G., Ginsberg, H.S. and Martin, M.A. (1987) *Proc. Natl. Acad. Sci U.S.A.* 83, 9759–9764.

Hattori, T., Koito, A., Takatsuki, K., Ikematsu, S., Matsuda, J., Mori, H., Fukui, M., Akashi, K. and Matsumoto, K. (1989) *J. AIDS* 2, 272–276.

Kulaga, H., Folks, T.M., Rutledge, R. and Kindt, T.J. (1988) *Proc. Natl. Acad. Sci. U.S.A.* 85, 4455–4459.

Kulaga, H., Folks, T., Rutledge, R., Truckenmiller, M.E., Gugel, E. and Kindt, T.J. (1989) *J. Exp. Med.* 169, 321–326.

Miyoshi, I., Yoshimoto, S., Taguchi, H., Kuboniski, I., Fujishita, M., Ohtsuky, Y., Shiraishi, Y. and Akagi, T. (1983) *Gann* 74, 1–4.

Mosca, J.D., Bednarik, D.P., Raj, N.B.K., Rosen, C.A., Sodroski, J.G., Haseltine, W.A. and Pitha, P.M. (1987) *Proc. Natl. Acad. Sci. U.S.A.* 84, 7408–7412.

Okamoto, T., Akagi, T., Shima, H., Miwa, M. and Shimotohno, K. (1987) *Gann* 78, 1297–1301.

Quinn, T.C., Piot, P. and McCormick, J.B. (1987) *J. Am. Med. Ass.* 257, 2617– 2621.

Rinsky, L., Hauber, J., Dukovich, M., Malim, M.H., Langlois, A., Cullen, B.R. and Green, W.C. (1988) *Nature* 335, 738–740.
Seto, A., Kawanishi, M., Matsuda, S., Ogawa, K., Eguchi, T. and Miyoshi, I. (1987) *Gann* 78, 1150–1155.
Seto, A., Kawanishi, M., Ogawa, K. and Miyoshi, I. (1988) *Gann* 79, 335–341.
Truckenmiller, M.E., Kulaga, H., Gugel, E. and Kindt, T.J. (1989) *J. Cell Biochem.* 13E, 309.
Truckenmiller, M.E., Kulaga, H., Gugel, E., Dickerson, D. and Kindt, T.J. (1989) *Res. Immunol.* 140, 527–544.
Uemura, Y., Kotani, S., Yoshimoto, S., Fujishita, M., Yano, S., Ohtsuki, Y. and Miyoshi, I. (1986) *Gann* 77, 970–973.
Zack, J.A., Cann, A.J., Lugo, J.P. and Chen, I.S.Y. (1988) *Science* 240, 1026–1029.

*Eds. H. Schellekens and M.C. Horzinek*
*Animal Models in AIDS*



# 11

# Establishment of a bioassay to determine serum levels of dextran sulfate, a potent inhibitor of human immunodeficiency virus

M. WITVROUW, M. BABA[1], J. BALZARINI, R. PAUWELS and E. DE CLERCQ

Rega Institute for Medical Research, Katholieke Universiteit Leuven, B-3000 Leuven, Belgium and [1] Department of Bacteriology, Fukushima Medical College, Fukushima 960-12, Japan

**Summary**

There is at present no reliable assay method to monitor blood drug levels in humans following the administration of dextran sulfate (DS). We have now developed a sensitive bioassay based on the inhibitory effect of DS against human immunodeficiency virus type 2 (HIV-2) in MT-4 cells. This method permits the detection in (rabbit) serum of DS (MW: 1000) and DS (MW: 5000) concentrations as low as 11 μg/ml. Pharmacokinetic studies in rabbits revealed that the concentrations of DS (MW: 1000) and DS (MW: 5000) after intravenous bolus injection declined biphasically with initial half-lives of approximately 10–30 min and 30–70 min, respectively.

## Introduction

Several sulfated polysaccharides (i.e., dextran sulfate, heparin, pentosan polysulfate) are potent and selective inhibitors of human immunodeficiency virus (HIV) in vitro (Ueno and Kuno, 1987; Ito et al., 1987; Baba et al., 1988b; Mitsuya et al., 1988). The mechanism of anti-HIV action appears to be due to inhibition of virus adsorption, as has been demonstrated by Mitsuya et al. (1988), Baba et al. (1988a), Schols et al. (1989) and Nakashima et al. (1989).

Because of the marked in vitro activity of the sulfated polysaccharides against HIV-1 (Table 1), dextran sulfate (Abrams et al., 1989) has been introduced in the clinic for the treatment of AIDS. However, there is no reliable assay method to monitor drug levels in blood. Chemical methods suffer from the drawback that they may also detect degradation products which are no longer active as anti-HIV agents. Clearly, the optimal detection method should be based on a bioassay that would allow to quantitate drug levels based on their biological activity.

We have now established a simple and sensitive bioassay system to measure serum concentrations of sulfated polysaccharides and, using this new procedure, we examined the pharmacokinetics of dextran sulfate (MW: 1000 and MW: 5000) following intravenous bolus injection in rabbits.

## Materials and methods

### Compounds

Dextran sulfate (molecular weight (MW) 5000) was purchased from Sigma Chemical Co. (St. Louis, MO, U.S.A.). Dextran sulfate (MW 1000) was obtained from Pfeifer & Langen (Dormagen, F.R.G.).

### Cells

MT-4 cells were grown in RPMI 1640 medium supplemented with 10% heat-inactivated fetal calf serum (FCS), 5 mM L-glutamine, 0.075% sodium bicarbonate, 100 IU/ml penicillin G and 20 μg/ml gentamicin.

### Viruses

HIV type 1 (HIV-1) was obtained from the culture supernatant of HUT-78 cells persistently infected with HTLV-$III_B$ (HUT-78/HTLV-$III_B$). HIV type 2 (HIV-2) was obtained from the culture supernatant of CEM cells persistently infected with LAV-$2_{ROD}$ (CEM/LAV-$2_{ROD}$). The titer of the stocks were $2 \times 10^5$ $CCID_{50}$ (50% cell culture infective dose) per ml for HIV-1 and $4 \times 10^5$ $CCID_{50}$ per ml for HIV-2.

### Rabbit experiments

Two rabbits (Leuven Animal Production Center) were used for the in vivo experiments. Each rabbit was given an intravenous injection (in the ear vein) of dextran sulfate MW 1000 or dextran sulfate MW 5000 at a dose of 0.1 g/kg. At different times after injection of the compound, blood was collected from the rabbit's other ear, and kept at 4°C for a period of 12 h, after which the serum was collected by centrifugation at low speed. The samples were stored at −20°C until assayed.

### Antiviral assay of serum samples

The antiviral assays were based on the inhibitory effect of the serum samples on virus-induced cytopathogenicity in vitro. Briefly, MT-4 cells were suspended

TABLE 1
Inhibitory effect of dextran sulfate MW 1000 and 5000 on the replication of HIV-1 and HIV-2 in MT-4 cells

| Compound | $IC_{50}$ [a] (μg/ml) | |
|---|---|---|
| | HIV-1 (HTLV-$III_B$) | HIV-2 (LAV-$2_{ROD}$) |
| Dextran sulfate | | |
| MW 1000 | 7.2 | 0.11 |
| MW 5000 | 0.5 | 0.11 |

[a] 50% Inhibitory concentration, based on the inhibition of the cytopathogenicity of HIV for MT-4 cells.
All data represent mean values for at least four separate experiments.

in culture medium at $2.5 \times 10^5$ cells/ml and infected with HIV-1 and HIV-2 at 100 $CCID_{50}$/ml. Immediately after infection, the cell suspension was transferred to microtiter tray wells (100 μl cell suspension per well) containing various dilutions of the serum samples (highest dilution: 1/100). After 5 days incubation at 37°C, the number of viable cells was assessed by the MTT (3′-(4,5-dimethylthiazol-2-yl)-2,5-diphenyltetrazolium bromide) method as described by Pauwels et al. (1988). The concentrations of the compounds in the rabbit serum samples were determined by comparison of their 50% inhibitory concentration ($IC_{50}$) with the $IC_{50}$ values of the compounds tested as such or in the presence of appropriate dilutions of control serum.

## Results

### Establishment of a bioassay for measuring dextran sulfate concentrations in serum

When dextran sulfate MW 1000 and dextran sulfate MW 5000 were examined for their inhibitory effects on HIV-1 and HIV-2 replication in MT-4 cells, HIV-2 was about 70- and 5-fold more sensitive to dextran sulfate MW 1000 or 5000, respectively than HIV-1 (Table 1). This result indicated that a sensitive bioassay could be developed using HIV-2 rather than HIV-1 as the challenge virus, since based on the $IC_{50}$ values of the compounds for the two virus types, it should be possible to detect lower drug levels with HIV-2 than HIV-1.

At concentrations of 10% and 5%, control rabbit serum was cytotoxic to MT-4 cells and inhibitory to HIV-2 replication, whereas no inhibitory effect on either HIV-2 replication or cell viability was observed at a serum concentration of 1%. The rabbit serum samples were assayed without previous inactivation at 56°C, starting from a 1:100 dilution. Under these assay conditions, the minimum detectable concentration of dextran sulfate MW 1000 and dextran sulfate MW 5000 was 11 μg/ml.

SERUM CONCENTRATIONS OF DEXTRAN SULFATE IN RABBITS

When dextran sulfate MW 1000 at a dose of 0.1 g/kg was administered intravenously to rabbits and its concentration in the serum samples was measured by the bioassay described above, a concentration of 1.3 mg/ml was found 15 min after injection (Fig. 1). Then the level of dextran sulfate decreased rapidly so that 3 h after injection, a concentration of 24 μg/ml was detected. At 24 h after injection, the concentration of dextran sulfate MW 1000 was below the minimum detection level (11 μg/ml).

When dextran sulfate MW 5000 was administered intravenously to rabbits, the serum concentration reached by the compound 15 min after injection was 0.56

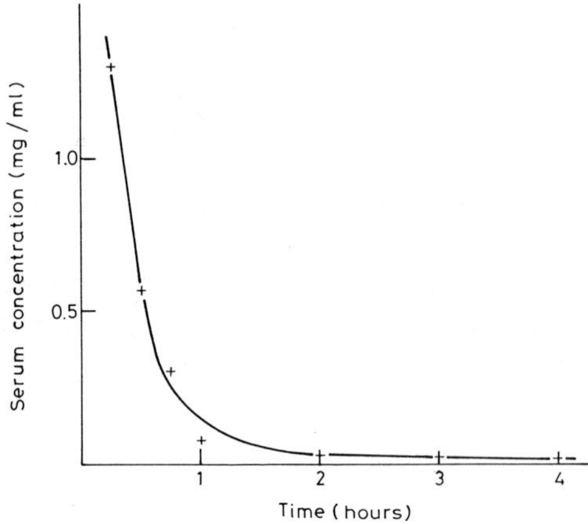


Fig. 1. Serum concentrations following intravenous injection of dextran sulfate (MW 1000) at 0.1 g/kg to rabbits. Data represent mean values of two separate experiments.

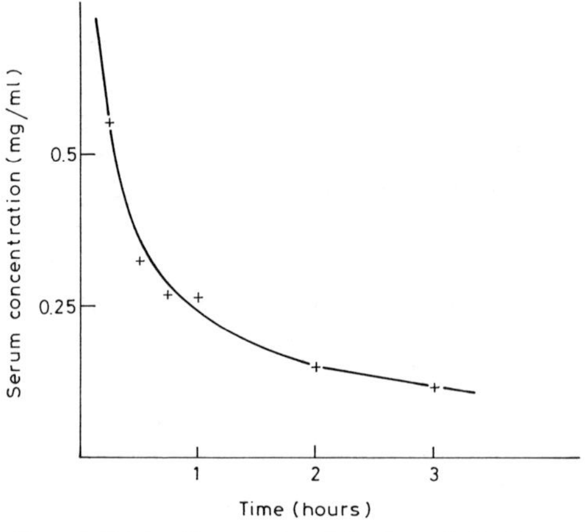


Fig. 2. Serum concentrations following intravenous injection of dextran sulfate (MW 5000) at 0.1 g/kg to rabbits. Data represent mean values of two separate experiments.

mg/ml (Fig. 2). This concentration was lower than that achieved by dextran sulfate MW 1000 at 15 min after injection. As for dextran sulfate MW 1000, the blood levels of dextran sulfate MW 5000 decreased rapidly. However, after 3 h, the serum concentration of dextran sulfate MW 5000 was still 119 $\mu$g/ml. The concentrations of dextran sulfate MW 1000 and dextran sulfate MW 5000 declined biphasically with initial half-lives of approximately 10–30 min and 30–70 min, respectively (Figs. 1 and 2).

## Discussion

The results of the clinical trials initiated with dextran sulfate in the treatment of patients with AIDS have so far been inconclusive. The compound has been administered orally, although it is not known to what extent dextran sulfate is absorbed from the gut. To gain better insight into the pharmacokinetics of dextran sulfate and related compounds, we have now developed a sensitive bioassay that permits measurement of dextran sulfate in the serum. This method should also be applicable to other sulfated polysaccharides and other biological specimens.

The assay is based on our observations that dextran sulfate (MW: 1000 or 5000) inhibits HIV-2 replication at a concentration that is markedly lower than that required for inhibition of HIV-1 replication. The minimum concentration (11 $\mu$g/ml) of dextran sulfate (MW: 1000 or 5000) that could be detected by this method is equivalent to approximately 0.02 and 0.11 heparin (anticoagulant) units per ml, respectively. This is well below the threshold at which bleeding complications occur.

Because of their high potency and selectivity as inhibitors of HIV replication in vitro, sulfated polysaccharides such as dextran sulfate (MW: 1000 and 5000) merit further investigations as potential anti-AIDS drugs. In any clinical studies that are undertaken with these compounds it would appear necessary to monitor the patient's blood drug levels. The bioassay described here may prove quite useful in this regard. When using serum samples of human origin, we could make the bioassay more sensitive by starting from a 1:50 dilution. At concentrations of 10% and 5%, human serum was slightly cytotoxic to MT-4 cells and inhibitory to HIV-2 replication, whereas no inhibitory effect of human serum on either HIV-2 replication or cell viability was observed at a concentration of 2% (data not shown). With the aid of this bioassay it should also be possible to establish the appropriate treatment regimens that are required to achieve and maintain sufficient levels of the compounds in the plasma.

## Acknowledgments

We thank Hilde Azijn for excellent technical assistance and Christiane Callebaut for fine editorial help.

## References

Abrams, D.I., Kuno, S., Wong, R., Jeffords, K., Nash, M., Molaghan, J.B., Gorter, R. and Ueno, R. (1989) Oral dextran sulfate (UA001) in the treatment of the acquired immunodeficiency syndrome (AIDS) and AIDS-related complex. *Ann. Intern. Med.* 110, 183–188.

Baba, M., Pauwels, R., Balzarini, J., Arnout, J., Desmyter, J. and De Clercq, E. (1988a) Mechanism of inhibitory effect of dextran sulfate and heparin on replication of human immunodeficiency virus in vitro. *Proc. Natl. Acad. Sci. U.S.A.* 85, 6132–6136.

Baba, M., Nakajima, M., Schols, D., Pauwels, R., Balzarini, J. and De Clercq, E. (1988b) Pentosan polysulfate, a sulfated oligosaccharide, is a potent and selective anti-HIV agent in vitro. *Antiviral Res.* 9, 335–343.

Ito, M., Baba, M., Sato, A., Pauwels, R., De Clercq, E. and Shigeta, S. (1987) Inhibitory effect of dextran sulfate and heparin on the replication of human immunodeficiency virus (HIV) in vitro. *Antiviral Res.* 7, 361–367.

Mitsuya, H., Looney, D.J., Kuno, S., Ueno, R., Wong-Staal, F. and Broder, S. (1988) Dextran sulfate suppression of viruses in the HIV family: inhibition of virion binding to CD4+ cells. *Science* 240, 646–649.

Nakashima, H., Yoshida, O., Baba, M., De Clercq, E. and Yamamoto, N. (1989) Anti-HIV activity of dextran sulfate as determined under different experimental conditions. *Antiviral Res.* 11, 233–246.

Pauwels, R., Balzarini, J., Baba, M., Snoeck, R., Schols, D., Herdewijn, P., Desmyter, J. and De Clercq, E. (1988) Rapid and automated tetrazolium-based colorimetric assay for the detection of anti-HIV compounds. *J. Virol. Methods* 20, 309–321.

Schols, D., Baba, M., Pauwels, R. and De Clercq, E. (1989) Flow cytometric method to demonstrate whether anti-HIV-1 agents inhibit virion binding to $T_4^+$ cells. *J. AIDS* 2, 10–15.

Ueno, R. and Kuno, S. (1987) Dextran sulfate, a potent anti-HIV agent in vitro having synergism with zidovudine. *Lancet* i, 1379.

# *Simian retroviruses*

*Eds. H. Schellekens and M.C. Horzinek*
*Animal Models in AIDS*



# 12

# SIV infection of rhesus macaques: in vivo titration of infectivity and development of an experimental vaccine

M.P. CRANAGE [1], N. COOK [1], P. JOHNSTONE [1], P.J. GREENAWAY [1], P.A. KITCHIN [2], E.J. STOTT [2], N. ALMOND [2] and A. BASKERVILLE [1]

[1] PHLS Center for Applied Microbiology and Research, Division of Pathology, Porton Down, Salisbury SP4 0JG, U.K. and [2] National Institute of Biological Standards and Control, Blanche Lane, South Mimms, Potters Bar EN6 3QG, U.K.

## Introduction

The simian immunodeficiency viruses (SIVs) are lentiviruses closely related to the human immunodeficiency viruses (Chakrabarti et al., 1987; Franchini et al., 1987; Schneider et al., 1987; Smith et al., 1988). Isolations of SIVs has been described from several monkey species including macaques (Daniel et al., 1985; Kanki et al., 1985; Benveniste et al., 1986; Gardner et al., 1988), sooty mangabeys (Fultz et al., 1986; Lowenstine et al., 1986; Murphey-Corb et al., 1986), African green monkeys (Daniel et al., 1988; Ohta et al., 1988) and mandrills (Tsujimoto et al., 1988). For recent reviews see Schneider and Hunsmann (1988) and Gardner and Luciw (1988). Information is still being gathered on the host range of these viruses and their ability to induce disease in infected monkeys. The primary aim of this work was to establish within the U.K., as part of the Medical Research Council's AIDS Directed Programme, a system that may be used for vaccine and chemotherapy evaluation and for the study of pathogenesis. In this report we describe our results using rhesus macaques and an accompanying paper (this volume) describes those obtained using cynomolgus macaques. Initial experiments were done to compare the infection of rhesus macaques with various isolates of SIV. $SIV_{mac}$ was chosen for further study and a pool of low passage virus established following isolation from an infected monkey. A minimum infectious dose ($MID_{50}$) was determined in two experiments by titration in rhesus macaques. A formalin inactivated whole virus experimental vaccine has been prepared and is now under investigation.

**Comparison of SIV strains**

A total of nine rhesus macaques and two vervet monkeys were inoculated i.v. variously with one of six strains of SIV (Table 1). Animals were monitored for infection by seroconversion using immunoblotting with $SIV_{mac251}$ crude virus pellet and/or by radioimmunoprecipitation assay (RIPA) using [$^{35}$S]-methionine-labelled infected cell lysates and uninfected controls. Immune complexes were detected in both assays using protein A-based reagents. Where done, virus isolation was attempted by co-cultivation of phytohaemagglutinin (PHA)-stimulated peripheral blood lymphocytes (PBL) from inoculated monkeys with PHA-stimulated pooled human cord blood lymphocytes (CBL) in the presence of interleukin 2. Cultures were monitored over 30 days for cytopathic effect and for cell-free reverse transcriptase (RT) activity. Cultures were only scored as positive when RT activity was at least two standard deviations above the mean activity of the control cultures, and showed an increase with time during part of the culture period. Full details of the procedures used are to be published elsewhere. $SIV_{mac251}$ and $SIV_{cyn186}$ were obtained from Dr R. Desrosiers. Two animals were each inoculated with 2 ml of supernatant fluid from high passage $SIV_{mac251}$ grown on the C8166 human T cell line. One animal received 0.5 ml of $SIV_{mac251}$ purified by equilibrium density gradient centrifugation on sucrose. This preparation was shown to include intact virions by electron microscopy and had an RT activity of $5 \times 10^5$ cpm/ml.

The two animals receiving high passage, non-purified virus failed to seroconvert and have shown no clinical evidence of infection. Whilst the animal receiving

TABLE 1
Comparison of SIV strains in rhesus macaques

| Virus | Animal | Time p.i. (months) | Sero-conversion | Culture | Disease |
|---|---|---|---|---|---|
| $SIV_{mac251}$ | Rh64H | 20 | – | NT | None |
| high pass | Rh72H | 20 | – | NT | None |
| $SIV_{mac251}$ | Rh15H | 19 | ± [b] | – | None |
| high pass pure | | | | | |
| $SIV_{mac251}$ | Rh32H | 18[a] | + | + | Wasting, 17.5 months |
| low pass | | | | | |
| $SIV_{cyn186}$ | Rh53H | 19 | + | + | Lymphadenopathy at 17 months |
| $SIV_{sm7}$ | Rh2H | 17 | + | NT | None |
| SIVpFLB10 | Rh67H | 15 | – | – | None |
| $SIV_{agm}$TY01 | Rh60H | 19 | – | NT | None |
| | Ver37728 | 19 | – | NT | None |
| $SIV_{agm}$TY02 | Rh40H | 19 | – | NT | None |
| | Ver37736 | 19 | –? [b] | NT | Gum lesions from 11 months |

[a] Killed in extremis at 18 months.
[b] See text for details.
NT: not tested.

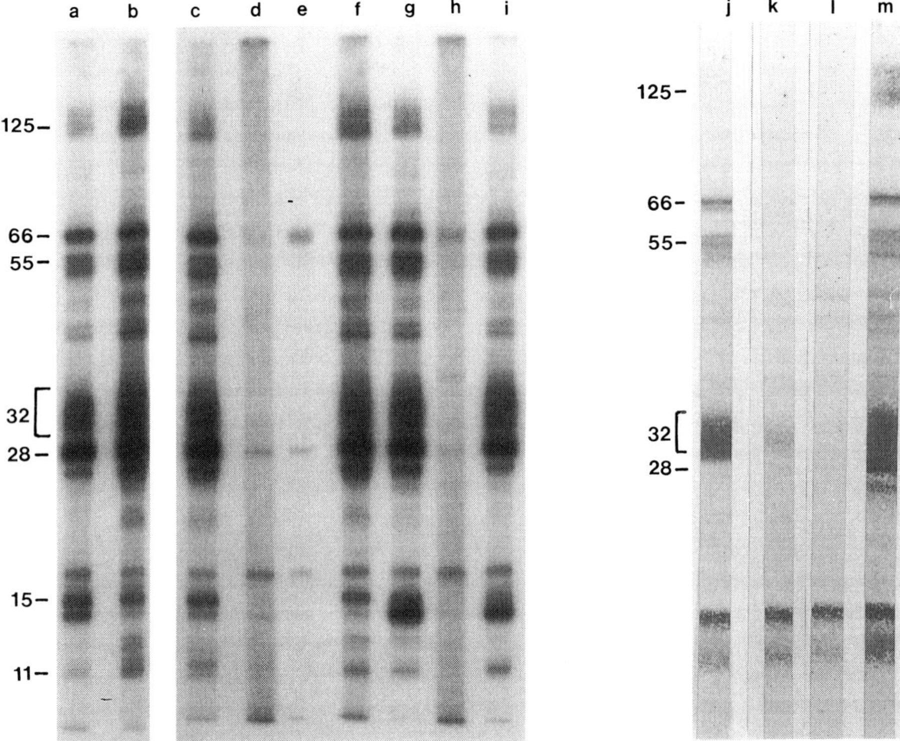


Fig. 1. Immunoblot profiles from SIV infected macaques. Crude virus pellet purified from the culture medium of $SIV_{mac251}$ 32H isolate infected C8166 cells was electrophoresed on 12.5% SDS polyacrylamide gels. Proteins were transferred to nitrocellulose. Sera were tested at a dilution of 1/100 and probed with either [$^{125}$I]protein A (tracks a–i) or peroxidase-conjugated protein A (tracks j–m). Sera tested were from (a) 32H infected with $SIV_{mac251}$; (b) 53H infected with $SIV_{cyn186}$. All other tracks show sera from monkeys inoculated with the 11/88 pool of $SIV_{mac251}$ 32H isolate; (c) 3H; (d) 5H; (e) 6H; (f) 27H; (g) 44H; (h) 71H; (i) 85H; (j) K8; (k) K33; (l) K69; (m) I67.

purified high passage $SIV_{mac251}$ has also shown no clinical signs and virus has not been recovered from PBL, a weak transient immune response has been seen by immunoblotting peaking at 4 months post inoculation (p.i.). The predominant reaction was to a 66 kD protein, with weaker reactivity seen to p28 (major *gag*-encoded core antigen), gp32 (*env*-encoded transmembrane protein) and gp125 (*env*-encoded external glycoprotein). Weak reactivity with gp160/gp125 was also observed with sera from this animal by radioimmunoprecipitation. It is not clear whether this weak response is due to infection, since this animal received inoculum with a much higher protein concentration than the others. Weak responses in the absence of other signs of infection have similarly been described in baboons inoculated with $SIV_{mne}$ (Benveniste et al., 1986). In contrast rhesus 32H receiving 100 $\mu$l of filtered cell-free supernatant from $SIV_{mac251}$ low passage infected H9 cells showed a rapid and strong seroconversion by immunoblotting (Fig. 1) and RIPA. Strong reactivity by immunoblotting was seen with bands of

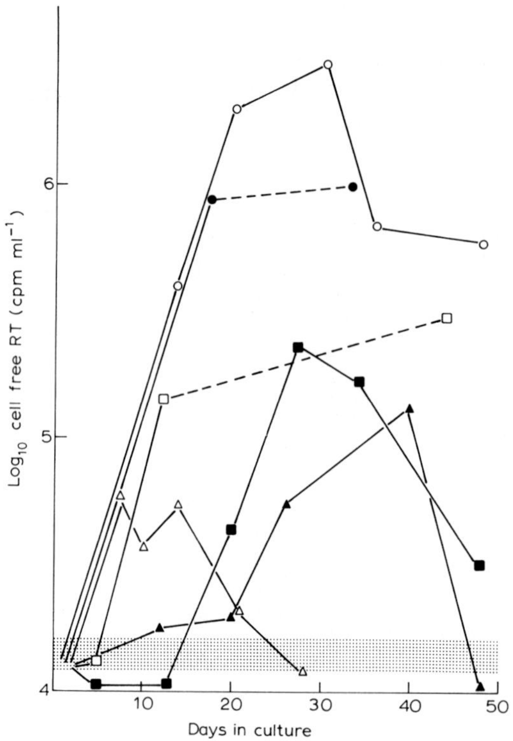


Fig. 2. Growth patterns of serial isolates of SIV from rhesus 32H measured by the production of cell-free reverse transcriptase in cultures of monkey PBLs cultured with human cord blood lymphocytes. The stippled area indicates ± one standard deviation of the mean RT activity in control cultures (n = 8). Monkey PBLs were taken post inoculation at 57 days (○), 89 days (●), 143 days (□), 185 days (■), 302 days (△) and 464 days (▲).

125 kD, 66 kD, multiple bands of about 55 kD, a diffuse region of approximately 32 kD, 28 kD, 15 kD, 14.5 kD and approximately 11 kD, whereas RIPA (data not shown) showed a predominant reaction with 160/125 kD and to a lesser extent with 28 kD. Reactivity to p28 was seen by the first bleed p.i. at day 18. By 1 month p.i. reactivity to gp32, gp125 and p66 (probably polymerase) was seen. Virus was recovered from PBL on each of seven occasions tested over a 17.5 month period. The variability in virus growth characteristics from six PBL samples taken serially from rhesus 32H over a 464 day period is shown in Fig. 2. Assay of virus recovered post mortem is still in progress. The levels of cell-free RT activity recovered generally declined with samples taken later in infection and there was no evidence for a change from so called slow/low to rapid/high, as described for HIV-1 isolates (Gardner et al., 1988). This result, however, may be influenced by our use of human primary cells in these assays and work is now being done to compare the growth properties of serial viral isolates on primary cells and cell lines of various origin. Rhesus 32H remained healthy until 17 months p.i. when it started to lose weight and condition rapidly. Lymphadenopa-

thy was not seen at any stage. The animal was killed in extremis at 18 months and post-mortem showed peritonitis and muscle wasting only. Histological examination however revealed loss of lymphoid tissue from lymph nodes and spleen. Virus was recovered from plasma, spleen and lymph nodes at the time of death. The rhesus macaque inoculated with 100 $\mu$l of $SIV_{cyn186}$ (a virus isolated from a cynomolgus monkey that died with lymphoma; R. Desrosiers, personal communication) showed a full pattern of seroconversion when serum was immunoblotted against $SIV_{mac251}$ virus antigen, with a pattern similar to the profile seen from rhesus 32H (Fig. 1). Virus has been recovered from this animal and it has developed persistent lymphadenopathy at 17 months. Seroconversion was also seen in the monkey inoculated with 0.5 ml $SIV_{smm7}$. This virus was isolated from a sooty mangabey and was kindly provided to us by Dr P. Fultz. No attempt at virus isolation has been made from this animal and no disease has been seen. Virus derived from tissue culture of a full length infectious molecular clone of SIV, pFLB10, kindly made available by Dr W. Haseltine, failed to infect the inoculated animal. Similarly no clear evidence of infection was seen when rhesus macaques and vervets were inoculated each with $SIV_{agmTYO1}$ and $SIV_{agmTYO2}$ (kindly provided by Dr M. Hayami) although a weak transient anti-gp 160/125 response was seen by RIPA in vervet 37736 six months after inoculation.

Since virus was easily recovered from rhesus 32H, and $SIV_{mac}$ has been reported to reproducibly induce AIDS type illness in rhesus macaques (Letvin et al., 1985; Daniel et al., 1987) we chose this virus to study in more detail.

### Establishment of a virus pool for vaccine/challenge studies

Briefly, virus was isolated from PBL taken from rhesus 32H 57 days after inoculation, by co-cultivation with human CBLs. The culture was supplemented with freshly stimulated CBLs on four occassions over a 17 day period after which time an extremely marked cytopathic effect was present and cell-free RT activity had reached $2 \times 10^6$ cpm/ml (Fig. 2). The virus was adapted to the C8166 human T cell line by addition of these cells to the adherent cell population present after draining the primary culture. Cultures were fed ("passaged") every 3–4 days by the addition of freshly diluted cells in a ratio of 1 volume to 3 volumes. Within 5 days of culture extensive formation of syncytia and ballooning of cytoplasm was seen in the C8166 cells. Cell-free supernatant was taken from a 250 ml culture at passage 4, passed through a 0.22 $\mu$m filter and aliquotted for storage in liquid nitrogen. This pool of the 32H isolate of $SIV_{mac251}$ (designated 11/88) was used for subsequent study. The reisolated virus was authenticated as SIV by electron microscopy, serological analysis and nucleotide sequence analysis of polymerase chain reaction (PCR) amplified proviral DNA from a 496 bp region of *gag* – and a 875 bp region of *env* – (Kitchin et al., 1990). No evidence of simian D-type retrovirus was seen, by electron microscopy of infected cells, immunoblot profiles or by culture on Raji cells (M. McClure, personal communication). Indeed none of the rhesus macaques used in the study reported here had evidence of antibodies to simian D-type retroviruses by a solid phase immunosorbent assay.

The reverse transcriptase activity of the 11/88 virus pool was $1.1 \times 10^6$ cpm/ml and the $TCID_{50}$ was $10^{-4.5}$/ml as determined by infectivity end point titration on C8166 cells. Immunoblotting showed that the transmembrane protein in this virus pool was full length and subsequent nucleotide sequence analysis has shown the absence of a premature stop codon in the carboxy terminal portion of *env* – (Cranage et al., 1989).

## Titration of 11/88 virus pool in rhesus macaques

In the first experiment (Table 2) 100-fold dilutions of virus pool from $10^{-1}$ to $10^{-7}$ were inoculated intravenously at 2 ml per animal into two rhesus macaques for each dilution. Animals were bled each month and seroconversion was monitored by immunoblotting and RIPA. PCR analysis was performed on DNA extracted from monkey PBLs (Kitchin et al., 1990) and virus culture was done either at the time of death or 4 months p.i., whichever was the soonest. Of the five animals with evidence of infection, three have died or have been killed in extremis. Proviral DNA was detected in lymphocytes from animals receiving $10^{-1}$ and $10^{-3}$ dilutions of virus and from one animal receiving $10^{-5}$ dilution of virus on each occasion tested at 1 month, 2 months and 3 months (where applicable) after inoculation. A weak PCR result was obtained from rhesus 6H only at 3 months p.i., all previous samples being negative. The significance of this result is not clear since this animal has no evidence of infection, either serologically or upon culture of PBLs and shows no disease. The other two animals receiving $10^{-7}$ and $10^{-5}$ dilutions of virus show no evidence of infection.

TABLE 2
Titration of $SIV_{mac251}$ 32H isolate, pool 11/88 in rhesus macaques (1)

| Animal | Inoculum | Seroconversion | | PCR | Culture | Disease [a] | Time to death (months) |
|---|---|---|---|---|---|---|---|
| | | Immunoblot | RIPA | | | | |
| Rh85H | $10^{-1}$ | + | + | + | + | + | 5.5 |
| Rh27H | $10^{-1}$ | + | + | + | + | + | >11 |
| Rh3H | $10^{-3}$ | + | + | + | + | None | >11 |
| Rh68H | $10^{-3}$ | – | – | + | + | + | 2 |
| Rh44H | $10^{-5}$ | + | + | + | NT | + | 4 |
| Rh5H | $10^{-5}$ | – | – | – | – | None | >11 |
| Rh71H | $10^{-7}$ | – | – | – | – | None | >11 |
| Rh6H | $10^{-7}$ | – | – | ± [b] | – | None | >11 |

[a] See text for details.
[b] Positive only at 3 months p.i.
NT: not tested.

Rhesus 85H ($10^{-1}$ virus) showed localised lymphadenopathy, hair loss and diarrhoea. By 5.5 months p.i. the animal had lost 33% of its weight and was killed in extremis. Post-mortem revealed enteritis, muscle wasting and very small lymph nodes. Histopathology showed extreme lymphoid depletion and fibrosis of the spleen. A more variable picture was seen with the lymph nodes, some showing depletion, whilst others showed paracortical enlargement. Enteropathy was also recorded.

Rhesus 27H ($10^{-1}$ virus) developed inguinal lymphadenopathy 4 months p.i. Gingivitis started at 7 months and has continued to the present (11 months p.i.). At last examination this animal showed enlargement of all superficial lymph nodes and splenomegaly. The animal has failed to gain weight.

Rhesus 3H ($10^{-3}$ virus) despite clear evidence of infection remained well and has shown a steady weight gain equivalent to that seen in uninfected animals.

Rhesus 68H ($10^{-3}$ virus) showed no evidence of a humoral immune response, however virus was cultured post mortem from PBL and a strong PCR was obtained directly from PBL. Two months p.i. the animal developed diarrhoea continuing for 5 days when it died, despite fluid therapy. At death the animal had lost 37% of its body weight. Autopsy revealed a necrotising enterocolitis and *Yersinia enterocolitica* was isolated. Histopathology showed lymphoid depletion in nodes and spleen, enterocolitis and an AIDS-type encephalopathy.

Rhesus 44H ($10^{-5}$ virus) had localised lymphadenopathy at 4 months p.i. when it developed diarrhoea. This continued for 1 week until death when the animal had lost 20% of its body weight. Histopathological findings included colitis with ulceration, lymphoid depletion of nodes and spleen and follicular fibrosis.

Where seroconversion occurred in this series of animals, reactivity was detected to all the major viral components, although some differences in reactivity to bands migrating at 15 kD and 11 kD were noted (Fig. 1). In a second experiment a closer range titration was performed with 10-fold dilutions of virus pool from $10^{-4}$ to $10^{-8}$ (Table 3). Both animals receiving $10^{-4}$ dilution of virus pool and one animal receiving $10^{-5}$ dilution became infected. Rhesus K33 ($10^{-4}$ virus) developed intermittent diarrhoea and became progressively thinner from 3 months p.i. The animal was killed in extremis at 4.5 months. At post-mortem the animal was found to have wasting muscles and small lymph nodes; histopathology is not yet available. Interestingly this animal made only a very weak humoral immune response, immunoblotting showing extremely weak reactivity only with gp32. Both of the other animals in this series with signs of infection have had single enlarged lymph nodes from 3 months p.i. Rhesus K8 has made only a weak antibody response, predominantly to gp32 with no evidence of anti-p28 reactivity. Others have reported that animals infected with $SIV_{mac}$ that make only low titer antibody responses, limited to anti-envelope activity, have a poor prognosis (Kannagi et al., 1986). In contrast, rhesus I67 showed responses to all the major viral components, giving a similar response to that seen in the seropositive animals in the first series described above.

TABLE 3
Titration of $SIV_{mac251}$ 32H isolate, pool 11/88 in rhesus macaques (2)

| Animal | Inoculum | Seroconversion immunoblot | Culture | Disease | Time to death (months) |
|---|---|---|---|---|---|
| K33 | $10^{-4}$ | wk | + | + | 4.5 |
| K8 | $10^{-4}$ | [+][a] | + | + | > 5 |
| I67 | $10^{-5}$ | + | + | + | > 5 |
| K69 | $10^{-5}$ | − | − | None | > 5 |
| K52 | $10^{-6}$ | − | − | None | > 5 |
| K24 | $10^{-6}$ | − | − | None | > 5 |
| K42 | $10^{-7}$ | − | − | None | > 5 |
| K32 | $10^{-7}$ | − | − | None | > 5 |
| K23 | $10^{-8}$ | − | − | None | > 5 |
| K44 | $10^{-8}$ | − | − | None | > 5 |

[a] Anti-*env* response only.

Taken together these data would indicate an $MID_{50}$ of $10^{-5}$ for this pool of virus. As well as its infection potential it is clear that this virus stock is also able to induce AIDS-like illness in the majority of infected animals, including some evidence of early neurological involvement. Fifty percent of seropositive and/or PCR positive animals died or were killed in extremis within the first 6 months after inoculation. The disease spectrum seen is similar to that reported by others (Letvin et al., 1985).

## Development of an experimental vaccine

We have recently prepared a formalin inactivated, whole virus preparation. Briefly, cell-free supernatant was harvested from 40 litres of SIV (11/88 virus pool pass 10–14) infected C8166 cells. Virus was concentrated by ultracentrifugation and low molecular weight components removed by gel filtration chromatography on Sepharose 4B (McGrath et al., 1970). Sixteen percent of the total protein applied to the column was recovered in the first two fractions which contained 86% of the total RT activity eluted. Silver staining of SDS PAGE preparations showed that serum albumin was depleted to undetectable levels from the virus containing fractions and an approximate 10-fold enrichment of major viral core antigen was seen. Sera from infected monkeys reacted with all the major viral components when the virus preparation was tested by immunoblotting and interestingly diffuse regions at both 32 kD and 41 kD were seen (Fig. 3). Evidence has been obtained to show that this preparation contains both full length and truncated transmembrane glycoprotein (Cranage et al., 1989). Finally, the virus preparation was treated with formaldehyde and is now undergoing inactivation validation experiments both in vitro and in vivo. We hope to

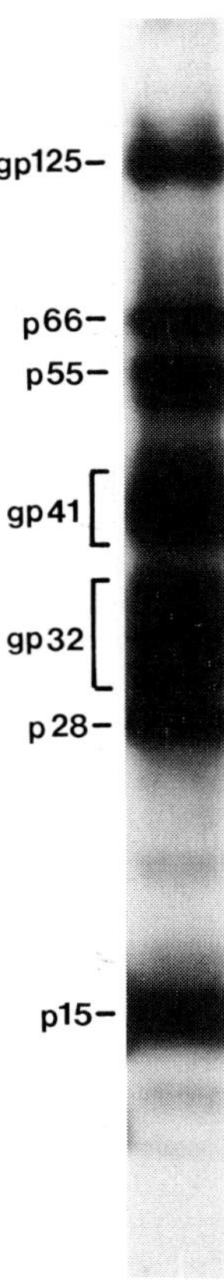


Fig. 3. Immunoblot profile of an experimental vaccine preparation. The immunoblot was probed with serum from rhesus 32H taken 12 months p.i.

start a vaccine trial in both rhesus macaques and cynomolgus monkeys within the next month.

## Conclusions

We have found rhesus macaques to be susceptible to infection with low passage $SIV_{mac251}$, $SIV_{cyn186}$ and $SIV_{sm7}$ but not with two isolates of $SIV_{agm}$, or with more highly passaged $SIV_{mac251}$ or with a molecular clone of $SIV_{mac}$. Virus from an animal infected with $SIV_{mac251}$ has been partially characterised and a pool of virulent virus, able to induce disease in macaques, has been established. The $MID_{50}$ has been found to be similar to the $TCID_{50}$. A vaccine trial with formalinised semi-purified virus is under way.

## Acknowledgements

This work was supported by the U.K. Medical Research Council's AIDS Directed Programme and the Public Health Laboratory Service. We are indebted to Dr G.H. Farrar for help with vaccine production. We are grateful to Mrs P.M. Lomas for preparation of the manuscript.

## References

Asjo, B., Morfeldt-Manson, L., Albert, J. et al. (1986) Replicative capacity of human immunodeficiency virus from patients with varying severity of HIV infection. *Lancet* ii, 660–662.

Benveniste, R.E., Arthur, L.O., Tsai, C.C. et al. (1986) Isolation of a lentivirus from a macaque with lymphoma. Comparison with HTLV-III/LAV and other lentiviruses. *J. Virol.* 60, 483–490.

Benveniste, R.E., Raben, D., Hill, R.W. et al. (1989) Molecular characterization and comparison of simian immunodeficiency virus isolates from macaques, mangabeys and African green monkeys. *J. Med. Primatol.* 18, 287–303.

Chakrabarti, L., Guyader, M., Alizon, M. et al. (1987) Sequence of simian immunodeficiency virus from macaque and its relationship to other human and simian retroviruses. *Nature* 328, 543–547.

Cranage, M.P., Almond, N., Jenkins, A. and Kitchin, P.A. (1989) Transmembrane protein of SIV. *Nature* 342, 349.

Daniel, M.D., Letvin, N.L., King, N.W. et al. (1985) Isolation of T-cell tropic HTLV-III-like retrovirus from macaques. *Science* 228, 1201–1204.

Daniel, M.D., Letvin, N.L., Sehgal, P.K. et al. (1987) Long-term persistent infection of macaque monkeys with the simian immunodeficiency virus. *J. Gen. Virol.* 68, 3183–3189.

Daniel, M.D., Li, Y., Naidu, Y.M. et al. (1988) Simian immunodeficiency virus from African green monkeys. *J. Virol.* 62, 4123–4128.

Franchini, G., Gurgo, C., Guo, H.G., et al. (1987) Sequence of simian immunodeficiency virus and its relationship to the human immunodeficiency viruses. *Nature* 328, 539–543.

Fultz, P.N., McClure, H.M., Anderson, D.C., Swenson, R.B., Anand, R. and Srinivasan, A. (1986) Isolation of a T-lymphotropic retrovirus from naturally infected sooty mangabey monkeys (*Cercocebus atys*). *Proc. Natl. Acad. Sci. U.S.A.* 83, 5286–5290.

Gardner, M.B., and Luciw, P.A. (1988) Simian immunodeficiency viruses and their relationship to the human immunodeficiency viruses. *AIDS* 2 (Suppl. 1), S3–S10.

Gardner, M., Luciw, P., Lerche, N. and Marx, P. (1988) Non-human primate retrovirus isolates and AIDS. In: K. Perk (Ed.), *Advances in Veterinary Science and Comparative Medicine,* Vol. 32. Academic Press, New York, NY, pp. 171–226.

Kanki, P.J., McLane, M.F., King, N.W. et al. (1985) Serological identification and characterization of a macaque T-lymphotropic retrovirus closely related to HTLV-III. *Science* 228, 1199–1201.

Kannagi, M., Kiyotaki, M., Desrosiers, R.C. et al. (1986) Humoral immune responses to T cell tropic retrovirus simian T lymphotropic virus type III in monkeys with experimentally induced acquired immune deficiency-like syndrome. *J. Clin. Invest.* 78, 1229–1236.

Kitchin, P.A., Almond, N., Szotyori, Z. et al. (1990) The use of the polymerase chain reaction for the detection of simian immunodeficiency virus in experimentally infected macaques. *J. Virol Methods* 28, 85–100.

Letvin, N.L., Daniel, M.D., Sehgal, P.K. et al. (1985) Induction of AIDS-like disease in macaque monkeys with T-cell tropic retrovirus STLV-III. *Science* 230, 71–73.

Lowenstine, N.L., Pedersen, N.C., Higgins, J. et al. (1986) Seroepidemiologic survey of captive Old World primates for antibodies to human and simian retroviruses, and isolation of a lentivirus from sooty mangabeys *(Cercocebus atys). Int. J. Cancer* 38, 563–575.

McGrath, M., Witte, O., Pincus, T. and Weissan, I.L. (1978) Retrovirus purification: method that conserves envelope glycoprotein and maximizes infectivity. *J. Virol.* 25, 923–927.

Murphey-Corb, M., Martin, L.N., Rangan, S.R.S. et al. (1986) Isolation of an HTLV-III related retrovirus from macaques with simian AIDS and its possible origin in asymptomatic mangabeys. *Nature* 321, 435–437.

Ohta, Y., Masuda, T., Tsujimoto, H. et al. (1988) Isolation of simian immunodeficiency virus from African green monkeys and seroepidemiologic survey of the virus in various non-human primates. *Int. J. Cancer* 41, 115–122.

Scheider, J. and Hunsmann, G. (1988) Simian lentiviruses—the SIV group. *AIDS* 2, 1–9.

Schneider, J., Jurkiewicz, E., Hayami, M., Desrosiers, R., Marx, P. and Hunsmann, G. (1987) Serological and structural comparison of HIV, SIVmac, SIVagm and SIVsm, four primate lentiviruses. In: J.C. Gluckman and E. Vilmer (Eds.), *Acquired Immunodeficiency Syndrome,* Elsevier, Paris, pp. 63–69.

Smith, T.F., Srinivasan, A., Schochetman, G., Marcus, M. and Myers, G. (1988) The phylogenetic history of immunodeficiency viruses. *Nature* 333, 573–575.

Tsujimoto, H., Cooper, R.W., Kodama, T. et al. (1988) Isolation and characterization of simian immunodeficiency virus from mandrills in Africa and its relationship to other human and simian immunodeficiency viruses. *J. Virol.* 62, 4044–4050.

*Eds. H. Schellekens and M.C. Horzinek*
*Animal Models in AIDS*



# 13

# Titration of $SIV_{mac251}$ (32H isolate) in cynomolgus macaques for use as a challenge in vaccination studies

P.A. KITCHIN [1], M.P. CRANAGE [2], N. ALMOND [1], A. BARNARD [1], A. BASKERVILLE [2], T. CORCORAN [1], C. FROMHOLC [1], P. GREENAWAY [2], C. GRIEF [1], A. JENKINS [1], K. KENT [1], C. LING [1], B. MAHON [1], K. MILLS [1], M. PAGE [1], P. SILVERA [1], Z. SZOTYORI [1], F. TAFFS [1] and E.J. STOTT [1]

[1] AIDS Collaborating Centre, National Institute of Biological Standards and Control, Blanche Lane, Potters Bar EN6 3QG, U.K. and [2] Division of Pathology, Centre for Applied Microbiology and Research, Porton Down, Salisbury SP4 0JG, U.K.

**Summary**

Preliminary experiments indicated that $SIV_{mac251}$ can infect and cause an AIDS-like syndrome in both rhesus and cynomolgus monkeys. A low passage pool, designated 11/88, was prepared from virus re-isolated from rhesus monkey number 32H (see Cranage et al., this volume). The titer of this virus was $10^{4.5}$ $TCID_{50}$/ml in C8166 cells. Dilutions of the 11/88 pool were each inoculated intravenously into cynomolgus macaques. Virus was re-isolated from some of the animals by 14 days post inoculation. Infection was confirmed by PCR, ELISA and immunoblot analyses. The $MID_{50}$ is $10^{4.75}$.

Cynomolgus monkeys were vaccinated with glutaraldehyde fixed SIV-infected cells, or vaccinia recombinants carrying the SIV genes for *env, gag* or *pol.* The immune responses of these animals are being assessed before challenge with 10 $MID_{50}$ of the 11/88 pool of $SIV_{mac251}$ (32H isolate). The degree of protection will be assessed by virological, serological and clinical criteria.

## Introduction

A variety of simian immunodeficiency virus (SIV) strains have been shown to infect rhesus macaques and cause an AIDS-like disease which ultimately leads to death (Fultz et al., 1986; Kannagi et al., 1986; Murphey-Corb et al., 1986). These primate models of human AIDS provide a valuable system in which the pathogenesis of immunodeficiency viruses can be studied. Furthermore, they offer the most appropriate model presently available in which AIDS vaccines can be developed and assessed (Desrosiers et al., 1989). The majority of these studies have been performed in rhesus macaques and relatively little information is available concerning the behaviour of such viruses in the more readily obtainable cynomolgus macaque (*Macaca fascicularis*).

As part of the United Kingdom's Medical Research Council's AIDS Directed Programme (ADP), we initiated a comparative study of six different strains of SIV in both rhesus and cynomolgus macaques (see also Cranage et al., this volume). Several of these viruses were pathogenic and a re-isolate, derived from $SIV_{mac251}$, was chosen for the ADP's first generation animal model.

We describe here the determination of an $MID_{50}$ for this virus stock as well as our initial assessment of the immune responses of cynomolgus macaques to a variety of SIV antigens.

## Materials and methods

### Source of viruses

$SIV_{mac251}$, high passage (HP), $SIV_{mac251}$, low passage (LP) and $SIV_{cyn186}$ (LP) were all obtained from Dr R. Desrosiers at the New England Regional Primate Research Centre, Boston, MA, U.S.A. $SIV_{sm7}$ was obtained from Dr P. Fultz, Yerkes Primate Centre, Atlanta, GA, U.S.A. $SIV_{agm}$ Tyo1 and $SIV_{agm}$ Tyo2 (high passage) were obtained from Dr M. Hayami, Institute of Medical Science, Tokyo, Japan. Virus derived from the molecular clone SIV pFLB10 was obtained from Dr W. Haseltine, Harvard Medical School, Boston, MA, U.S.A.

### Preparation and inoculation of viruses

$SIV_{mac251}$ (LP) and $SIV_{cyn186}$ (LP) were received as frozen vials of cell-free virus containing $4 \times 10^5$ cpm/ml and $2 \times 10^5$ cpm/ml reverse transcriptase counts respectively. The vials were thawed and 100 $\mu$l immediately injected intravenously. $SIV_{mac251}$ (HP) was received as persistently infected HUT78 cells. These were propagated for several weeks and a 1:50 concentration of cell-free supernatant was prepared by centrifugation. This preparation contained many virus particles (Grief et al., 1989) and about $10^6$ reverse transcriptase counts/ml. Animals received 100 $\mu$l intravenously. $SIV_{agm}$ Tyo1 and Tyo2 were received as persistently infected Molt-4 cells. Animals received 100 $\mu$l intravenously. SIV pFLB10 was received as a frozen vial of cell-free virus. Animals received 100 $\mu$l intravenously (about $2.3 \times 10^4$ reverse transcriptase counts).

### Virus re-isolations from monkeys

Peripheral blood mononuclear cells were isolated on Percoll gradients and co-cultivated with C8166 cells in RPMI 1640 medium containing 10% heat-inactivated foetal calf serum (HFCS) and 10 $\mu$g/ml purified phytohaemagglutinin (Wellcome). Cultures were fed twice weekly with medium containing 5 IU/ml of recombinant human interleukin-2 (IL-2). The appearance of large syncytia in these cultures indicated the presence of SIV, which was confirmed by a p24 antigen assay (Dupont).

### Source of monkeys

Cynomolgus macaques (*Macaca fascicularis*) were from a U.K.-bred colony obtained from Shamrock Farms, Dorset, U.K.

### SIV ELISA

C8166 cells infected with $SIV_{mac251}$ (32H isolate) were resuspended in 0.5% Nonidet P40 in distilled water at $10^7$ cells per ml. After centrifugation at $10{,}000 \times g$ for 1 min the supernatant constituted viral antigen. Control antigen was derived in the same way from uninfected C8166 cells. The wells of micro-ELISA plates (Falcon Plastics) were coated with antigen diluted 1:100 in distilled water and allowed to dry overnight at 37°C. Plates were blocked for 30 min in phosphate-buffered saline containing 5% pig serum and 0.05% Tween 20. After washings, serial dilutions of monkey sera were added and plates incubated for 1 h. Bound antibody was detected using goat anti-human antibody coupled to horseradish peroxidase and tetramethyl benzidine as substrate. After stopping the reaction with 2 M sulphuric acid, optical density was measured at 450 nm using a Titertek plate reader. The readings with control antigen were subtracted from those with viral antigen to obtain specific anti-SIV values. These were plotted against serum dilutions and the end point calculated by regression analysis. Titers were taken as the reciprocal of the serum dilution giving an $OD_{450}$ of 0.15.

### Immunoblots

The immunoblots were carried out as described by Thorpe et al. (1987), except that 5% skimmed milk powder (Marvel, Premier Brands U.K. Ltd) was substituted for bovine haemoglobin in the blocking and washing steps. An $^{125}$I-labelled anti-human IgG monoclonal antibody was used to detect bound monkey antisera. The antigen used for the analysis was a 50-fold concentrate of C8166 cells persistently infected with $SIV_{mac251}$ (32H isolate).

### Polymerase chain reaction

This was performed exactly as described by Kitchin et al. (1990).

### Lymphocyte surface markers

Cytofluorographic analysis of lymphocyte sub-populations were performed on whole blood samples using a direct staining technique employing anti-human CD4 and CD8 monoclonal antibodies which cross-reacted with macaque lymphocytes. Peripheral blood samples (50 μl) were incubated for 20 min at 20°C with fluorescein isothiocyanate (FITC) conjugated anti-CD4 (OKT4, Ortho) and phycoerythrin (PE) conjugated anti-CD8 (Leu 2a, Becton Dickinson), diluted according to the manufacturer's instructions. Red blood cells were lysed with FACS lysing solution (Becton Dickinson). After washing in phosphate-buffered saline, the remaining cells were fixed in 0.5% formaldehyde in physiological saline. Green (FITC) and red (PE) fluorescence of the gated lymphocyte population was measured on a FACscan (Becton Dickinson) and analysed by a Consort 30 computer system (Becton Dickinson).

### Electron microscopy

Virus-infected C8166 cells were fixed in 2% glutaraldehyde for 2 h at room temperature. The cells were then washed in cacodylate buffer, and embedded in 1% low melting point agarose. The agarose embedded material was post-fixed in 1% osmium tetroxide in isotonic buffer and then treated with 0.5% aqueous uranyl acetate, dehydrated in ethanol and embedded via epoxy propane in Araldite resin. Sections were stained with uranyl acetate and lead citrate and examined with a Philips CM12 EM.

### Preparation of fixed SIV-infected cell vaccine

C8166 cells infected with SIV were pelleted at $400 \times g$ for 5 min and resuspended in ice-cold Earle's balanced salt solution (EBSS) at $2 \times 10^6$ cells/ml. An equal volume of cold 0.15% glutaraldehyde in EBSS was added and the mixture held on ice for 5 min. After adding an equal volume of 0.1 M glycine, the cells were pelleted at $400 \times g$ for 5 min and then resuspended in RPMI 1640 medium containing 10% HFCS, 0.05 M Tris buffer, pH 7.5, and 0.015% fresh β-propiolactone. After incubating at 37°C for 4 h, the cells were pelleted, resuspended at $10^7$ cells/ml in medium containing 10% dimethyl sulphoxide and stored at −70°C. Inactivation of virus infectivity was validated by co-cultivating $2 \times 10^6$ fixed cells with C8166 cells for 4 weeks. The absence of viral cytopathic effect or antigen production indicated that infectivity had been destroyed. A vaccine dose consisted of $2 \times 10^6$ fixed cells resuspended in 0.5 ml phosphate-buffered saline containing 100 μg of Quil A (Superfos, Denmark), injected subcutaneously.

### Recombinant vaccinia virus vaccines

Recombinant vaccinia viruses PJ VV-*env* and PJ VV*gag-pol* containing the genes for SIV *env,* or *gag* and *pol* respectively were the generous gift of Dr Philip Johnson (NIH, Bethesda, MD, U.S.A.). The recombinant SK VV-*env* was kindly donated by Dr C. Thiriart (Smith Kline Biologicals, Rixensart, Belgium). Monkeys were injected intradermally with $10^7$ pfu of virus.

## Results

### $SIV_{mac251}$ (HP), $SIV_{agm}$ Tyo1, $SIV_{agm}$ Tyo2 AND SIV pFLB10

A summary of the results obtained from the comparison of six different SIV strains is shown in Table 1. The animals receiving $SIV_{mac251}$ (HP), $SIV_{agm}$ Tyo1, $SIV_{agm}$ Tyo2 and SIV pFLB10 failed to seroconvert, were not viraemic and showed no overt signs of pathology 14–18 months post inoculation (p.i). These animals were considered to be uninfected and were not studied further.

### $SIV_{sm7}$

Macaque number 7250 (Table 1) seroconverted between 53 and 86 days p.i. as judged by immunoblot analysis (Fig. 1a) and ELISA (Fig. 2). The response to p27 was observed before the response to gp125. Maximal responses were seen to both *gag* (p27 + p59) and *env* (gp125 + gp32) between 191 and 244 days p.i. However, antibody responses declined thereafter. The animal developed persistently enlarged inguinal lymph glands from about 180 days p.i. It continued to lose condition and developed persistent diarrhoea at about 380 days p.i. It was killed in extremis at 421 days p.i. Post-mortem analysis revealed a mild colitis and both the spleen and lymph nodes showed hyperplasia and involution.

### $SIV_{cyn186}$

Macaque number 630C (Table 1) seroconverted between 58 and 114 days p.i. during which time antibody responses to p27 and gp125 were detected (Figs. 1B

TABLE 1
Summary of disease status in cynomolgus macaques

| Number | Virus received | Sero-conver-sion [a] | Virus isola-tion | Clinical signs |
|---|---|---|---|---|
| 705B | $SIV_{mac251}$ (LP) | + | + | Weight loss; CD4 depletion; Died 305 days p.i. Pneumocystis. |
| 613B | $SIV_{mac251}$ (HP) | – | – | None seen at 18 months p.i. Killed. |
| 630C | $SIV_{cyn186}$ | + + | + | Lymphadenopathy; weight loss; skin tumour; killed in extremis 355 days p.i. Retroperitoneal fibromatosis. |
| 725O | $SIV_{sm7}$ | + + | + | Persistent diarrhoea; killed in extremis 421 days p.i. Mild colitis. |
| 713C | $SIV_{agm}$ Tyo1 | – | NT | None seen at 14 months; killed. |
| 523A | $SIV_{agm}$ Tyo2 | – | NT | None seen at 14 months; killed. |
| 095B | SIV pFLB10 | – | – | None seen at 14 months; killed. |

[a] Tested by ELISA and immunoblotting.
NT: not tested.

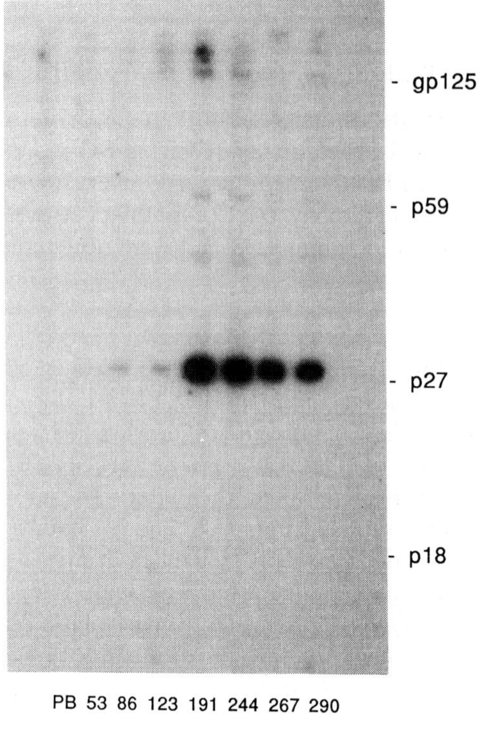


Fig. 1. Immunoblot analyses of antibody responses of cynomolgus macaques infected with $SIV_{sm7}$ (panel A) or $SIV_{cyn186}$ (panel B).

and 2). Antibody responses to gp120 and gp32 continued to increase thereafter and the response to *gag* (p27 and p59) was maximal between 142 and 301 days p.i. Antibodies to p27 subsequently declined to undetectable levels, in contrast to the p59 antibodies which remained high. The animal developed persistent generalised lymphadenopathy and a skin tumour at about 300 days p.i. It subsequently (about 315 days p.i.) developed a gross abdominal distortion and was eventually killed in extremis at 355 days p.i. Post-mortem analysis revealed extensive retroperitoneal fibromatosis.

## $SIV_{mac251}$ (LP)

Macaque number 705B (Table 1) developed a comparatively weak antibody response that was detectable only by ELISA (Fig. 2) or RIPA (*env* only; data not shown) and not by immunoblotting. Virus was recovered from this animal up to 141 days p.i. but not thereafter. The animal began to lose weight and CD4

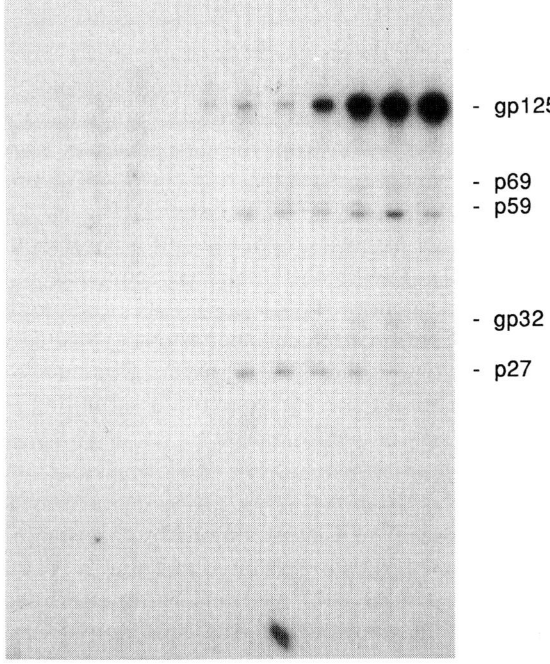


Fig. 1 (continued).

positive lymphocytes from about 180 days p.i. and died from a severe wasting syndrome at 305 days p.i. Post-mortem analysis revealed completely atrophied lymph nodes and the presence of Pneumocystis.

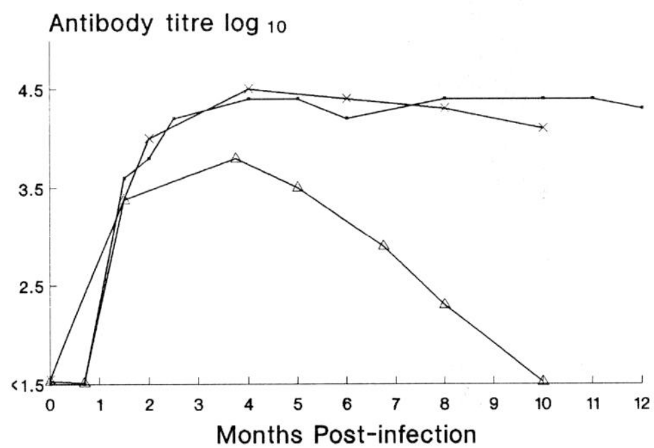


Fig. 2. SIV ELISA of antibody responses of cynomolgus macaques infected with $SIV_{cyn186}$ (■———■), $SIV_{mac251}$ LP (△———△) and $SIV_{sm7}$ (×———×).

## SEQUENCE ANALYSIS OF $SIV_{mac251}$ (32H ISOLATE)

Virus was re-isolated from a rhesus macaque (number 32H) originally infected with $SIV_{mac251}$ (LP) as described by Cranage et al. (this volume). An aliquot of this low passage isolate (11/88 pool) was taken for characterisation and authentication. The p18/p27 junction region from the *gag* gene was amplified with SIV specific primers by the polymerase chain reaction (PCR) (Kitchin et al., 1990). A single band of the expected size (496 bp) was observed (Fig. 3). This material was directly sequenced by primer extension analysis and a continuous region of 336 bases was found to be identical to the published sequence for $SIV_{mac251}$ (Los Alamos 1989 AIDS database entry SIVMM251). Additional PCR and sequence analysis of DNA extracted from C8166 cells persistently infected with this isolate confirmed a > 98% homology in the full-length *gag* gene and > 95% homology in the transmembrane portion of the *env* gene (data submitted for publication).

## $MID_{50}$ DETERMINATION FOR THE 11/88 POOL

The $MID_{50}$ for this virus isolate was determined by titration in 20 cynomolgus macaques. A summary of the results is presented in Table 2. All animals receiving doses of virus at $10^{-1}$, $10^{-3}$ and $10^{-4}$ dilutions became infected, as judged by seroconversion (Fig. 4), ability to re-isolate virus, detection of viral DNA by PCR and persistent lymphadenopathy. One out of four animals receiving the $10^{-5}$

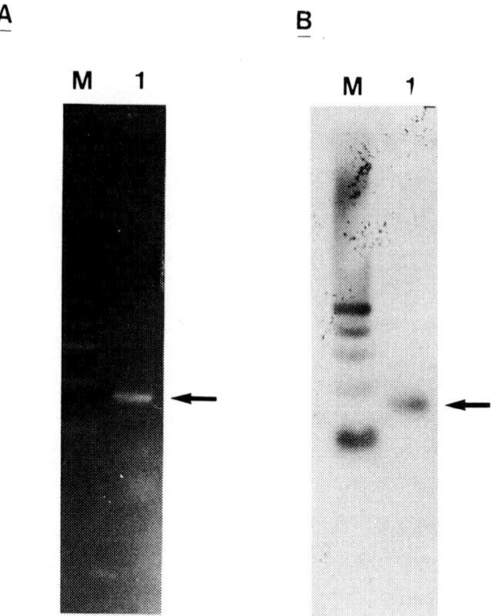


Fig. 3. PCR amplification of a region from the SIV *gag* gene from DNA extracted from the 11/88 pool of $SIV_{mac251}$ (32H isolate). (A) Products from the PCR were analysed by agarose gel electrophoresis, stained with ethidium bromide and photographed under ultraviolet illumination. (B) The DNA shown in panel A was transferred to a nylon membrane and simultaneously probed with a radiolabelled internal SIV *gag* specific oligonucleotide and radiolabelled $\phi$X174/*Hae*III DNA. Lane 1, product from the SIV *gag* PCR. M, $\phi$X174 DNA digested with *Hae*III.

TABLE 2
Summary of $MID_{50}$ determination

| Animal number | Dilution inoculated | Test Positive by Weeks p.i. | | | | CD4/CD8 decrease | Clinical signs |
|---|---|---|---|---|---|---|---|
| | | ELISA | Virus isolation | PCR | Western blotting | | |
| I15 | $10^{-1}$ | 2 | 2 | 2 | 10 | 64%(24) | PGL + LOC |
| I16 | $10^{-1}$ | 2 | 2 | 2 | 8 | 45%(24) | PGL |
| I17 | $10^{-3}$ | 2 | 2 | 2 | 10 | 86%(24) | PGL + LOC |
| I18 | $10^{-3}$ | 4 | 2 | 2 | 6 | 22%(24) | PGL |
| I114 | $10^{-3}$ | 4 | 2 | 2 | 6 | - | L + D |
| I115 | $10^{-3}$ | 4 | 2 | 2 | 8 | - | L + D |
| I116 | $10^{-4}$ | 4 | 2 | 2 | 6 | Slight(6) | L |
| I117 | $10^{-4}$ | 8 | 2 | 2 | −(8) | - | D + LOC |
| I118 | $10^{-4}$ | 4 | 2 | 2 | 8 | - | Healthy |
| I119 | $10^{-4}$ | 4 | 2 | 2 | 6 | - | Healthy |
| I120 | $10^{-5}$ | 4 | 2 | 2 | 8 | - | Healthy |
| I121 | $10^{-5}$ | – | – | – | – | - | Healthy |
| I19 | $10^{-5}$ | – | – | – | – | - | Healthy |
| I20 | $10^{-5}$ | – | – | – | – | - | Healthy |
| I21 | $10^{-7}$ | – | – | – | – | - | Healthy |
| I22 | $10^{-7}$ | – | – | – | – | - | Healthy |
| I23 | $10^{-9}$ | – | – | – | – | - | Healthy |
| I24 | $10^{-9}$ | – | – | – | – | - | Healthy |
| I25 | Medium | – | – | – | – | - | Healthy |
| I26 | Medium | – | – | – | – | - | Healthy |

Numbers in parentheses are weeks p.i.
D: diarrhoea; PGL: persistent generalised lymphadenopathy; LOC: loss of condition; L: lymphadenopathy.
- Normal value.

dilution became infected. None of the other animals that received greater dilutions of virus ($10^{-7}$–$10^{-9}$), nor the controls, became infected by 190 days p.i.

Antibody responses to specific viral proteins were variable, but generally the antibodies to p27 appeared first and were detectable between 28 and 42 days p.i. (Fig. 4). Responses to *env* (gp125, gp32), *pol* (p69) and other *gag* proteins (p18, p59) developed between 70 and 112 days p.i. Antibody responses in three animals (I15, I17 and I117) were poor (see Table 2). The former two animals, in contrast to all others, have shown a persistent decrease in their CD4/CD8 lymphocyte ratio as well as their absolute CD4 positive lymphocyte count (Fig. 5). Monkey number I17 has lost "condition" although it and all other animals remain apparently healthy at this time. The $MID_{50}$ for this isolate is thus $10^{4.75}$ when administered intravenously to cynomolgus macaques.

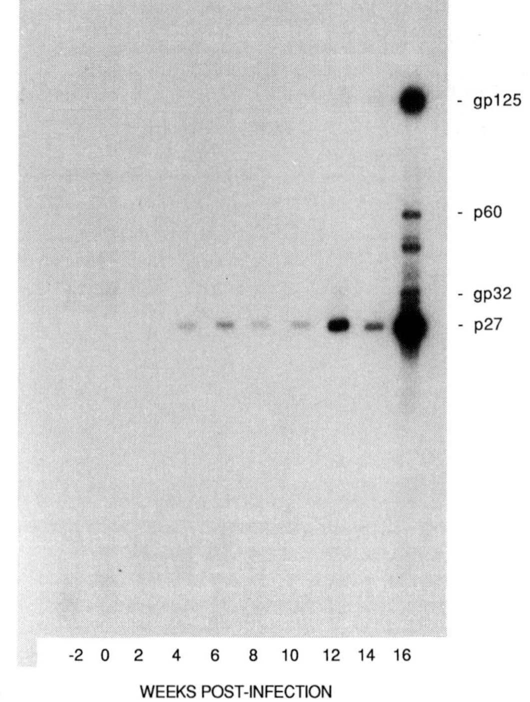


Fig. 4. Immunoblot analyses of antibody responses of cynomolgus macaques infected with the 11/88 pool of $SIV_{mac251}$ (32H isolate). (A) Macaque number I16 which received the $10^{-1}$ dilution of virus. (B) Macaque number I18 which received the $10^{-3}$ dilution of virus.

## Immune responses to SIV antigens

Table 3 presents a summary of the initial antibody responses of cynomolgus macaques to SIV antigens. Animals immunised with glutaraldehyde fixed, SIV-infected C8166 cells (Fig. 6) seroconverted to *env* (gp120 + gp32) and *gag* proteins (p27 and p59) after the first booster injection (Fig. 7). This response had declined at 8 weeks post boost, but 2 weeks later, following a second boost, antibody responses to *env, gag* and *pol* proteins were observed. No responses to cellular proteins were seen. The levels of these antibodies, as judged by ELISA, are about an order of magnitude lower than those produced during an experimental infection (data not shown).

Four macaques (I54–57) were infected with recombinant vaccinia viruses containing the *env* or *gag* and *pol* genes from SIV. These animals developed pustular lesions 15–25 mm in diameter after the first vaccination, slight reddening after the second vaccination and virtually no dermal response to the final dose. No antibodies to SIV were detected by ELISA 28 days after the first dose (Table 3). However, animals I108 and I109 were primed to *env,* since *env* antibodies were detected 4 weeks after a second vaccination with a recombinant carrying the *env* gene. Further analysis of these responses is in progress.

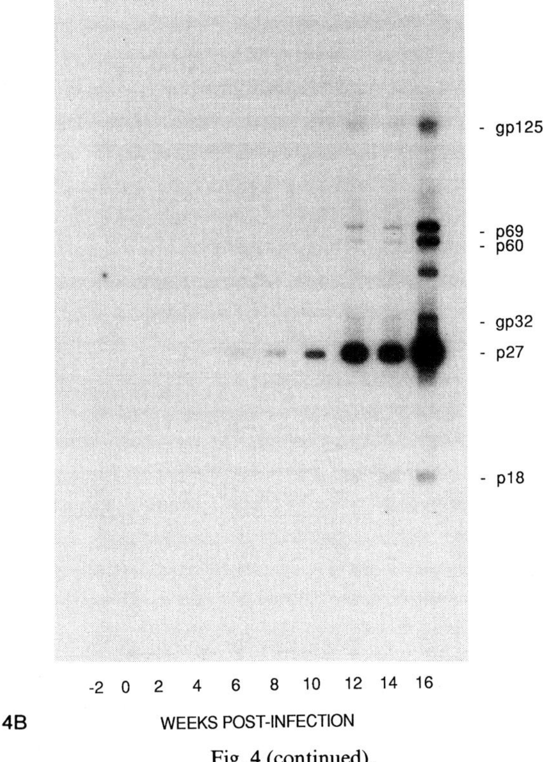


Fig. 4 (continued).

## Discussion

The comparison of six different strains of SIV demonstrated that $SIV_{mac251}$, $SIV_{cyn186}$ and $SIV_{sm7}$ were all capable of infecting cynomolgus macaques (Table

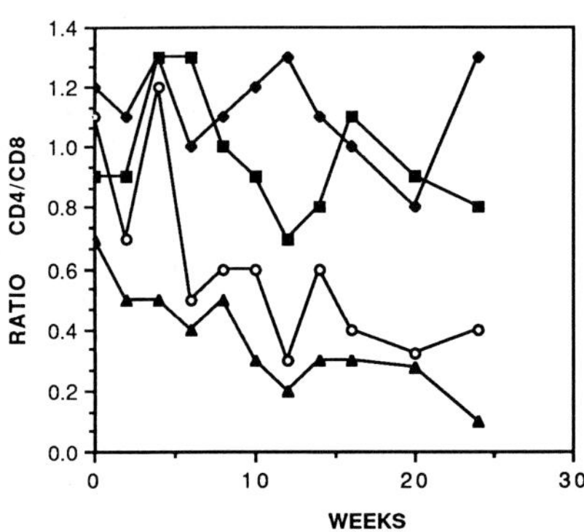


Fig. 5. CD4/CD8 ratio of cynomolgus macaques infected with the 11/88 pool of $SIV_{mac251}$ (32H isolate). I25, ■———■; I26, ◆———◆; I15, ○———○; I17, ▲———▲.

TABLE 3
Immune responses to SIV antigens

| Monkey | Vaccine regime [a] | | | SIV ELISA titer ($\log_{10}$) | | | | Immunoblot | | | |
|---|---|---|---|---|---|---|---|---|---|---|---|
| | D0 | D28 | D56 | D0 | D28 | D56 | D70 | D0 | D28 | D56 | D70 |
| I54 | $2\times10^6$ | $2\times10^6$ | $2\times10^6$ | <1.5 | <1.5 | 2.2 | 2.4 | − | − | + | ++ |
| I55 | cells | cells | cells | <1.5 | <1.5 | 2.1 | 2.8 | − | − | ++ | ++ |
| I56 | with | with | with | <1.5 | <1.5 | 2.0 | 2.3 | − | − | +/− | + |
| I57 | Quil A | Quil A | Quil A | <1.5 | <1.5 | 2.6 | 2.9 | − | − | + | + |
| I106 | SKVV*env* | PJVV*gag* | PJVV*env* | <1.5 | <1.5 | <1.5 | | | | | |
| I107 | | + *pol* | | <1.5 | <1.5 | <1.5 | | | | | |
| I108 | PJVV*env* | SKVV*env* | PJVV*gag* | <1.5 | <1.5 | 2.2 | | | | | |
| I109 | | | + *pol* | <1.5 | <1.5 | 2.4 | | | | | |
| I110 | PJVV*gag* | PJVV*env* | SKVV*env* | <1.5 | <1.5 | <1.5 | | | | | |
| I111 | + *pol* | | | <1.5 | <1.5 | <1.5 | | | | | |

[a] See Materials and methods.
D: days post injection.

1). The cynomolgus macaques have all subsequently died or have developed various symptoms of an AIDS-like disease requiring them to be killed on ethical grounds. However, the macaques are known to have antibodies to type D retroviruses and the role of these endogenous retroviruses in the disease course of experimentally infected macaques remains to be determined.

The difference in the ability of low passage and high passage variants of the $SIV_{mac251}$ isolate to infect cynomolgus macaques is striking (Table 1). The inability of the high passage isolate to infect macaques is probably due to an accumulation of defective and non-pathogenic, tissue culture adapted forms of SIV, during the extended passage in vitro. The accumulation of such defectives has been well documented for HIV-1 (Meyerhans et al., 1989) and there is every reason to believe the same will occur for SIV. The inability of the high passage $SIV_{agm}$ Tyo1 and 2 isolates to infect macaques is probably due to a similar reason.

The authenticity of the $SIV_{mac251}$ (32H isolate) chosen for further study was confirmed by sequence analysis of PCR amplified regions of the *gag* gene (Fig. 3). This isolate proved to be capable of reproducibly infecting cynomolgus macaques and this allowed the determination of an accurate $MID_{50}$. Previous studies of SIV vaccines have indicated that an accurately determined challenge dose may be crucial in identifying potentially protective products (Desrosiers et al., 1989). Evidence for infection can be reproducibly obtained by 2 weeks p.i. in all cases (Table 2). This allows the model to be used to assess the potency of vaccine and chemotherapeutic regimes against SIV infection. To date, only one animal has shown signs of disease (I17). Consequently, it is still too early to obtain a clear indication of the time course of progression from infection to disease in these animals.

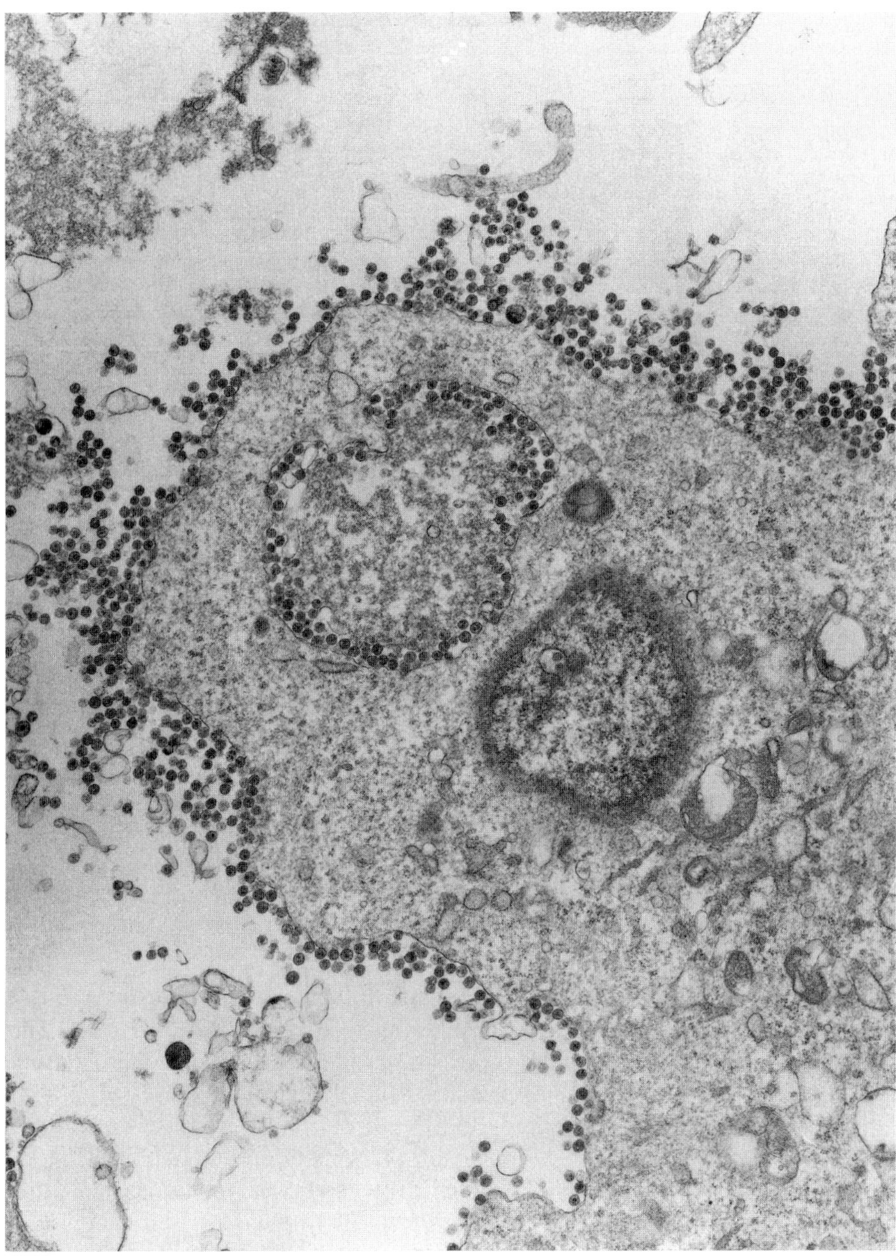

Fig. 6. Electron micrograph of fixed, whole C8166 cells infected with $SIV_{mac251}$ (32H isolate). Magnification $\times$16,000.

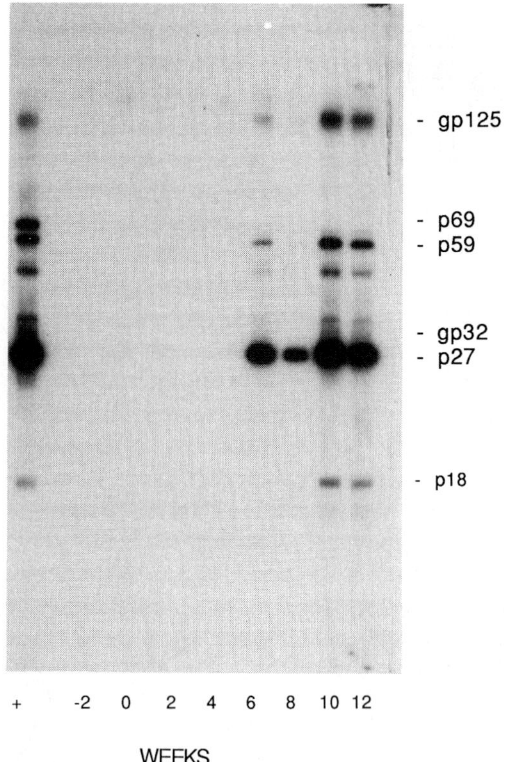


Fig. 7. Immunoblot analysis of the antibody response of a cynomolgus macaque (I55) injected with a preparation of fixed, whole C8166 cells infected with $SIV_{mac251}$ (32H isolate).

The initial studies on the immune responses of cynomolgus macaques to SIV antigens were based on the use of whole, inactivated, SIV-infected cells. This approach has previously been used successfully with other enveloped viruses such as Marek's disease virus and respiratory syncytial virus (Stott et al., 1984). Although only low levels of antibody to SIV were detected by ELISA (Table 3), they reacted strongly with the *env* and *gag* proteins in an immunoblot (Fig. 7). Challenge studies will indicate whether protection can be induced by this approach.

The initial antibody responses to recombinant vaccinia viruses were disappointing. However, it is clear that a primary vaccination does not totally prevent the replication of virus given subsequently. Thus, repeated doses of recombinant viruses may enhance the response to the inserted gene. It is also possible that the parent viruses used to produce the recombinants are not the most appropriate for use in cynomolgus monkeys.

### Acknowledgements

We are grateful to Drs R. Desrosiers, P. Fultz, M. Hayami, W. Haseltine, P. Johnson and C. Thiriart, for the generous gifts of viruses. We would like to acknowledge the technical assistance of Ms L. McAlpine and Mr M. Macartney. Thanks are also due to Mr A. Davis and Miss S. Prime for preparation of the manuscript.

This work is supported in part by grants from the MRC AIDS Directed Programme and the European Community.

### References

Desrosiers, R.C., Wyand, M.S., Kodama, T., Ringler, D.J., Arthur, L.O., Sehgal, P.K., Letvin, N.L., King, N.W. and Daniel, M.D. (1989) Vaccine protection against simian immunodeficiency virus infection. *Proc. Natl. Acad. Sci. U.S.A.* 86, 6353–6357.

Fultz, P., McClure, H., Anderson, D., Swenson, R., Anand, R. and Srinivasan, A. (1986) Isolation of a T-lymphocyte retrovirus from naturally infected sooty mangabey monkeys *(Cercocebus atys). Proc. Natl. Acad. Sci U.S.A.* 83, 5286–5290.

Grief, C., Hockley, D.J., Fromholc, C.E. and Kitchin, P.A. (1989) The morphology of simian immunodeficiency virus as shown by negative staining electron microscopy. *J. Gen. Virol.* 70, 2215–2219.

Kannagi, M., Kiyotaki, M., Desrosiers, R.C., Reimann, K.A., King, N.W., Waldron, L.M. and Letvin, N.L. (1986) Humoral immune responses to T-cell tropic retrovirus simian T-lymphotropic virus type III in monkeys with experimentally induced acquired immune deficiency-like syndrome. *J. Clin. Invest.* 78, 1229–1236.

Kitchin, P.A., Almond, N., Szotyori, Z., Fromholc, C.E., McAlpine, L., Silvera, P., Stott, E.J., Cranage, M., Baskerville, A. and Schild, G. (1990) The use of the polymerase chain reaction for the detection of simian immunodeficiency virus in experimentally infected macaques. *J. Virol. Methods* 28, 85–100.

Meyerhans, A., Cheynier, R., Albert, J., Seth, M., Kwok, S., Sninsky, J., Morfeldt-Manson, L., Asjo, B. and Wain-Hobson, S. (1989) Temporal fluctuations in HIV quasispecies in vivo are not reflected by sequential HIV isolations. *Cell* 58, 901–910.

Murphey-Corb, M., Martin, L.N., Rangan, S.R.S., Baskin, G.B., Gormus, B.J., Wolf, R.H., Andes, W.A., West, M. and Moantelaro, R.C. (1986) Isolation of an HTLV-III related retrovirus from macaques with simian AIDS and its possible origin in asymptomatic mangabeys. *Nature* 321, 248–250.

Stott, E.J., Thomas. L.H., Taylor, G., Collins, A.P., Jebbett, J. and Crouch, S. (1984) A comparison of three vaccines against respiratory syncytia virus in calves. *J. Hygiene* 93, 251–261.

Thorpe, R., Brasher, M.D.R., Bird, C.R., Garrett, A.J., Jacobs, J.P., Minor, P.D. and Schild, G.C. (1987) An improved immunoblotting procedure for the detection of antibodies against HIV. *J. Virol. Methods* 16, 87–96.

*Eds. H. Schellekens and M.C. Horzinek*
*Animal Models in AIDS*



# 14

# Potent anti-simian immunodeficiency virus (SIV) activity and pharmacokinetics of 9-(2-phosphonylmethoxyethyl)adenine (PMEA) in rhesus monkeys

J. BALZARINI [1], L. NAESENS [1], J. SLACHMUYLDERS [2], H. NIPHUIS [2], I. ROSENBERG [3], A. HOLY [3], H. SCHELLEKENS [2] and E. DE CLERCQ [1]

[1] Rega Institute for Medical Research, Katholieke Universiteit Leuven, B-3000 Leuven, Belgium, [2] TNO Primate Center, 2280 HV Rijswijk, The Netherlands and [3] Institute of Organic Chemistry and Biochemistry, Czechoslovak Academy of Sciences, 16610 Prague, Czechoslovakia

**Summary**

9-(2-Phosphonylmethoxyethyl)adenine (PMEA) is a potent and selective inhibitor of the in vitro replication of a number of retroviruses, including human immunodeficiency virus (HIV) type 1 and type 2, simian immunodeficiency virus (SIV), simian AIDS-related virus (SRV) and Moloney murine sarcoma virus (MSV). At a dose of 20 or 10 mg/kg/day, PMEA causes a marked suppression of the induction of anti-$SIV_{MAC}$ gp120 antibodies in $SIV_{MAC}$-infected rhesus monkeys. No marked toxic side effects were noted following a PMEA treatment period of 30 days. Our data suggest that PMEA should be pursued for its potential in the treatment of AIDS and other retrovirus infections.

## Introduction

At present, only 3′-azido-2′,3′-dideoxythymidine (AZT, zidovudine), which has proved to prolong survival of patients with advanced AIDS (Yarchoan et al., 1986, 1987; Fischl et al., 1987), has been officially licensed for the treatment of human immunodeficiency virus (HIV) infection. The principal toxicity associated with the administration of AZT is bone marrow suppression (Richman et al., 1987). 2′,3′-Dideoxycytidine (ddCyd) has also shown benefit in AIDS patients, but this compound causes severe peripheral neuropathy as a major toxic side effect (Yarchoan et al., 1988). Clearly, novel anti-HIV drugs are needed that are less toxic than AZT or ddCyd.

Recently, we described a new group of acyclic nucleoside phosphonate derivatives (De Clercq et al., 1986), of which several congeners were found to selectively

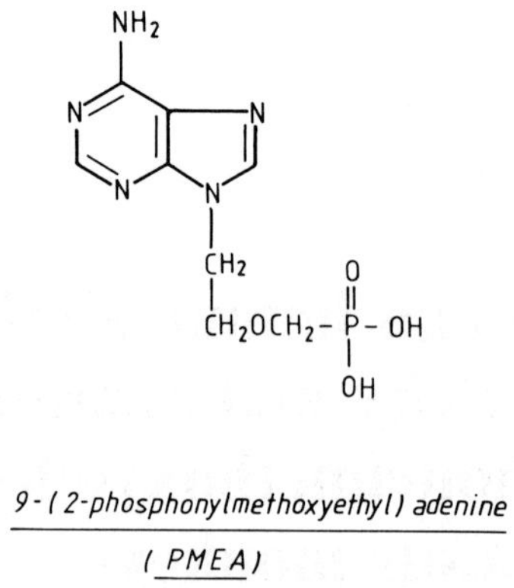

*9-(2-phosphonylmethoxyethyl) adenine*

*(PMEA)*

Fig. 1. Structural formula of 9-(2-phosphonylmethoxyethyl)adenine (PMEA).

inhibit HIV replication in vitro (Pauwels et al., 1988). The prototype compound, 9-(2-phosphonylmethoxyethyl)adenine (PMEA), inhibits HIV-induced cytopathogenicity in MT-4 cells (Pauwels et al., 1988; Balzarini et al., 1989a) and is also effective in inhibiting Moloney murine sarcoma virus (MSV)-induced transformation of murine C3H/3T3 embryo fibroblasts (Pauwels et al., 1988; Balzarini et al., 1989a). PMEA causes a dose-dependent suppression of tumor formation and associated mortality in MSV-infected newborn NMRI mice (Balzarini et al., 1989a). In this respect, PMEA is 25-fold more potent as an anti-retrovirus agent than AZT (Balzarini et al., 1989a). We have now evaluated the effectiveness of PMEA against a number of retroviruses in vitro, including the lentiviruses HIV-1, HIV-2 and $SIV_{MAC}$, and the simian AIDS-related virus (SRV). We also evaluated the effect of PMEA on simian immunodeficiency virus infection in rhesus monkeys.

## Materials and methods

### Compound

PMEA was synthesized according to a previously published procedure (Holý and Rosenberg, 1987).

### Antiviral assays

The methodology of the anti-HIV-1 assays has been described previously (Balzarini et al., 1987, 1988; Mitsuya et al., 1985) and is based on the examination of the protective activity of PMEA against HIV-1-induced cytopathogenicity in MT-4 cells. Anti-HIV-2 and -SIV assays in MT-4 cells were performed according to the same methodology. The 50% effective dose ($ED_{50}$) and 50% cytotoxic (cytostatic) dose ($CD_{50}$) were defined as the compound concentrations required to reduce by 50% the number of viable cells in the virus-infected and mock-infected cell cultures, respectively.

Infection of Raji cells with SRV was carried out according to a previously published procedure (Balzarini et al., 1989b). The total number of SRV-induced giant cells present in the infected cell cultures was estimated on day 12 of the experiment and the $ED_{50}$ of the test compounds was defined as the compound concentration that caused a 50% reduction in the number of giant cells.

CEM cells were suspended at 250,000 cells/ml culture medium and infected with HIV-1 or HIV-2 at 5 $CCID_{50}$/ml and 500 $CCID_{50}$/ml, respectively. Then, 100 $\mu$l of the infected cell suspension was added to 200-$\mu$l microtiter plate wells, containing 100 $\mu$l of an appropriate dilution of the test compound. After 4 days incubation at 37°C, cell cultures were examined for giant cell formation.

C3H/3T3 cells were seeded at 20,000 cells/ml into wells of Tissue Culture Cluster Plates (48 wells/plate). Following a 24-h incubation period, cell cultures were infected with 80 focus-forming units of MSV during 120 min, after which the culture medium was replaced by 1 ml fresh medium containing appropriate concentrations of the test compound. After 6 days, transformation of the cells was examined microscopically.

## Determination of the cytostatic effect of PMEA

The cytostatic effect of PMEA was assessed by measuring the inhibition of cell proliferation on day 3 after the addition of the compound to the cells. The number of viable cells was counted on day 7 (ATH8 cells) or day 5 (MT-4 cells). Selectivity index is expressed as the ratio 50% cytostatic dose to 50% effective dose.

## Pharmacokinetics of PMEA

The rhesus monkeys 2BJ and 1WW used in the experiments weighed 3.1 and 2.8 kg, respectively. PMEA in phosphate-buffered saline (PBS) at 250 mg/ml was administered as an intravenous (i.v.) bolus injection at a dose of 250 mg/kg *via* the saphenous vein. Blood was collected from the iliac vein. PMEA plasma levels were determined by high-performance liquid chromatography (HPLC), using an anion exchange Partisil SAX-10 column (particle size 10 $\mu$m) (Whatman, Chemical Separation Inc., Clifton, NJ, U.S.A.).

Plasma concentrations of PMEA as a function of time were fitted to a bi-exponential equation ($C_t = A_e^{-\alpha t} + B_e^{-\beta t}$) (two-compartment model). Pharmacokinetic parameters were then calculated by standard methods. The plasma area under the curve (AUC) was determined by the linear trapezoidal rule including all samples from 0 to 7 h after i.v. administration. The terminal elimination half-life in plasma was obtained by calculating the elimination constant, $k_e$, from the formula $C_t = C_o \cdot e^{-k_e t}$ and using the equation $t_{1/2} = 0.693/k_e$. The total body clearance ($Cl_{tot}$) was calculated from the relationship

$Cl_{tot}$ = Dose/AUC. The distribution volume $V_d$ was calculated from the formula $V_d$ = Dose/$C_o$.

### Tissue distribution of PMEA

A rhesus monkey (designated KX), weighing 6.6 kg, was given an i.v. bolus injection of 1 g PMEA per kg. PMEA was injected as a solution in 5% glucose (20 ml) in the left leg. The monkey was killed at 5.5 h post injection; specimens of organs and tissues were removed and immediately frozen at −80°C. The amounts of PMEA in the different organs and tissues were determined by HPLC.

## Results and discussion

### In vitro anti-retrovirus effect of PMEA

In all in vitro systems, PMEA showed a marked anti-retrovirus activity (Table 1). The 50% effective doses of PMEA for HIV-1-, HIV-2- and $SIV_{MAC}$-induced cytopathogenicity in MT-4 cells and HIV-1- and HIV-2-induced giant cell formation in CEM cells ranged from 7.0 to 17 μM. PMEA also exerted a potent inhibitory effect on SRV-induced giant cell formation in Raji cells, as well as

TABLE 1
Antiretroviral activity of PMEA in vitro

| Retrovirus system | $ED_{50}$ (μM) | $CD_{50}$ (μM) | Selectivity index [a] |
|---|---|---|---|
| HIV-1-induced cytopathogenicity in | | | |
| ATH8 cells | 2.5 | 80 | 32 |
| MT-4 cells | 7.0 | 144 | 21 |
| HIV-1-induced giant cell formation in | | | |
| CEM cells | 7.0 | 69 | 10 |
| HIV-1 antigen expression in | | | |
| MT-4 cells | 1.6 | 144 | 90 |
| H9 cells | 0.4 | 81 | 203 |
| HIV-2-induced cytopathogenicity in | | | |
| MT-4 cells | 7.5 | 144 | 19.7 |
| HIV-2-induced giant cell formation in | | | |
| CEM cells | 10 | 69 | 7 |
| $SIV_{MAC}$-induced giant cell formation in | | | |
| HUT-78 cells | 4 | 103 | 26 |
| $SIV_{MAC}$-induced cytopathogenicity in | | | |
| MT-4 cells | 17 | 144 | 8.5 |
| SRV-induced giant cell formation in | | | |
| Raji cells | 0.7 | 32 | 46 |
| MSV-induced transformation of | | | |
| murine C3H/3T3 cells | 2.2 | > 40 | > 15 |

[a] Selectivity index or ratio of $CD_{50}$ to $ED_{50}$.

Moloney murine sarcoma virus (MSV)-induced transformation of murine C3H/3T3 embryo fibroblasts ($ED_{50}$: $\pm 1$ $\mu$M). Thus, in vitro PMEA proved effective against a wide variety of retroviruses, i.e., HIV-1, HIV-2, SRV and MSV, irrespective of the choice of the assay system or cell line.

## In vivo anti-retrovirus effect of PMEA

Eight rhesus monkeys were included in the in vivo study. Four monkeys were inoculated with a molecular clone of $SIV_{MAC}$ (designated $SIV_{BK28}$), and the course of the virus infection was followed for 180 days after virus inoculation by determining the titer of anti-SIV gp120 antibodies. Under parallel conditions, two sets of 2 $SIV_{MAC}$-infected monkeys were treated daily intramuscularly with PMEA at $2 \times 5$ or $2 \times 10$ mg/kg for 29 consecutive days, starting 1 day before virus inoculation.

Treatment of $SIV_{MAC}$-infected rhesus monkeys with PMEA at $2 \times 5$ or $2 \times 10$ mg/kg/day significantly delayed the appearance of anti-SIV gp120 antibodies in the serum. In fact, at both PMEA doses no antibodies against $SIV_{MAC}$ gp120 could be detected during the PMEA treatment period (day 0–29) (Fig. 2). In control animals, however, anti-SIV gp120 antibodies appeared as early as 15–29 days after virus infection, and the titer of anti-SIV gp120 antibodies increased progressively with time (Fig. 2). In the PMEA-treated animals, the antibody response to SIV gp120 did not occur until 35–42 days post infection. Moreover, the higher the PMEA dose, the later the anti-SIV gp120 antibody appeared. Virus replication must have been completely suppressed since no anti-SIV gp120 antibody could be detected during the whole treatment period (29 days). Thus, PMEA achieved a dose-dependent inhibition of SIV replication as evidenced by the delay in the appearance of anti-SIV gp120 antibodies as well as the slower rise in antibody titer (Fig. 2). Our results indicate that PMEA may prevent retrovirus replication in vivo, if administered immediately before and/or after virus exposure. Although a 1-month treatment regimen with PMEA starting immediately before virus inoculation completely suppressed SIV replication, it did not totally eradicate the infection. It is possible that with prolonged PMEA treatment, virus replication may remain suppressed.

## Pharmacokinetics of PMEA in rhesus monkeys

The PMEA plasma concentrations following a single i.v. bolus injection of PMEA (250 mg/kg) in rhesus monkeys are shown in Fig. 3. Mean plasma drug levels ranged from 633–850 $\mu$g/ml ($\pm$2.7 mM) at 3 min to about 1.7–5.2 $\mu$g/ml ($\pm$13 $\mu$M) at 7 h. The $\beta$-phase half-life $t_{1/2}$ was 120 min. A total body clearance of 1594 (ml/h)/kg was calculated from the AUC (535 ($\mu$g/ml)/h) (average values for two monkeys) (Table 2). The pharmacokinetic parameters following i.v. administration of PMEA are presented in Table 2. Thus, the major features of PMEA disposition in rhesus monkeys are: a relatively short plasma half-life ($\pm$2 h), yet longer than that observed for AZT in man ($1.55 \pm 0.35$ h) (Klecker et al.,

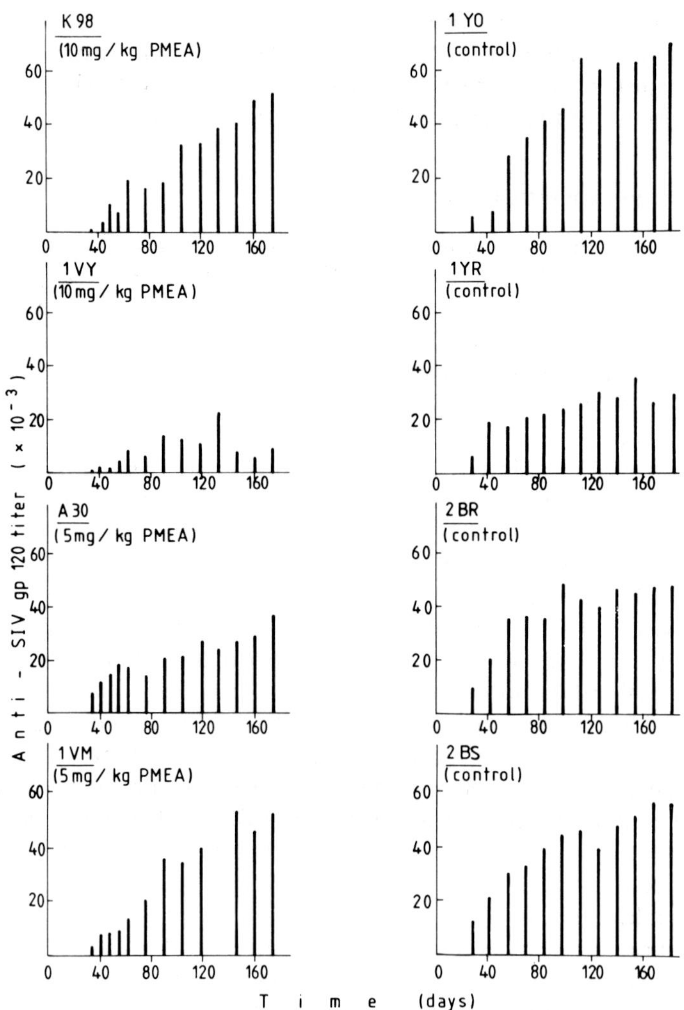


Fig. 2. Anti-SIV gp120 antibody titers in rhesus monkeys infected with $SIV_{MAC}$, and not treated with PMEA (monkeys 1YO, 1YR, 2BR and 2BS), treated intramuscularly with PMEA at 5 mg/kg twice a day (monkeys A30 and 1VM), or treated intramuscularly with PMEA at 10 mg/kg twice a day (monkeys K98 and 1VY). The reciprocal dilution of the serum concentration corresponding to the anti-SIV gp120 titer is plotted as a function of time.

1987); and a plasma clearance of 1.59 l/kg/h, which is similar to that observed for AZT in man (1.3 l/kg/h) (Klecker et al., 1987).

## Tissue distribution of PMEA

Various organs and tissues of a rhesus monkey were examined for the presence of PMEA after an i.v. bolus injection of 1000 mg/kg. The monkey was killed 5.5

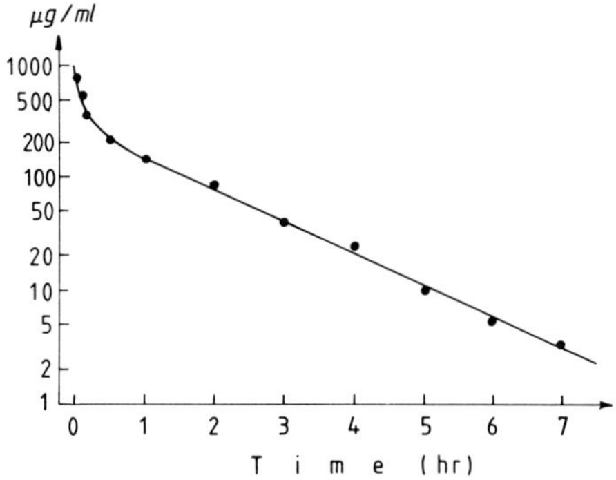


Fig. 3. Plasma concentrations of PMEA following i.v. administration of PMEA at 250 mg/kg. The data correspond to the mean values obtained for two rhesus monkeys (1WW and 2BJ).

TABLE 2
Pharmacokinetic parameters following administration of PMEA to rhesus monkeys

| Monkey | Total dose (mg) | Concentration range in plasma (μg/ml) | $t_{1/2}$ (h) | AUC ((μg/ml)×h) | $Cl_{tot}$ ((ml/h)/kg) | Distribution volume (ml) |
|---|---|---|---|---|---|---|
| 2BJ | 770 | 633 − 1.74 | 3.07 | 314 | 2253 | 9994 |
| 1WW | 700 | 850 − 5.24 | 1.09 | 756 | 935 | 1471 |

h after administration of the drug. The highest drug content was found in the kidney (1.68 g/kg), followed by the liver (0.95 g/kg), prostate (0.75 g/kg) and lung (0.53 g/kg). Low but significant levels of PMEA were detected in the brain (cerebrum and cerebellum) suggesting that PMEA is able to cross the blood-brain barrier, albeit relatively poorly.

## Conclusion

PMEA is a potent broad-spectrum anti-retrovirus (i.e., HIV-1, HIV-2, SIV, SRV, MSV) agent in vitro. It is clearly superior to AZT in inhibiting MSV-induced disease in mice (Balzarini et al., 1989a). We have now demonstrated that PMEA also exerts a significant antiviral effect in SIV-infected rhesus monkeys. This is the first demonstration of anti-retroviral efficacy of a potential anti-AIDS drug in a retrovirus model that is very close to and representative of the human situation. From our studies, PMEA emerged as a compound that should be able to prevent HIV infection in humans.

## References

Balzarini, J., Cooney, D.A., Dalal, M., Kang, G.-J., Cupp, J.E., De Clercq, E., Broder, S. and Johns, D.G. (1987) 2′,3′-Dideoxycytidine: regulation of its metabolism and anti-retroviral potency by natural pyrimidine nucleosides and by inhibitors of pyrimidine nucleotide synthesis. *Mol. Pharmacol.* 32, 798–806.

Balzarini, J., Baba, M., Pauwels, R., Herdewijn, P. and De Clercq, E. (1988) Anti-retrovirus activity of 3′-fluoro- and 3′-azido-substituted pyrimidine 2′,3′-dideoxynucleoside analogues. *Biochem. Pharmacol.* 37, 2847–2856.

Balzarini, J., Naesens, L., Herdewijn, P., Rosenberg, I., Holý, A., Pauwels, R., Baba, M., Johns, D.G. and De Clercq, E. (1989a) Marked in vivo antiretrovirus activity of 9-(2-phosphonylmethoxyethyl)adenine, a selective anti-human immunodeficiency virus agent. *Proc. Natl. Acad. Sci. U.S.A.* 86, 332–336.

Balzarini, J., Van Aerschot, A., Herdewijn, P. and De Clercq, E. (1989b) 5-Chloro-substituted derivatives of 2′,3′-didehydro-2′,3′-dideoxyuridine, 3′-fluoro-2′,3′-dideoxyuridine and 3′-azido-2′,3′-dideoxyuridine as anti-HIV agents. *Biochem. Pharmacol.* 38, 869–874.

De Clercq, E., Holý, A., Rosenberg, I., Sakuma, T., Balzarini, J. and Maudgal, P.C. (1986) A novel selective broad-spectrum anti-DNA virus agent. *Nature* 323, 464–467.

Fischl, M.A., Richman, D.D., Grieco, M.H., Gottlieb, M.S., Volberding, P.A., Laskin, O.L., Leedom, J.M., Groopman, J.E., Mildvan, D., Schooley, R.T., Jackson, G.G., Durack, D.T., Phil, D., King, D. and The AZT Collaborative Working Group (1987) The efficacy of azidothymidine (AZT) in the treatment of patients with AIDS and AIDS-related complex. *N. Engl. J. Med.* 317, 185–191.

Holý, A. and Rosenberg, I. (1987) Synthesis of 9-(2-phosphonylmethoxyethyl)adenine and related compounds. *Collect. Czech. Chem. Commun.* 52, 2801–2809.

Klecker, R.W., Collins, J.M., Yarchoan, R., Thomas, R. and Jenkins, J.F. (1987) Plasma and cerebrospinal fluid pharmacokinetics of 3′-azido-3′-deoxythymidine: a novel pyrimidine analog with potential application for the treatment of patients with AIDS and related diseases. *Clin. Pharmacol. Ther.* 41, 407–412.

Mitsuya, H., Weinhold, K.J., Furman, P.A., St. Clair, M.H., Nusinoff-Lehrman, S., Gallo, R.C., Bolognesi, D., Barry, D.W. and Broder, S. (1985) 3′-Azido-3′-deoxythymidine (BW A509U): an antiviral agent that inhibits the infectivity and cytopathic effect of human T-lymphotropic virus type III/lymphadenopathy-associated virus in vitro. *Proc. Natl. Acad. Sci. U.S.A.* 82, 7096–7100.

Pauwels, R., Balzarini, J., Schols, D., Baba, M., Desmyter, J., Rosenberg, I., Holý, A. and De Clercq, E. (1988) Phosphonylmethoxyethyl purine derivatives, a new class of anti-human immunodeficiency virus agents. *Antimicrob. Agents Chemother.* 32, 1025–1030.

Richman, D.D., Fischl, M.A., Grieco, M.H., Gottlieb, M.S., Volberding, P.A., Laskin, O.L., Leedom, J.M., Groopman, J.E., Mildvan, D., Hirsch, M.S., Jackson, G.G., Durack, D.T., Nusinoff-Lehrman, S. and The AZT Collaborative Working Group (1987) The toxicity of azidothymidine (AZT) in the treatment of patients with AIDS and AIDS-related complex. *N. Engl. J. Med.* 317, 192–197.

Yarchoan, R., Klecker, R.W., Weinhold, K.J., Markham, P.D., Lyerly, H.K., Durack, D.T., Gelmann, E., Nusinoff-Lehrman, S., Blum, R.M., Barry, D.W., Shearer, G.M., Fischl, M.A., Mitsuya, H., Gallo, R.C., Collins, J.M., Bolognesi, D.P., Myers, C.E. and Broder, S. (1986) Administration of 3′-azido-3′-deoxythymidine, an inhibitor of HTLV-III/LAV replication, to patients with AIDS or AIDS-related complex. *Lancet* i, 575–580.

Yarchoan, R., Berg, G., Brouwers, P., Fischl, M.A., Spitzer, A.R., Wichman, A., Grafman, J., Thomas, R.V., Safai, B., Brunetti, A., Perno, C.F., Schmidt, P.J., Larson, S.M., Myers, C.E. and Broder, S. (1987) Response of human-immunodeficiency-virus-associated neurological disease to 3′-azido-3′-deoxythymidine. *Lancet* i, 132–135.

Yarchoan, R., Perno, C.F., Thomas, R.V., Klecker, R.W., Allain, J.-P., Wills, R.J., McAtee, N., Fischl, M.A., Dubinsky, R., McNeely, M.C., Mitsuya, H., Pluda, J.M., Lawley, T.J., Leuther, M., Safai, B., Collins, J.M., Myers, C.E. and Broder, S. (1988) Phase I studies of 2′,3′-dideoxycytidine in severe human immunodeficiency virus infection as a single agent and alternating with zidovudine (AZT). *Lancet* i, 76–81.

*Eds. H. Schellekens and M.C. Horzinek*
*Animal Models in AIDS*



# 15

# Immunobiology of SIV in rhesus macaques

THOMAS P. McGRAW [1], BENJAMIN R. VOWELS [1], MURRAY B. GARDNER [1] and M. ERIC GERSHWIN [2]

[1] Department of Medical Pathology and [2] Department of Internal Medicine, Division of Rheumatology/Allergy/Clinical Immunology, University of California, Davis, CA 95616, U.S.A.

## Introduction

The relentless spread of AIDS since its initial recognition has mandated studies of animal models of lentivirus infection in an effort to gain an understanding of the natural history and immunobiology of human immunodeficiency virus (HIV) infection in humans.

Following infection with a viral pathogen, a complex series of cellular interactions occur resulting in an immune response which should control the spread of the agent and induce resistance to further challenges. Viral antigens are expressed on the cell surface in association with major histocompatibility complex (MHC) gene products where they can be recognized by T cells bearing antigen specific receptors (Davis and Bjorkman, 1988). The generation of a specific immune response requires processing of viral antigens presented in association with MHC class II determinants on the surface of antigen presenting cells (APC) to CD4+ helper T cells (Berzofsky, 1988; Unanue and Allen, 1987) and the production of the cytokine interleukin-1 (IL-1) by the APC (Unanue and Allen, 1987). This results in the activation of virus-specific CD4+ cells, as evidenced by their proliferation and production of lymphokines including IL-2 (Kishimoto, 1985; Takatsu et al., 1987), which mediate activation and differentiation of many other cells involved in the immune response. The activation of virus-specific CD4+ cells results in the differentiation of CD4+ T cells into effectors mediating delayed-type hypersensitivity (Mosmann and Coffman, 1989), CD8+ T cells into cytotoxic T lymphocytes (CTL) or suppressor T cells (Mosmann and Coffman, 1989), and the activation of monocytes/macrophages (Kelso and Glasebrook, 1984). In contrast to class II MHC restriction requirements of CD4+ helper T cells, the generation of CD8+ CTL from precursors requires recognition of viral antigen in association with class I MHC determinants (Berzofsky, 1988) and appropriate CD4+ helper T cell soluble mediators (Mosmann and Coffman,

1989; Takatsu et al., 1987). Infected target cell recognition and CTL effector function occur in the same context (Berzofsky, 1988). The important role that CTL play in anti-viral immunity has been firmly established by adoptive transfer experiments using CTL lines or clones.

The ultimate goal of these investigations is to develop the means to control and prevent AIDS. Historically vaccines are the safest, easiest, most economical, and most effective means of preventing infectious disease. Therefore, this investigation focused on establishing methods to assess both proliferative and cytotoxic T cell responses of simian immunodeficiency virus (SIV)-infected rhesus macaques. Future investigations will use the methods described in this communication to define the immunodominant T cell epitopes of SIV since they will undoubtedly be the foundation for a successful lentivirus vaccine.

## Materials and methods

### Animals

Eight healthy juvenile (< 2.5 years) rhesus macaques (*Macaca mulatta*) (six males and two females) that were seronegative for $SIV_{mac}$, simian type D retrovirus (SRV), and simian T-leukemia virus-I (STLV-1) by Western blot analysis (Damato et al., 1988) were selected for these studies. Animal husbandry practices and procedures at the California Primate Research Center allowed for definitive identification of both sire and dam of the animals used in these studies. All animals were maintained in accordance with recommendations of the Committee on the Care and Use of Laboratory Animals, National Research Council and the Guide for Care and Use of Laboratory Animals, Health and Human Services.

### Experimental protocol

Four animals (23099, 23476, 23838, 23866) were infected i.v. with 1 ml of $SIV_{mac}$ which had a titer of $10^{-1.7}$ $TCID_{50}$ and four animals were used as uninfected controls. This dose has been demonstrated to be uniformly effective in causing clinical disease at the California Primate Research Center. Each animal was tested monthly over the course of this study.

### $SIV_{mac}$ production and isolation

$SIV_{mac}$ was produced in the HUT78 cell line and isolated as previously described (McGraw et al., 1990). Western blot analysis, as described below, confirmed that virus purified by this method retained all major proteins. The protein content of the band was assessed using the BCA protein analysis kit (Pierce Chem., Rockford, IL). Virus (100 $\mu$g) was inactivated by incubation at 56°C for 1 h prior to assay.

### Western blot and viral culture

Western blot analysis was performed according to the method of Damato (1988). Viremia was demonstrated by incubating $3 \times 10^6$ peripheral blood mononuclear cells (PBMC), from infected animals or uninfected controls, with 1.5 $\mu$g of staphylococcal enterotoxin A (SEA, Toxin Technology, Madison, WI) for a period of 72 h. PBMC were then co-cultivated with HUT78 cells and examined for syncytia formation and reverse transcriptase activity every 3 days for 6 weeks.

### Simian leukocytes

Monkeys were anesthetized with ketamine on the day of assay and peripheral blood collected in heparinized tubes. Plasma was removed after centrifugation. The buffy coat was collected, diluted 1:3 with phosphate-buffered saline (PBS), pH 7.2, and layered on a Ficoll-Hypaque gradient (Lymphocyte Separation Media (LSM), Organon-Teknica, Durham, NC). The gradient was centrifuged at $800 \times g$ for 30 min at room temperature and the PBMC band collected and washed twice in PBS. Prior to the assay, cells were separated into T and non-T cells by rosetting PBMC with 2-aminoethyl-isothiouronium bromide (AET, Sigma Chemical, St. Louis, MO)-treated sheep red blood cells (SRBC, Colorado Serum Co., Denver, CO) (Kaplan and Clark, 1974).

### CTL assay

Assays for CTL were performed as previously described (Vowels et al., 1989).

### T cell proliferation assay

Assays for T cell proliferation were performed as previously described (McGraw et al., 1990).

### Characterization of antigen presenting cells

Adherent cells were removed by incubation on polystyrene tissue culture flasks. Following incubation in RPMI 1640 (JR Scientific, Woodland, CA) + 10% fetal calf serum (Hyclone Laboratories, Logan, UT) for 60 min at 37°C, non-adherent cells were removed by aspiration. The adherent cell populations were washed thoroughly prior to their removal from the flask by incubating at 4°C in the presence of divalent cation-free PBS.

### Monoclonal antibodies (mAb)

The reagents used in phenotyping were monoclonal anti-CD4 (Leu 3a), anti-CD8 (Leu 2a), anti-CD14 (Leu M3), anti-CD16 (Leu 11a), anti-CD20 (Leu 16) (Becton-Dickinson (BD), Mountain View, CA) and goat anti-monkey surface immunoglobulin (GAM-sIg) (Tago, Burlingame, CA). Anti-MHC class II mAb (anti-DR, BD) and anti-MHC class I mAb (anti-HLA A, B, C, clone W6/32, Dako Industries, Carpinteria, CA) were used in MHC blocking experiments. For T cell subset depletion, OKT4 (ATCC, Rockville, MD) and OKT8 (ATCC) were used. Anti-CD16 (Leu 11b, BD) was used in NK cell depletion experiments.

### T cell subset depletion

T cells were depleted by treatment with mAb + C as previously described (Vowels et al., 1989).

### MHC blocking of target cells

Immediately following $^{51}$Cr and SIV labeling, target cells were incubated with a predetermined optimal concentration of anti-MHC class I or class II mAb for 30 min at 37°C. Target cells were washed once in culture medium prior to assay.

### Characterization of target cells

Immediately following $^{51}$Cr and prior to SIV pulsing, target cells were incubated with a predetermined optimal concentration of anti-CD4 (Leu 3a or OKT4) mAb for 30 min at 37°C. Target cells were washed once in culture medium and then pulsed with SIV prior to assay.

### Statistics

The data were analyzed using a paired sample, two-tailed $t$ test for determination of $P$ values.

## Results

### Clinical and serological findings

Sera and PBMC from the four rhesus macaques that were experimentally infected with $SIV_{mac}$ were analyzed for antibody reactivity and for the presence of virus as outlined in the Materials and methods section. All four infected macaques were seropositive by Western blot analysis and SIV-infected by virus culture (data not shown) whereas all four uninfected animals were seronegative and virus culture negative. Virus cultures remained positive throughout the course of this study.

### CTL response of SIV-infected rhesus macaques

T cells from infected animals demonstrated consistent levels of significant CTL activity against $SIV_{mac}$-pulsed, MHC compatible target cells over the course

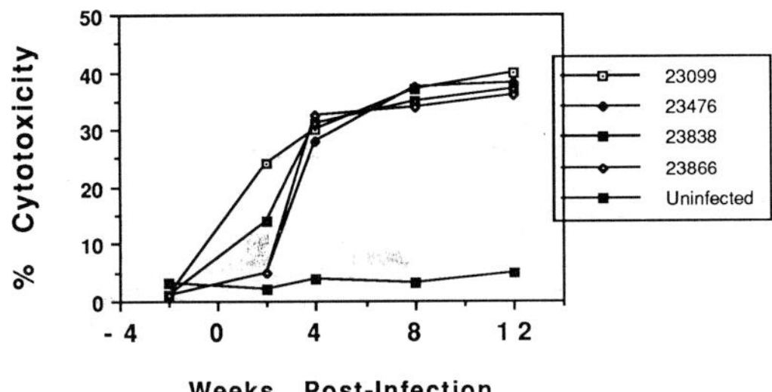


Fig. 1. Serial CTL activity of SIV-infected rhesus macaques. E-rosette positive T cells were obtained and were assayed at an E/T ratio of 100:1.

of this study (Fig. 1). CTL activity was detectable in two animals at 2 weeks post infection and all animals demonstrated significant CTL activity at 4 weeks post infection ($P < 0.02$).

### Characterization of T cells mediating CTL activity

Treatment of E-rosette positive T cells with anti-CD16 + C had no effect on the cytotoxic activity against SIV target cells, in contrast, CD8 + C treatment resulted in a significant decrease in cytotoxic activity ($P < 0.01$, Fig. 2).

### Demonstration of CD4 + , MHC class II restricted CTL

Incubation of CD4-enriched T cells with anti-MHC class II mAb resulted in a significant decrease in cytotoxic activity ($P < 0.05$) against SIV target, whereas anti-MHC class I mAb had no effect on cytotoxic activity (Fig. 3).

### Characterization of target cell phenotype

Incubation of target cells with Leu 3a, which blocks the SIV binding site, significantly inhibited target cell generation ($P < 0.02$), however, incubation with

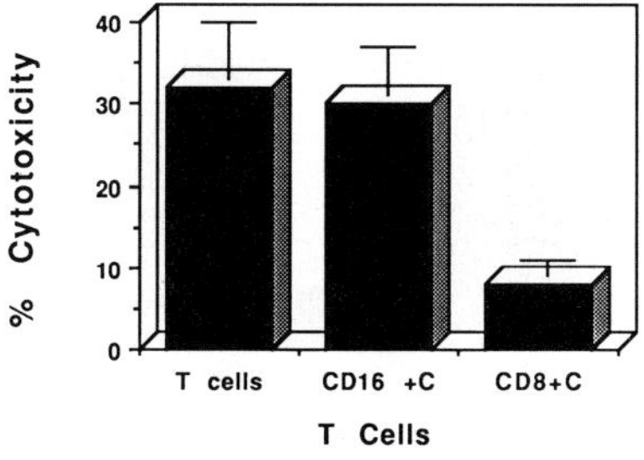


Fig. 2. CTL activity of T cells from SIV-infected rhesus macaques (n = 3) treated with anti-CD16 + C or anti-CD8 + C. T cells were assayed at an E/T ratio of 100:1. There is a significant decrease ($P < 0.01$) in cytotoxic activity following treatment with anti-CD8 + C, however, there is no significant decrease ($P > 0.5$) after treatment with anti-CD16 + C.

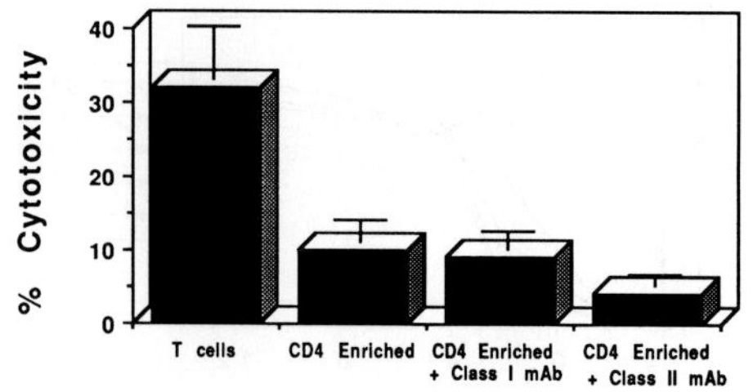


Fig. 3. CTL activity of CD4-enriched T cells from SIV-infected rhesus macaques (n = 3) in the presence of anti-MHC class I or class II mAb. CD4-T cells were enriched by treatment of the T cell population with anti-CD8 + C and were assayed at an E/T ratio of 100:1. There is a significant ($P < 0.05$) decrease in cytotoxic activity in the presence of anti-MHC class II mAb as compared to the untreated CD4-enriched population.

OKT4, which binds to an epitope on the CD4 molecule distinct from the SIV binding site, did not result in inhibition of target cell generation (Fig. 4).

## T cell proliferation studies

Significant T cell proliferative responses ($P < 0.02$) to both heat-inactivated (Fig. 5) and infectious SIV (Fig. 6) were demonstrated as early as 2 weeks post infection. Higher levels of T cell proliferation to infectious SIV were obtained compared to responses to heat-inactivated SIV. Responses to both heat-inactivated and infectious SIV were at their peak level by 2 weeks post infection and declined in subsequent studies.

## Characterization of non-T, antigen presenting cells

Significant T cell proliferation responses ($P < 0.02$) were demonstrated when $2 \times 10^5$ purified monocytes were used as antigen presenting cells (Fig. 7). This

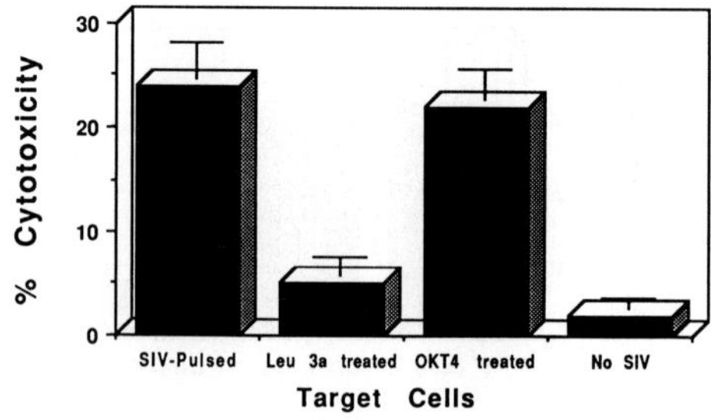


Fig. 4. Effect of anti-CD4 mAb added prior to SIV on target cell generation. When target cells are treated with Leu 3a, which blocks the SIV binding site, a significant decrease ($P < 0.02$) in cytotoxic activity is observed. When target cells are treated with OKT4, which does not block SIV binding, no significant decrease ($P > 0.5$) in cytotoxic activity is observed.

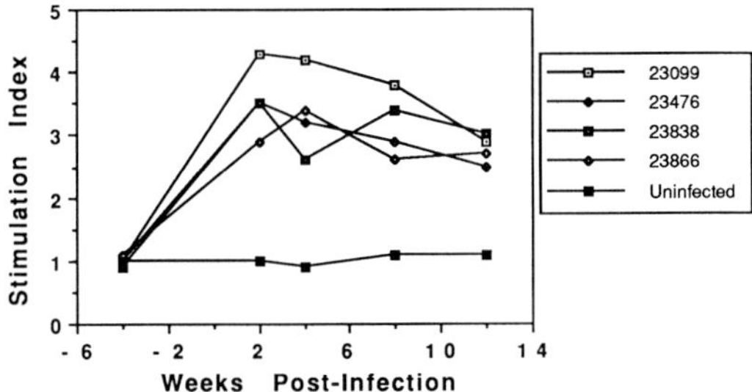


Fig. 5. Serial T cell proliferative response of SIV-infected rhesus macaques to heat-inactivated SIV. PBMC were separated into T and non-T cells by rosetting with AET-treated sheep red blood cells. Non-T cells were pulsed with heat-inactivated SIV for 18 h prior to their addition to T cells. Assay wells were pulsed with $^3$H after 5 days and harvested 18 h later.

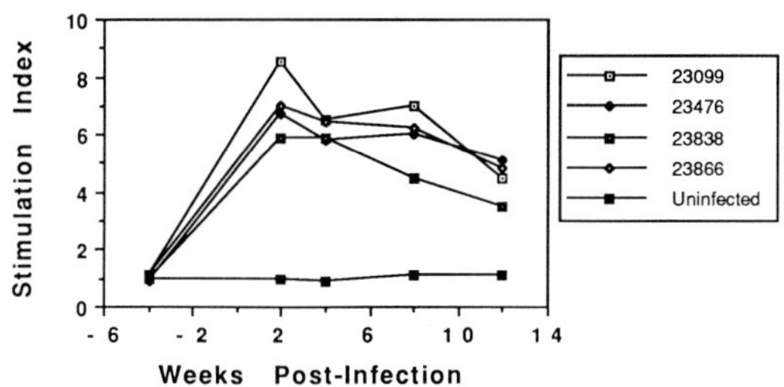


Fig. 6. Serial T cell proliferative response of SIV-infected rhesus macaques to infectious SIV. PBMC were separated into T and non-T cells by rosetting with AET-treated sheep red blood cells. Non-T cells were pulsed with infectious SIV for 18 h prior to their addition to T cells. Assay wells were pulsed with $^3$H after 5 days and harvested 18 h later.

response is equivalent to T cell proliferation responses elicited by E-rosette negative, non-T cells. Flow cytometric studies using mAbs specific for B cells (CD20), T cells (CD4 and CD8), NK (CD16), and monocytes (CD14) indicate

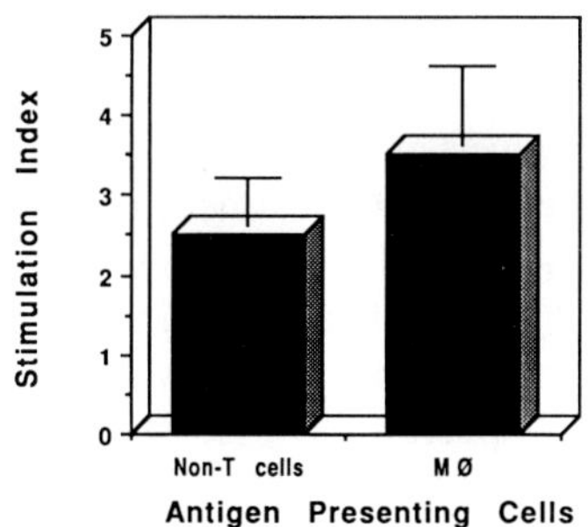


Fig. 7. Characterization of APC in T cell proliferative response to heat-inactivated SIV. E-rosette negative, non-T cells were obtained and adherent cells (MØ) were removed from an aliquot by plastic adherence. $5\times10^5$ non-T cells or $2\times10^5$ MØ were pulsed with SIV and then added back to $4\times10^5$ T cells.

that the adherent cell population is highly enriched (> 90%) for monocytes (data not shown).

## Discussion

Previous studies have defined the optimal conditions for the assessment of T cell proliferation (McGraw et al., 1990) and CTL (Vowels et al., 1989) responses specific for primate lentivirus. T cells from SIV-infected monkeys failed to proliferate in response to SIV added directly to the culture. However, when SIV is processed by autologous antigen presenting cells (APC) prior to culture with purified T cells, proliferative responses can be uniformly demonstrated by SIV-infected monkeys but not uninfected controls. There is no proliferation in response to non-MHC compatible, SIV-pulsed APC. Proliferation in response to killed SIV has been demonstrated to be mediated by CD4+ T cells and is MHC class II restricted. The proliferative response to live SIV is mediated by both CD4+ and CD8+ T cells and is either MHC class I or II restricted. As disease progressed, a progressive decline in the T cell proliferative response was observed. Demonstration of CTL activity required MHC compatible target cells that had been pulsed with SIV. No CTL activity was observed when target cells were pulsed with SRV. Incubation of target cells with leupeptin prior to the cytotoxic assay inhibited target cell generation suggesting that active processing is required. The majority of CTL activity was demonstrated to be mediated by MHC class I restricted, CD8+ T cells. There was no detectable cytotoxic activity against cells which had not been pulsed with SIV or were MHC incompatible. In contrast, the non-T (E-rosette negative) mononuclear cell population from infected monkeys demonstrated no cytotoxic activity against MHC compatible cells regardless of SIV pulsing. Neither T or non-T cells from uninfected animals demonstrated detectable cytotoxic activity against MHC compatible or incompatible cells regardless of SIV pulsing. As disease progressed, a progressive decline in the CTL response was observed.

The current study shows that CTL activity could be demonstrated as early as 2 weeks post infection with all animals showing significant CTL response by 4 weeks post infection. Furthermore, levels of killing are higher than those observed in previous studies (Vowels et al., 1989). This CTL activity is not mediated by natural killer cells since anti-CD16 treatment of the T cell population did not result in a significant decrease in CTL activity. In contrast, anti-CD8 treatment of the E-rosette positive T cells significantly diminishes CTL activity ($P < 0.01$). Previous studies suggested the presence of a low frequency of CD4+ CTL. This study demonstrates that SIV-specific CD4+ , MHC class II restricted CTL are observed when T cells are enriched for CD4+ cells. This observation is similar to in vitro studies in other viral diseases which demonstrate CD4+ CTL after elimination of CD8+ T cells (Bourgault et al., 1989). The level of cytotoxic activity observed with CD4-enriched T cells indicates that either they are less efficient in killing of SIV target cells or there is a lower frequency of these effectors compared to CD8+ T cells. This study also demonstrates that the target cells are phenotypically CD4 positive by blocking experiments using anti-CD4 mAb (Leu 3a) which binds to the same epitope of CD4 as SIV (Parnes, 1989).

In this investigation, the response to either heat-inactivated or infectious SIV has been examined in serial studies of each individual animal. Furthermore, as expected, these studies demonstrate that the monocytes are the primary antigen presenting cells in the E-rosette negative, non-T cell fraction. It should be emphasized that demonstration of T cell proliferative responses required processing of SIV by antigen presenting cells prior to their addition to T cells (McGraw et al., 1990).

In summary, these methods will help establish the natural history of the immune response to primate lentiviral infection and delineate the role that cell mediated immunity plays in AIDS. Immunodominant epitopes for CTL and T cell proliferative response will be defined in subsequent studies. The information obtained by these investigation will undoubtedly be critical to the development of an effective lentiviral vaccine (Berzofsky, 1988).

## Acknowledgements

We wish to acknowledge the assistance of Dr. Renan Acevado and Dr. Norman Levy who designed and performed the flow cytometric analysis for this study. We also thank Lawrence J.T. Young for his technical assistance in preparing and purifying the $SIV_{mac}$. This work was supported by Grants NCI-FOD-1020, NIAID AI 26471, NIH-DRR-RR 00169, and NIAID AI 25900.

## References

Berzofsky, J.A. (1988) Structural basis of antigen recognition by T lymphocytes. Implications for vaccines. *J. Clin. Invest.* 82, 1811–1817.

Bourgault, I., Gomez, A., Gomrad, E., Picard, F. and Levy, J.P. (1989) A virus-specific CD4+ cell-mediated cytolytic activity revealed by CD8+ cell elimination regularly develops in uncloned human antiviral cell lines. *J. Immunol.* 242, 252–256.

Damato, J.J., Kim, H., Fipps, D.R., Wylie, N. and Burke, D.S. (1988) High resolution HIV Western blot methodology using Bio Rad mini protein II test system. *Lab. Med.* 19, 753–756.

Davis, M.M. and Bjorkman, P.J. (1988) T-cell antigen receptor genes and T-cell recognition. *Nature* 334, 395–402.

Kaplan, M. and Clark, C. (1974) Improved rosetting assay for detection of human T lymphocytes. *J. Immunol. Methods* 5, 131–135.

Kelso, A. and Glasebrook, A. (1984) Secretion of interleukin 2, macrophage-activating factor, interferon, and colony-stimulating factor by alloreactive T lymphocyte clones. *J. Immunol.* 132, 2924–2931.

Kishimoto, T. (1985) Factors affecting B-cell growth and differentiation. *Annu. Rev. Immunol.* 3, 133–157.

McGraw, T.P., Vowels, B.R., Gardner, M.B., Ahmed-Ansari, A.A. and Gershwin, M.E. (1990) SIV-specific T cell-mediated proliferative response of infected rhesus macaques. *AIDS* 4, 191–198.

Mosmann, T.R. and Coffman, R.L. (1989) TH1 and TH2 cells: different patterns of lymphokine secretion lead to different functional properties. *Annu. Rev. Immunol.* 7, 145–173.

Parnes, J.R. (1989) Molecular biology and function of CD4 and CD8. *Adv. Immunol.* 44, 265–311.

Takatsu, K., Kikuchi, Y., Takahashi, T., Honjo, T., Matsumoto, M., Harada, N., Yamaguchi, N. and Tominaga, A. (1987) Interleukin 5, a T-cell-derived B-cell differentiation factor also induces cytotoxic T lymphocytes. *Proc. Natl. Acad. Sci. U.S.A.* 84, 4234–4238.

Unanue, E.R. and Allen, P.M. (1987) The basis for the immunoregulatory role of macrophages and other accessory cells. *Science* 236, 551–557.

Vowels, B.R., Gershwin, M.E., Gardner, M.B., Ahmed-Ansari, A.A. and McGraw, T.P. (1989) Characterization of SIV-specific T cell-mediated cytotoxic response of infected rhesus macaques. *AIDS* 3, 785–792.

*Eds. H. Schellekens and M.C. Horzinek*
*Animal Models in AIDS*



# 16

# Humoral immune response of rhesus monkeys vaccinated with the external glycoprotein gp130 of a simian immunodeficiency virus isolated from an African green monkey

W. LÜKE [1], F. POLZIEN [1], D. SCHREINER [1], K. KARJALAINEN [2], A. TRAUNECKER [2] and G. HUNSMANN [1]

[1] German Primate Center, Abteilung Virologie und Immunologie, 3400 Göttingen, F.R.G. and
[2] Basel Institute for Immunology, 4058 Basel, Switzerland

**Summary**

The external glycoprotein gp130 of a simian immunodeficiency virus (SIV) obtained from an African green monkey (agm) was isolated as micelles. With these gp130 micelles different vaccines were prepared and three rhesus monkeys were immunized with each preparation. All vaccinated animals developed an antibody titer of more than $10^6$. The antisera inhibited the binding of gp130 to the CD4 bearing cells with the same efficiency as an antiserum from a naturally SIV infected green monkey, an anti-CD4 murine monoclonal antibody and soluble CD4. The antiserum showing the highest inhibitory efficiency and the serum from a naturally SIV infected green monkey neutralized $SIV_{agm}$ and SIV isolated from a rhesus macaque (mac). The anti-CD4 monoclonal antibody neutralized both SIV isolates as well as HIV-2ben. The highest neutralization titers for all three isolates were obtained with the soluble CD4.

## Introduction

Chimpanzees and gibbons are the only animal species that can be infected with the human immunodeficiency virus type 1 (HIV-1). Attempts to protect chimpanzees with monomers, fragments or peptides of the external glycoprotein gp120 have so far failed (Alter et al., 1984; Francis et al., 1984; Fultz et al., 1986a; Arthur et al., 1987; Hu et al., 1987; Berman et al., 1988).

In recent years more than 30 isolates of immunodeficiency viruses were obtained from non-human primates such as the rhesus monkey (*Macaca mulatta;*

$SIV_{mac}$; Daniel et al., 1985), the African green monkey (*Cercopithecus aethiops;* $SIV_{agm}$; Ohta et al., 1988), the sooty mangabey (*Cercocebus atys;* $SIV_{smm}$; Fultz et al., 1986b), the pig-tailed macaque (*Macaca nemestrina;* $SIV_{mne}$; Benveniste et al., 1988) and mandrill (*Papio sphinx;* $SIV_{mnd}$; Tsujimoto et al., 1988). An AIDS-like disease was described in rhesus monkeys after infection with $SIV_{mac}$ (Letvin et al., 1985), $SIV_{smm}$ (McClure et al., 1989) and $SIV_{mne}$ (Benveniste et al., 1988). The latter virus is also pathogenic to pig-tailed macaques (Benveniste et al., 1988). First attempts to protect rhesus monkeys against experimental infection with $SIV_{mac}$ and $SIV_{mne}$ by immunization with the respective preparation of whole inactivated viruses have failed (Daniel et al., 1988; Gardner et al., 1989). Recent results however have demonstrated that a partial protection of rhesus monkeys against $SIV_{mac}$ was achieved with detergent treated whole virus (Desrosiers et al., 1989). Protection of monkeys with SIV subunit vaccines has not yet been described.

The efficiency of such subunit vaccines critically depends on the preservation of native antigenic sites and also on their presentation as multimeric forms which are much more immunogenic than monomers (Morein and Simons, 1985). Earlier investigations have shown that protective immunity against Friend virus-induced murine leukemia or against feline leukemia/sarcoma virus-induced tumors in young kittens was obtained by immunization with micellar complexes of purified viral envelope glycoproteins (Hunsmann et al., 1981, 1982, 1983; Kleiser, 1986). Therefore we have developed a procedure to prepare such micellar complexes of immunodeficiency virus envelope glycoproteins. The immunogenicity of such complexes was evaluated in rhesus monkeys.

## Methods

### Isolation of gp130 micelles and preparation of vaccines

The external glycoprotein of $SIV_{agm}$ TYO-7 was isolated to homogeneity as micellar complexes by four consecutive steps which comprised lysis of the virus with non-ionic detergent, chromatography on DEAE-cellulose, affinity chromatography on lentil lectin as well as sucrose gradient centrifugation.

For vaccine preparation gp130 micelles were linked by glutaraldehyde to keyhole limpet hemocyanin (gp130/GA/KLH) or the gp130 micelles were just mixed with KLH (gp130/KLH). A third vaccine was prepared by Tween-ether treatment of purified $SIV_{agm}$ (SIV/TE).

### Vaccination of rhesus monkeys and their immune response

The vaccine preparations were emulsified in incomplete Freund's adjuvant (ICFA). Three rhesus monkeys were vaccinated four times with each vaccine 4 weeks apart with a total of 80 $\mu$g of gp130 micelles per animal. The serological response was examined by ELISA with whole virus or purified gp130 as antigen.

### Inhibition of gp130 binding and virus neutralization

Purified gp130 micelles were radiolabelled with $^{125}I$ to a specific activity of 2 $\times$ $10^6$ cpm/$\mu$g protein. The radioactive micelles were incubated with the human Molt-4 clone 8 T4 cell line in the presence or absence of antisera from animals 222z, 5279 and 5265, from the naturally SIV infected African green monkey 6115, the anti-CD4 monoclonal antibody 30F16H5 or the soluble CD4 (sCD4). Thereafter cells were lysed and the gp130 bound to the CD4 was detected by radioimmunoprecipitation (RIPA).

The virus neutralization activity of these antisera as well as of the sCD4 was analyzed in the MT-4 cell test (Harada et al., 1986).

## Results

### Purification of gp130 micelles

SDS PAGE demonstrated that the isolated gp130 micelles were about 90% pure. On electron micrographs the micelles appeared as roundish particles with a mean diameter of 10–20 nm (Fig. 1). The molecular mass of the gp130 micelles

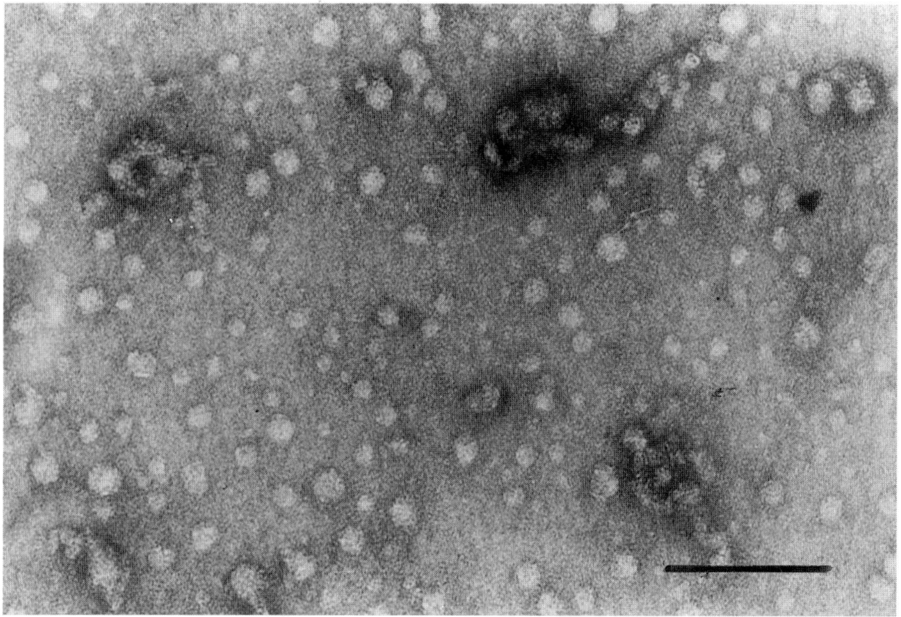

Fig. 1. Electron microscopy of the gp130 micelles. Electron micrographs of gp130 micelles were obtained after sucrose gradient centrifugation and negative staining with uranyl acetate. The bar represents 100 nm.

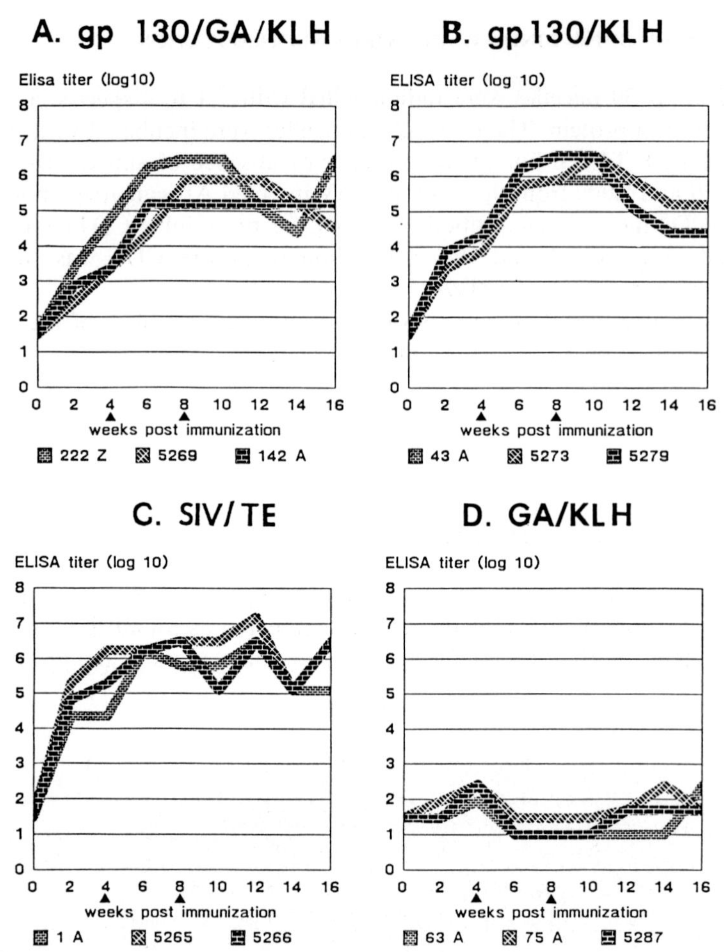


Fig. 2. Antibody response of rhesus monkeys immunized with different vaccine preparations of the gp130 micelles. The antibody reaction was measured in an ELISA using whole virus as antigen. Triangles represent the dates of first and second boost.

was 700 kDa as determined by velocity sedimentation in glycerol gradients. Thus gp130 micelles appeared to be composed of about five monomers.

### Antibody response of immunized animals

All vaccine preparations induced a strong humoral immune response. After the second boost antibodies measured in the ELISA with whole virus as antigen reached plateau levels extending over more than 10 weeks (Fig. 2). Animals with the strongest response were 222z of the gp130/GA/KLH group, 5279 of the gp130/KLH group, and 5265 of the SIV/TE group. These antisera were also titrated in an ELISA using purified gp130 micelles as antigen. In this test the

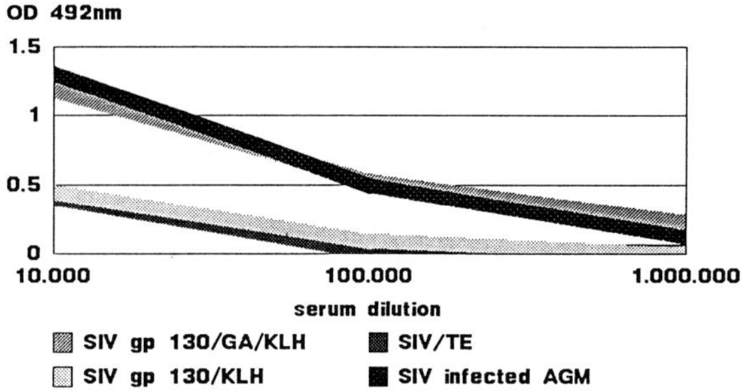


Fig. 3. Titration in an ELISA with purified gp130 micelles of the antisera from animals 222z, 5279 and 5265 showing the strongest immune response of each vaccine group.

antiserum obtained from animal 222z exhibited the highest titer in the range of $10^6$ comparable to an antiserum obtained from the naturally infected African green monkey 6115 (Fig. 3).

The strongest antisera of each vaccine group (222z, 5279, 5265) were further examined for their ability to inhibit the binding of radioiodinated gp130 to CD4 bearing cells. Both gp130 vaccine preparations as well as the Tween-ether extracted $SIV_{agm}$TYO-7 induced antibodies which inhibited the binding of gp130 to CD4 bearing cells with a similar efficiency as obtained with the antiserum from the naturally infected African green monkey 6115, the anti-CD4 monoclonal antibody (30F16H5) and the sCD4 (Table 1).

The three sera differed markedly in their ability to neutralize virus. Only the antiserum obtained from animal 222z showed significant neutralization. This antiserum neutralized $SIV_{agm}$ up to a dilution of 140 and cross-neutralized $SIV_{mac}$

TABLE 1
Inhibition of $^{125}$I-gp130 binding to CD4 bearing cells

| Serum | Species | Antigen | % Binding inhibition |
|---|---|---|---|
| No serum | – | – | 0 |
| Preimmune serum | Rhesus monkey | – | 2 |
| 6115[a] | African green monkey | SIV | 95 |
| 222z[b] | Rhesus monkey | gp130/GA/KLH | 96 |
| 5279[b] | Rhesus monkey | gp130/KLH | 93 |
| 5265[b] | Rhesus monkey | SIV/TE | 88 |
| 30F16H5[c] | Mouse | CD4 | 95 |
| sCD4[d] | – | – | 96 |

[a] Serum of an African green monkey naturally infected with SIV.
[b] Animal number.
[c] Murine anti-CD4 monoclonal antibody.
[d] Recombinant soluble CD4.

TABLE 2
Neutralization of $SIV_{agm}$, $SIV_{mac}$ and HIV-2

| Virus | Virus neutralization [a] | | | |
|---|---|---|---|---|
| | sCD4 [b] | 30F16H5 [c] | 6115 [d] | 222z [e] |
| $SIV_{agm}$ TYO-7 | 1,500 | 140 | 120 | 140 |
| $SIV_{mac251}$ | 8,000 | 520 | 80 | 60 |
| HIV-2ben | 12,000 | 800 | < 5 | < 5 |

[a] The neutralization titer was defined as 75% reduction of viral infectivity determined in the MT-4 cell assay.
[b] Recombinant soluble CD4.
[c] Murine anti-CD4 monoclonal antibody.
[d] Serum of an African green monkey naturally infected with SIV.
[e] Serum of rhesus monkey 222z after immunization with gp130/GA/KLH.

with a titer of 60, whereas it did not neutralize HIV-2ben (Table 2). The antiserum of the naturally infected African green monkey neutralized $SIV_{agm}$ up to a dilution of 90 and $SIV_{mac}$ with a titer of 80 but also not HIV-2ben. As expected the anti-CD4 monoclonal antibody (30F16H5) and the sCD4 showed neutralizing activity for all three isolates with the highest efficiency for HIV-2ben followed by $SIV_{mac}$ and $SIV_{agm}$.

## Discussion

Protective vaccines against retroviral diseases in mice and cats have been developed (Hunsmann et al., 1975; Hunsmann, 1985; Osterhaus et al., 1985). Comparing various vaccine preparations we have observed that micellar complexes of external glycoproteins of Friend leukemia virus and feline leukemia virus induced a protective immunity (Hunsmann et al., 1981, 1983). Protected animals developed high-titered neutralizing and cytotoxic antibodies. However, cytotoxic T-cell and natural killer cell activity was not recorded. These data encouraged us to develop a similar subunit vaccine against immunodeficiency virus infection. With a modification of the original technique the external glycoprotein gp130 from $SIV_{agm}$ TYO-7 could be isolated as micelles. These micelles induced a strong immune response in vaccinated rhesus monkeys. Sera of these animals inhibited binding of gp130 to CD4 bearing cells as did a serum from the naturally SIV infected green monkey 6115, the anti-CD4 monoclonal antibody (30F16H5) and the sCD4. In spite of the binding inhibition obtained with the sera from the immunized monkeys, only the antiserum from animal 222z immunized with gp130 micelles cross-linked to KLH and the antiserum from the green monkey 6115 neutralized $SIV_{agm}$ TYO-7 and $SIV_{mac251}$ but not HIV-2ben. In addition to binding inhibition, the anti-CD4 monoclonal antibody and sCD4 showed intermediate to high neutralizing activity against all three isolates.

Thus sCD4, the anti-CD4 monoclonal antibody and the antisera from animals 222z and 6115 inhibit the interaction of gp130 to CD4 with similar efficiency but are markedly different in their neutralizing and cross-neutralizing activity. Antisera directed against HIV-1 have been described which neutralize HIV-1 but do not interfere with the CD4 binding of the external glycoprotein gp120 (Skinner et al., 1988). Such antisera could interact with post-CD4 binding events, e.g., membrane fusion. However, we have found antisera which inhibit CD4 binding but cannot neutralize virus. Such antisera might mediate antibody-dependent infection via Fc receptors which were found on T4 cells (Ling et al., 1988). Alternatively, the conformation of the purified gp130 might differ from that of the intact virus particle. In this case our sera might not inhibit binding of virus to the CD4 bearing cells or neutralizing epitopes on gp130 might have been destroyed during purification and vaccine preparation.

Genetically HIV-2ben is more closely related to $SIV_{mac251}$ than to $SIV_{agm}$ TYO-1 (Kirchhoff, personal communication). Thus we were surprised to find that sera from monkey 222z immunized with $SIV_{agm}$ TYO-7 gp130 and from the naturally SIV infected African green monkey did not neutralize HIV-2ben but cross-neutralized $SIV_{mac251}$. Since $SIV_{agm}$ TYO-7 has not yet been sequenced it could still be closer to HIV-2ben and $SIV_{mac251}$ than to $SIV_{agm}$ TYO-1.

The discrepancy between the high CD4 binding inhibition and the low neutralizing activity observed with sera from immunized monkeys is a potential problem for vaccine development. A better understanding of this phenomenon could help to improve vaccines against immunodeficiency viruses.


## Acknowledgements

We thank Dr. R. Desrosiers, New England Regional Primate Research Center, Southborough, MA, U.S.A. for the gift of $SIV_{mac251}$ and Dr. M. Hayami, Kyoto University, Kyoto, Japan, for the gift of $SIV_{agm}$ TYO-7 and Molt-4 clone 8 cells.


## References


Alter, H., Eichberg, J., Masur, H., Saxinger, W., Gallo, R., Macer, A., Lane, H. and Fauci, A. (1984) Transmission of HTLV-III infection from human plasma to chimpanzees: an animal model for AIDS. *Science* 226, 549–552.

Arthur, L., Pyle, S., Nara, P., Bess, J., Gonda, M., Kelliher, J., Gilden, R., Robey, W., Bolognesi, D., Gallo, R. and Fishinger, P. (1987) Serological responses in chimpanzees inoculated with human immunodeficiency virus glycoprotein (gp120) subunit vaccine. *Proc. Natl. Acad. Sci. U.S.A.* 84, 8583–8587.

Benveniste, R.E., Morton, W.R., Clark, E.A., Tsai, C.C., Ochs, H.D., Ward, J.M., Kuller, L., Knott, W.B., Hill, R.W., Gale, M.J. and Thouless, M.E. (1988) Inoculation of baboons and macaques with simian immunodeficiency virus/mne, a primate lentivirus closely related to human immunodeficiency virus type 2. *J. Virol.* 62, 2091–2101.

Berman, P., Groopman, J., Gregory, T., Clapham, P., Weiss, R., Ferriani, R., Riddle, L., Shimasaki, C., Lucas, C., Lasky, L.A. and Eichberg, J.W. (1988) Human immunodeficiency virus type 1 challenge of chimpanzees immunized with recombinant envelope glycoprotein gp120. *Proc. Natl. Acad. Sci. U.S.A.* 85, 5200–5204.

Daniel, M., Letvin, N., King, M., Kannagi, M., Sehgal, P., Hunt, R., Kanki, P., Essex, M. and Desrosiers, R. (1985) Isolation of T-cell tropic HTLV-III like retrovirus from macaques. *Science* 228, 1201–1204.

Daniel, M., Sehgal, P., King, N., Wyand, M., Schmidt, D. and Desrosiers, R. (1988) Protection of macaques against simian immunodeficiency virus infection by inactivated whole virus. *IV International Conference on AIDS*, Stockholm, Abstract 3062.

Desrosiers, R., Wyand, S., Kodama, T., Ringler, D., Arthur, L., Sehgal, P., Letvin, N., King, N. and Daniel, M. (1989) Vaccine protection against simian immunodeficiency virus infection. *Proc. Natl. Acad. Sci. U.S.A.* 86, 6353–6357.

Francis, D., Feorino, P., Broderson, J., McClure, H., Getchell, J., McGrath, C., Swenson, B., McDougal, J., Palmer, E., Harrison, A., Barre-Sinoussi, F., Chermann, J., Montagnier, L., Curran, J., Cabradialla, C. and Kalyanaraman, V. (1984) Infection of chimpanzees with lymphadenopathy-associated virus. *Lancet* ii, 1276–1277.

Fultz, P., McClure, H., Swenson, R., McGrath, C., Brodie, A., Getchell, J., Jensen, F., Anderson, D., Broderson, R. and Francis, D. (1986a) Persistent infection of chimpanzees with human T-lymphotrophic virus type III/lymphadenopathy-associated virus: a potential model for acquired immunodeficiency syndrome. *J. Virol.* 58, 116–124.

Fultz, P., McClure, H.M., Anderson, D.C., Swenson, R.B., Anand, R. and Srinivasan, A. (1986b) Isolation of a T-lymphotrophic retrovirus from naturally infected sooty mangabey monkeys (*Cercocebus atys*). *Proc. Natl. Acad. Sci. U.S.A.* 83, 5286–5290.

Gardner, M.B., Pedersen, N., Hanson, C.V., Miller, C., Gettie, A. and Jennings, M. (1989) Immunization of rhesus macaques with inactivated SIV fails to protect against mucosal or i.v. challenge. *V. International Conference on AIDS,* Montreal, Abstract Th.C.O.45.

Harada, S., Purtilo, D., Koyanagi, Y., Sonnabend, J. and Yamamoto, N. (1986) Sensitive assay for neutralizing antibodies against AIDS-related viruses (HTLV-III/LAV). *J. Immunol. Methods* 92, 177–181.

Hu, S., Fultz, P., McClure, P., Eichberg, J., Thomas, E., Zarling, J., Singhal, M., Kosowske, S., Swenson, B., Anderson, D. and Torado, G. (1987) Effect of immunization with a vaccinia-HIV *env* recombinant on HIV infection of chimpanzees. *Nature* 328, 721–723.

Hunsmann, G. (1985) Subunit vaccines against exogeneous retroviruses: overview and perspectives. *Cancer Res.* 45, 4691–4693.

Hunsmann, G. and Schneider, J. (1982) Immunoprevention of type-C virus-induced murine leukemias by vaccination with viral envelope polypeptides. In: D.S. Yohn and J.R. Blakeslee (Eds.), *Advances in Comparative Leukemia Research*. Elsevier, New York, NY, pp. 209–210.

Hunsmann, G., Moening, V. and Schäfer, W. (1975) Properties of mouse leukemia viruses. IX. Active and passive immunization of mice against Friend leukemia with isolated viral gp71 glycoprotein and its corresponding antiserum. *Virology* 66, 327–329.

Hunsmann, G., Schneider, J. and Schulz, A. (1981) Immunoprevention of Friend virus-induced erythroleukemia by vaccination with viral envelope glycoprotein complexes. *Virology* 113, 602–612.

Hunsmann, G., Pedersen, N., Thielen, G. and Bayer, H. (1983) Active immunization with feline leukemia virus envelope glycoprotein suppresses growth of virus-induced feline sarcoma. *Microbiol. Immunol.* 171, 233–241.

Kleiser, C., Schneider, J., Bayer, H. and Hunsmann, G. (1986) Immunoprevention of Friend leukemia virus-induced erythroleukemia by vaccination with aggregated gp70. *J. Gen. Virol.* 67, 1901–1907.

Letvin, N., Daniel, M., Sehgal, P., Desrosiers, R., Hunt, R., Waldron, L., Mackey, J., Schmidt, D., Chalifoux, L. and King, N. (1985) Induction of AIDS-like disease in macaque monkeys with T-cell tropic retrovirus STLV-III. *Science* 230, 71–73.

Ling, N., Johnson, G. and McLennan, I. (1988) Leukocyte typing. *Lancet* i, 249–250.

McClure, H., Anderson, D., Fultz, P., Ansari, A., Lockwood, E. and Brodie, A. (1989) Spectrum of disease in macaque monkeys chronically infected with $SIV_{smm}$. *Vet. Immunol. Immunopathol.* 21, 13–24.

Morein, B. and Simons, K. (1985) Subunit vaccines against enveloped viruses: virosomes, micelles and other protein complexes. *Vaccine* 3, 83–93.

Ohta, Y., Masuda, T., Tsujimoto, H., Ishikawa, K., Kodama, T., Morikawa, S., Nakai, M., Honjo, S. and Hayami, M. (1988) Isolation of simian immunodeficiency virus from African green monkeys and seroepidemiologic survey of the virus in various non-human primates. *Int. J. Cancer* 41, 115–122.

Osterhaus, A., Weijer, K., Uytdehaag, O., Jarrett, O., Sundquist, B. and Morein, B. (1985) Induction of protective immune response in cats by vaccination with feline leukemia virus ISCOM. *J. Immunol.* 135, 591–596.

Skinner, M., Langlois, A., McDanal, C., McDougal, S., Bolognesi, D. and Matthews, T. (1988) Neutralizing antibodies to an immunodominant envelope sequence do not prevent gp120 binding to CD4. *J. Virol.* 62, 4195–4200.

Tsujimoto, H., Cooper, R., Kodama, T., Fukasawa, M., Miura, T., Ohta, Y., Ishikawa, K., Nakai, M., Frost, E., Roelants, G., Roffi, J. and Hayami, M. (1988) Isolation and characterization of simian immunodeficiency virus from mandrills in Africa and its relationship to other human and simian viruses. *J. Virol.* 62, 4044–4050.

# *Feline retroviruses*

*Eds. H. Schellekens and M.C. Horzinek*
*Animal Models in AIDS*



# 17

# Pathogenic mechanisms of feline leukemia virus induced immunodeficiency syndrome

EDWARD A. HOOVER[1], SANDRA L. QUACKENBUSH[1], MARY L. POSS[1], JULIE M. OVERBAUGH[2], PETER R. DONAHUE[3] and JAMES I. MULLINS[4]

[1] Colorado State University, Fort Collins, CO 80523, U.S.A., [2] University of Washington, Seattle, WA 98195, U.S.A., [3] Children's Hospital of St. Paul, St. Paul, MN 55102, U.S.A. and [4] Stanford University, Stanford, CA 94305, U.S.A.

It is increasingly clear that naturally occurring retrovirus isolates are mixtures of multiple viral genotypes. Molecular cloning of these genomes has provided the opportunity to characterize retroviral genetic determinants of pathogenicity. The feline leukemia viruses (FeLV) have been associated with a spectrum of disease which includes: immunodeficiency syndrome, aplastic anemia, myeloproliferative diseases, lymphoma, neurologic disease, reproductive failure, glomerulonephritis, and fibrosarcoma under natural and experimental conditions. Probably the most universal and significant manifestation of FeLV infection, however, is induction of immunodeficiency (Hardy, 1980, 1982). We have been studying the molecular pathogenesis of a naturally occurring strain of FeLV, designated FeLV-FAIDS, which induces fatal immunodeficiency syndrome in virtually all animals which develop persistent infection (Mullins et al., 1986; Hoover et al., 1987). We have used restriction mapping, nucleotide sequencing, envelope glycoprotein analysis, cytopathicity for T lymphocyte and bone marrow progenitor cells, and viral chimeric constructs to examine the molecular determinants of FeLV-FAIDS pathogenesis in vivo and in vitro (Overbaugh et al., 1988; Donahue et al., 1988; Poss et al., 1989).

The original FeLV-FAIDS isolate was found to consist of at least two major viral genomes in Southern blotting analyses of cellular DNA from infected cats (Mullins et al., 1986). These were: (1) a highly replication-competent but minimally pathogenic ecotropic FeLV, originally designated the *common form* virus (the prototype clone obtained from intestinal DNA of animal No. 1161 has been designated 61E) (Overbaugh et al., 1988); and (2) a replication-defective but highly pathogenic *variant form* virus (clone 61C) obtained from the intestinal DNA of the same animal and recognized by two signature restriction sites (*Kpn*I

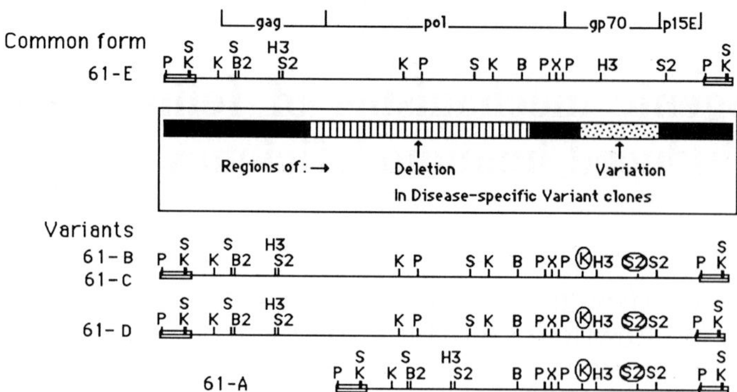


Fig. 1. FeLV-FAIDS "common form" and "major variant" genome restriction maps. Prototype clones are each 61E and 61C, respectively. The circled *Kpn*I and *Sst*II sites in the surface glycoprotein gene distinguish the variant family of viruses; the former is responsible for generation of the signature 2.1 kb fragment in Southern blots.

and *Sac*II) in the extracellular glycoprotein coding domain of the envelope gene (Fig. 1) (Overbaugh et al., 1988). The common form clone 61E has proven highly replication-competent, non-cytopathic or cytotropic for T cells, and fails to induce immunodeficiency syndrome, although animals infected for more than 400 days may develop lymphoma (Donahue et al., 1988). FeLV-FAIDS clone 61E thus appears representative of the ubiquitous, highly conserved, highly replication-competent, long latency lymphomagenic subgroup A FeLVs (Donahue et al., 1988). By contrast, the major FeLV-FAIDS variant virus, represented by clone 61C, although replication-defective in all of its molecularly cloned full-length versions, has proven both highly T cell cytotropic and cytopathic and capable of consistently inducing fatal immunodeficiency syndrome in all animals which develop persistent viremia after inoculation (Overbaugh et al., 1988; Donahue et al., submitted). The two unique restriction sites in the 61C variant were found to correspond to an 18 bp (six amino acid) deletion and an 18 bp (six amino acid) insertion, respectively, within the surface glycoprotein (gp70)-encoding region of *env*. In addition, 17 other scattered individual nucleotide substitutions distinguished the gp70 genes of clones 61E and 61C (Overbaugh et al., 1988). While three substitutions were found in the variant long terminal repeat (LTR), the transmembrane proteins had identical predicted primary sequences. Thus, mapping and sequence analysis pointed to the surface glycoprotein as the probable primary determinant of the striking differences in biologic properties between the FeLV-FAIDS genomes.

A series of in vitro and in vivo studies designed to examine the above thesis and identify the pathogenic determinants of FeLV-FAIDS were then conducted using specific-pathogen-free cats and the feline T cell line 3201 (Hardy and

TABLE 1
Experimental transmission of immunodeficiency syndrome in SPF cats with molecularly cloned viruses

| Virus inoculum FeLV-FAIDS clone(s) | Tissue of origin | Age of cats at infection (days) | Number with persistent viremia/ total | Number with acute FAIDS (days p.i.) | Number with chronic FAIDS (days p.i.) | Number with lymphoma (days p.i.) | Number without evidence of disease |
|---|---|---|---|---|---|---|---|
| 61E[a] | Intestine | 64–67 | 4/4 | 0 | 0 | 1 (611) | 3 |
| 61C + 61E[b] | Intestine | 57–66 | 12/12 | 10 (105 ± 49) | 1 (369) | 0 | 1 |
| 61C + 1Q[c] | Intestine | 55–58 | 2/8 | 2 (42,195) | – | 0 | – |
| 61B + 61E[d] | Intestine | 66 | 4/4 | – | 2 (231,294) | 2 (716,950) | – |
| 61D + 61E[e] | Bone marrow | 63–66 | 3/4 | 1 (86) | 1 (220) | 1 (556) | 0 |
| 82-11 + 61E[f] | Bone marrow | 64–67 | 4/4 | 1 (71) | 1 (209) | 1 (716) | 1 |

[a] Common form virus clone 61E obtained from intestine of cat 1161 (chronic FAIDS).
[b] Variant clone 61C from intestine of cat 1161 rescued by common form clone 61E.
[c] Variant clone 61C from intestine of cat 1161 rescued by a non-subgroup A FeLV.
[d] Variant clone 61B obtained from intestine rescued by common form clone 61E.
[e] Variant clone 61D obtained from bone marrow rescued by common form clone 61E.
[f] Variant clone 82-11 obtained from bone marrow of cat 1082 (chronic FAIDS) rescued by common form clone 61E.

Zuckerman). These experiments have demonstrated that while each of several separate molecular clones of the major FeLV-FAIDS variant obtained from different tissues of different animals proved replication-defective, each was fully capable of inducing severe immunodeficiency disease when co-infected or co-transfected with common form clone 61E (or another FeLV) serving as helper viruses (Table 1, Fig. 2). Moreover, more recent work employing viral chimeras constructed between 61E and 61C has localized the genetic elements essential for T cell cytopathicity in vitro and capacity for acute disease induction in vivo within the 61C *env* gene (Donahue et al., submitted).

To correlate the predicted alterations in the primary structure of the FeLV-FAIDS variant vs. common form *env* glycoprotein coding sequences with differences in the properties of the viral glycoproteins in infected cells, we conducted a series of radioimmunoprecipitation analyses in cells infected with either 61E or 61C (represented as a replication-competent chimera containing with entire *env*-3′ LTR of 61C) (Poss et al., 1989). These studies (Poss et al., 1989) demonstrated that the gp70 and precursor gp85 of 61C could be distinguished from those of 61E by both immune feline sera and a murine monoclonal antibody which reacts with an epitope on the p15E transmembrane protein. In

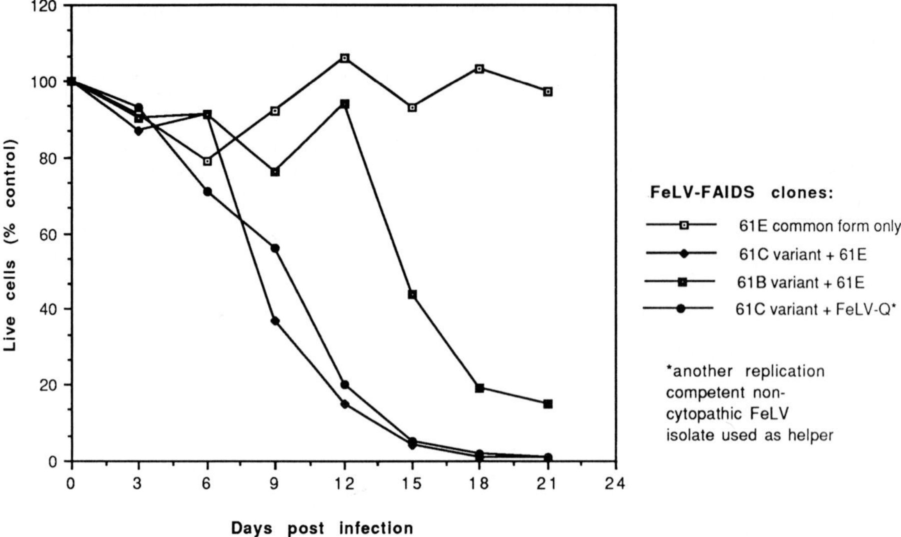


Fig. 2. In vitro cytopathic effect of cloned FeLV-FAIDS viruses in 3201 feline T lymphocyte cells.

addition, the molecular weights of the variant gp85 and gp70 were greater than those of the common form virus, despite the equal length of their predicted primary polypeptide sequences. When *env* gp glycosylation was precluded by treatment of the infected cells with tunicamycin, both the antigenic distinction and the molecular weight differences could be abolished. Finally, the processing of 61C gp85 to gp70 was substantially delayed relative to that observed for the 61E virus. Moreover, both the processing delay and antigenic recognition by 61C immune cat sera could be imparted to the 61E virus by inhibiting the processing of high-mannose oligosaccharide side chains with *N*-methyldeoxynojirmycin. The envelope glycoprotein of the FeLV-FAIDS pathogenic variant was therefore distinguishable from its probable parent virus (61E) by altered kinetics of posttranslational processing, glycosylation, size, and antigenic recognition. Thus, the *env* sequence divergence between the low and high pathogenicity FeLV-FAIDS viruses imparts distinct structural properties to their surface glycoproteins and divergent pathogenic properties to these closely related viruses.

In summary, studies conducted thus far in the FeLV-FAIDS system have demonstrated that: (a) acutely pathogenic retroviruses may themselves be replication-defective but complemented by coexistent replication-competent viruses; (b) the chief pathogenic determinants of a T cell cytopathic, immunosuppressive feline retrovirus reside in the extracellular glycoprotein gene; (c) differences in the surface glycoprotein structure probably mediate differences in cell receptor interactions, cell tropism, glycoprotein processing pathways, and other potentially cytopathogenic mechanisms.

## Acknowledgements

These studies were supported by Grants CA-43216 and AI-25273 from the National Institutes of Health, U.S. Public Health Service. We thank Michael Gallo for help with this work.

## References

Donahue, P.R., Hoover, E.A., Beltz, G.A., Hirsch, V.M., Overbaugh, J. and Mullins, J.I. (1988) Strong sequence conservation among horizontally transmissible, minimally pathogenic feline leukemia viruses. *J. Virol.* 62, 722–731.

Hardy, W.D. Jr. (1980) Feline leukemia virus diseases. In: W.D. Hardy, Jr., M. Essex and A.J. McCelland (Eds.), *Feline Leukemia Virus.* Elsevier/North Holland, Amsterdam, pp. 3–31.

Hardy, W.D. Jr. (1982) Immunopathology induced by the feline leukemia virus. *Springer Semin. Immunopathol.* 5, 75–106.

Hoover, E.A., Mullins, J.I., Quackenbush, S.L. and Gasper, P.W. (1987) Experimental transmission and pathogenesis of immunodeficiency syndrome in cats. *Blood* 70, 1880–1892.

Mullins, J.I., Chen, C.S. and Hoover, E.A. (1986) Tissue- and disease-specific production of unintegrated feline leukemia virus variant DNA in feline AIDS. *Nature* 319, 333–336.

Overbaugh, J., Donahue, P.R., Quackenbush, S.L., Hoover, E.A. and Mullins, J.I. (1988) Molecular cloning of a feline leukemia virus that induces fatal immunodeficiency disease in cats. *Science* 239, 906–910.

Poss, M.L., Mullins, J.I. and Hoover, E.A. (1989) Posttranslational modifications distinguish the envelope glycoprotein of the immunodeficiency disease-inducing feline leukemia virus retrovirus. *J. Virol.* 63, 189–195.

# 18

# Feline immunodeficiency virus infection

N.C. PEDERSEN

Department of Medicine, School of Veterinary Medicine, University of California, Davis, CA 95616, U.S.A.

**Summary**

Feline immunodeficiency virus (FIV) was first isolated from a large multiple cat household in 1986, but has probably been present in cats throughout the world for eons. The virus is a typical lentivirus in gross and structural morphology. It replicates preferentially but not exclusively in feline T-lymphoblastoid cells, where it causes a characteristic cytopathic effect. The major structural proteins are 50 (precursor core polyprotein), 10, 15 (small core proteins), 24 (major core protein), 31 (integrase), 14 (protease), 62 (reverse transcriptase), 41 (transmembrane glycoprotein) and 120 (major envelope glycoprotein) kDa in size. The various proteins are antigenically distinguishable from those of the lentiviruses, although some sera from EIAV-infected horses and V-MV-, EIAV- and CAEV-immunized rabbits will cross-react with some FIV antigens.

Kittens experimentally infected with FIV manifest a transient fever and neutropenia beginning 4–8 weeks after inoculation that lasts for 1–2 weeks. This is associated with a generalized lymphadenopathy that persists for up to 9 months. Most cats recover from this initial phase of the disease and become lifelong carriers of the virus. A terminal AIDS-like phase of the illness has been seen mainly in naturally infected cats. It appears 1–5 years or more following the initial exposure in an unknown proportion of infected animals.

Feline immunodeficiency virus infection is most prevalent in high density populations of free roaming cats (feral and pet), and is very uncommon in closed purebred catteries. Male cats are twice as likely to become infected as females. Older male cats adopted as feral or stray animals are at the highest risk of infection. Intimate, non-traumatic contact (mutual grooming or shared use of food, water and litter pans) is inefficient in transmitting the infection. In utero and venereal transmission could not be demonstrated in laboratory settings. Experimental and seroepidemiologic studies suggest that FIV is transmitted mainly by bites.

The infection rate among the general cat population rises throughout life, and reaches levels ranging from less than 1% to 12% or more depending on the area. From 3 to 30% or more of chronically ill cats will be infected, depending on the area and composition of the group being tested. Clinically affected cats tend to be 5 years or older at the time of hospitalization.

There does not appear to be a strong statistical linkage between FIV and feline leukemia virus (FeLV) infections in nature. The FeLV infection rate in FIV-infected animals is nearly the same as it is for non-FIV-infected cats, reflecting differences in the modes of transmission of FeLV and FIV. However, cats with both infections tend to die more quickly and at a younger age than animals infected with FIV alone. There is a statistical linkage between FIV infection and infection with a third retrovirus of cats, feline syncytium-forming virus (FeSFV). This is probably due to the common mode of transmission of FIV and FeSFV.

The clinical manifestations of terminal FIV infection in nature are varied. One group of cats succumbs over a period of months or years to progressive secondary or opportunistic infections of the oral cavity, upper respiratory tract, gastrointestinal tract, skin, or urinary tract. Others suffer from vague signs of illness, unexplainable anemias, FeLV negative myeloproliferative or lymphoproliferative neoplasms, or neurologic disorders. Neurologic signs are usually of a cortical nature, with dementia and behavioral abnormalities predominating.

Similarities between FIV infection of cats and HIV infection of man are striking, making FIV infection of cats a good model for human AIDS. There is no evidence that FIV is a health hazard to man or other species of animals, which further enhances its value as a small laboratory animal model.

## Introduction

Feline immunodeficiency virus (FIV) was first isolated from a large multiple cat household in Petaluma, CA in 1986 (Pedersen et al., 1987). The discovery was prompted by an outbreak of acquired immunodeficiency-like disease among a group of feline leukemia virus (FeLV) negative cats (Pedersen et al., 1987). The outbreak of disease arose shortly after the death of a recently acquired cat and seemed to spread in a horizontal manner among animals that were housed together in the same pen. Plasma and whole blood from three cats in this group were inoculated into two specific-pathogen-free cats. The inoculated cats developed fever, leukopenia, and generalized lymphadenopathy after 4–6 weeks. A lentivirus was isolated in normal feline T-lymphocyte enriched peripheral blood mononuclear cell cultures co-cultivated with similar cells from the two experimentally infected animals.

Feline immunodeficiency virus has been subsequently identified in many regions of the United States and Canada (Grindem et al., 1989; Shelton et al., 1989d; Witt et al., 1989; Yamamoto et al., 1989), Europe (Bennett et al., 1989; Harbour et al., 1988; Gruffyd-Jones et al., 1988; Lutz et al., 1988), South Africa (van der Riet et al., 1988), Japan (Ishida et al., 1988, 1989), China (Chan and Pedersen, unpublished observation, 1989), Australia (Belford et al., 1989; Sabine et al., 1988), and New Zealand (Swinney et al., 1989). Domestic cats spread from Europe to these various countries with the early traders and explorers hundreds of years ago, suggesting that FIV has also been in cats for at least a comparable period of time. Seropositive cats have been identified as far back as stored sera are available, which is 1975–1976 in Europe (Gruffyd-Jones et al., 1988), 1972 in Australia (Sabine et al., 1988), and 1968 in the United States (Shelton et al., 1990).

### Morphology of FIV

Feline immunodeficiency virus is morphologically identical to lentiviruses that cause acquired immunodeficiency syndrome (AIDS) in man and primates (Pedersen et al., 1987; Yamamoto et al., 1988a,b). The virus buds from the plasma membrane of infected cells in the same manner as other retroviruses. The complete virion is 105–125 nm in diameter, spherical to ellipsoid in shape, and possesses short poorly defined envelope projections. Budding viruses have the typical crescent-shaped appearance of C- and D-type retroviruses and lentiviruses, except that the developing viral core is separated from the overlying plasma membrane by an electron-lucent space. The viral core is composed of a conical shell that is surrounded by an electron-dense nucleoid. A polygonal electron-lucent space is seen between core shell and the granular layer just inside the outer viral membrane.

### In vitro growth characteristics of FIV

Feline immunodeficiency virus replicates in primary feline blood mononuclear cells, thymus cells, and spleen cells that have been stimulated initially with concanavalin A (ConA) and then maintained on human recombinant interleukin-2 (IL-2) (Pedersen et al., 1987; Yamamoto et al., 1988b). It will also replicate on permanent FeLV-infected cat T-lymphoblastoid cell lines such as LSA-1 and FL-74 (Yamamoto et al., 1988b). Some isolates can be adapted to replicate on Crandell feline kidney cells (Yamamoto et al., 1988b). Feline immunodeficiency virus will not replicate in non-feline cell lines such as the Raji continuous human B-lymphoblastoid cells, primary ConA- and IL-2-stimulated canine blood mononuclear or BALB/c mouse spleen cells, mouse IL-2-dependent HT-2c T-lymphoblastoid cells, or in sheep normal fibroblast cultures sensitive to Visna-Maedi virus (Yamamoto et al., 1988b).

### Reverse transcriptase

The reverse transcriptase (RT) gene has 40–65% genetic homology with human immunodeficiency virus (HIV), simian immunodeficiency virus (SIV), Visna-Maedi virus (V-MV), caprine arthritis encephalitis virus (CAEV) and equine infectious anemia virus (EIAV) (Olmsted et al., 1989; Talbot et al., 1989). The RT enzyme of FIV utilizes the cation $Mg^{2+}$, a feature of all lentiviruses, and the molar requirement for this ion is identical to that of HIV and SIV (Pedersen et al., 1987; Yamamoto et al., 1988b). The activity of the FIV reverse transcriptase is inhibited by the same antiviral compounds that inhibit HIV reverse transcriptase and at equal concentrations, making it a good model for anti-HIV drug studies (North et al., 1989).

### Genetic structure of FIV

Infectious molecular clones of FIV have been recently reported, and the genetic sequence of the virus elucidated (Olmsted et al., 1989; Talbot et al., 1989). The virus has the typical genetic structure of lentiviruses and a genome of about 9.4 kb. Phylogenetic analysis of the conserved polymerase gene indicates that FIV differentiated from other lentiviruses relatively early in evolution, i.e., shortly after the divergence of primate and non-primate lentiviruses, and before the divergence of EIAV from V-MV and CAEV (Talbot et al., 1989). The genomic structure of FIV, especially in the intergenomic regions, is more closely aligned with V-MV than other lentiviruses.

The precursor polyprotein of the viral core proteins migrates as a 47,000–52,000 Da protein by polyacrylamide gel electrophoresis (PAGE) (Yamamoto et al., 1988b; O'Connor et al., 1989). The predicted molecular weight based on genetic sequence data is 49,500 Da (Talbot et al., 1989). The major core protein has a molecular weight by PAGE of 26,000–28,000 Da (Yamamoto et al., 1988b; O'Connor et al., 1989). Based on sequencing data, the actual size of this protein is 24,493 Da (Talbot et al., 1989). Smaller viral core proteins of 15,000–17,000 and 10,000 Da have also been identified by PAGE (Yamamoto et al., 1988b; O'Connor et al., 1989). The actual sizes of these proteins are 14,900 and 9640 Da, respectively (Talbot et al., 1989).

The major envelope protein of FIV is around 120 kDa by radioimmunoprecipitation in its glycosylated form (Egberink et al., 1989; O'Connor et al., 1989). The entire FIV major envelope gene consists of approximately 750 base pairs, and contains 17 potential sites for N-linked glycosylation prior to the predicted processing site for the transmembrane glycoprotein (Talbot et al., 1989). The potential size of the non-glycosylated major envelope protein based on sequence data and tunicamycin inhibition studies is 75,000 Da (Egberink et al., 1989; Talbot et al., 1989). The transmembrane glycoprotein of FIV has a molecular weight by PAGE of around 41,000 Da (O'Connor et al., 1989; Yamamoto et al., 1988b). The genetic coding region of the transmembrane protein contains four potential N-linked glycosylation points and a hydrophobic spanning region of 71 bases (Talbot et al., 1989).

The entire polymerase gene region of FIV is comprised of 3371 bases and overlaps the 3′ end of the gene coding for the core proteins (Talbot et al., 1989). The predicted sizes of the protease and RT are 13,493 and 61,490 Da, respectively. The 3′ end of the polymerase gene is predicted to encode an integrase of 30,690 Da. A region of approximately 400 base pairs between RT and integrase would code for an additional unknown protein of approximately 14,600 Da (Talbot et al., 1989).

A putative viral infectivity factor (VIF) gene is present as an open reading frame overlapping the 3′ end of the polymerase gene (Talbot et al., 1989). Although this gene corresponds in position to the VIF of the primate lentiviruses, there is no significant genetic similarity. An intragenic region that is 3′ to the putative VIF gene has the potential to encode three overlapping reading frames unique to FIV and not found in other lentiviruses (Talbot et al., 1989). The significance of this region is unknown at this time.

The genetic structure of the long terminal repeats (LTRs) of FIV has been reported by Olmsted and coworkers (1989) and Talbot and associates (1989). Attempts to align the FIV LTR sequence with that of known lentiviruses were unsuccessful, and there were no significant similarities to any other reported viral sequences. The length of the LTR is similar to that of CAEV, V-MV and EIAV, but much shorter than that of HIV or SIV. The LTR contains a purine rich region for the initiation of plus-strand DNA synthesis and a primer binding site for the initiation of minus-strand DNA synthesis. Transcription signals present in the LTR of FIV include two TATA boxes, one similar to that of HIV and the second identical to that reported for CAEV, V-MV and EIAV. A consensus polyadenylation signal is present in the LTR, and a potential enhancer sequence similar to what is found in the B site of the *K* immunoglobulin gene enhancer. Feline immunodeficiency virus LTR-CAT gene constructs will produce high levels of choline acetyltransferase (CAT) in response to transcription signals produced by lectin-stimulated human T-cells, indicating that this site may be functional (Sparger and Luciw, personal communication, 1989). The 5′ LTR is immediately followed by an 18 base sequence that corresponds to the tRNA-lys primer binding site typical of all known lentiviruses (Talbot et al., 1989).

A transactivating (TAT) gene similar to that of HIV has not been identified in FIV, but a possible TAT gene is seen in the intragenic region 3′ to the putative VIF gene. Preliminary experiments suggest that the transactivating activity of the putative FIV TAT protein is low compared to the HIV TAT gene product (Sparger and Luciw, personal communication, 1989).

## Antigenic structure of FIV

The proteins of FIV are not recognized by human antisera to HIV-1 or HIV-2, rhesus monkey antisera to SIV (macaque and sooty mangabey isolates), goat antisera to CAEV, sheep antisera to V-MV, or bovine serum to bovine immunodeficiency-like virus (BIV) (Pedersen et al., 1987; Steinman et al., 1989). Horse antisera to EIAV will immunoprecipitate to some extent the major core protein (p24), the *core* precursor polyprotein (pr50), and the major envelope glycoprotein (gp120) (Steinman et al., 1989). Rabbit antiserum to EIAV will precipitate all of the *gag* proteins and *gag* precursor polyproteins of FIV (Egberink et al., 1989; Steinman et al., 1989). Rabbit antiserum to CAEV and V-MV will react with FIV-p24, while rabbit antisera to BIV and HIV-1 are non-reactive (Olmsted et al., 1989).

## Epidemiologic factors

The FIV infection rate among the general cat populations is less than 1% in Switzerland, 1–5% in North America (Grindem et al., 1989; Shelton et al., 1989c; Yamamoto et al., 1989), 9% in New Zealand (Swinney et al., 1989), and as high as 12% in Japan (Ishida et al., 1989). Among cats that are showing chronic signs of illness, the infection rate is around 3% in Switzerland and The Netherlands (Lutz et al., 1989), 10 to 14% in North America (Grindem et al., 1989; Shelton et al., 1989c; Yamamoto et al., 1989), 10–27% in the United Kingdom, France, and New Zealand (Bennett et al., 1989; Lutz et al., 1989; Swinney et al., 1989), and 14–30% or more in Japan and Australia (Belford et al., 1989; Ishida et al., 1988, 1989; Sabine et al., 1989).

The rate of infection appears to be greatly influenced by several different environmental factors. Cats that are allowed to roam freely between the indoors and outdoors are at the highest risk. The ratio of outdoor:indoor cats in the FIV-infected population is 19:1 in Japan (Ishida et al., 1989) and 7.2:1 in North America (Yamamoto et al., 1989). Feral cats have an even higher incidence of disease than owned free-roaming cats. The incidence in purebred catteries and households where cats are kept strictly indoors from kittenhood is extremely low (less than 0.1%). Male cats are infected twice or more frequently than females, even adjusting for a slight excess of males in the population (Grindem et al., 1989; Ishida et al., 1989; Shelton et al., 1989; Swinney et al., 1989; Yamamoto et al., 1989). The infection rate is also proportional to the density of the cat population that is freely roaming. Japan, with the highest density of free-roaming cats, has over three times the incidence of FIV infection that the United States has (Ishida et al., 1989; Yamamoto et al., 1989). Infected cats have been as young as a few months of age and as old as 18 years of age. The infection rate rises progressively after the first few months of life and plateaus around 5–6 years (Grindem et al., 1989; Ishida et al., 1989; Shelton et al., 1989c; Yamamoto et al., 1989). However, clinical disease tends to appear from 5 years of age onward. This is different from FeLV infection, which tends to affect cats younger than 6 years of age.

The epidemiologic relationship between FIV infection and the two other major retrovirus infections of cats, FeLV and feline syncytium-forming virus (FeSFV), has been studied. About one-sixth of the FIV-infected cats with clinical signs of immunodeficiency that were tested in North America and Japan were co-infected with FeLV (Ishida et al., 1989; Yamamoto et al., 1989). Cats co-infected with FeLV were about a year younger than those infected with FIV alone and tended to have more severe disease and died sooner. It is still not certain whether co-infection with FIV and FeLV occurs more frequently than chance infection with either virus. Large studies in North America and Japan indicated that the two infections occur independently of each other (Ishida et al., 1989; Yamamoto et al., 1989). A third smaller study from the United States showed only a weak positive relationship between FIV and FeLV infections (Grindem et al., 1989). Shelton and coworkers (1990) found that 14.4% of FeLV-infected cats were co-infected with FIV, which was virtually identical to the incidence of FIV infection among a similar group of cats reported by Yamamoto and associates (1989). In a second study by the same group, the incidence of FIV infection was 4.1% in a group of 587 pet cats in the Pacific Northwest of the United States; 6.6% of the group were infected with FeLV, and 0.7% with both FIV and FeLV (vs. an 0.27% anticipated incidence if the two infections were transmitted independently) (Shelton et al., 1989c). Sabine and associates (1988) found 14% of cat sera to be positive for FIV, 25% for FeLV, and 0.9% for both. Hosie and coworkers (1989) also concluded that FIV and FeLV infections were transmitted independently of each other.

There is some experimental and field evidence that dually infected cats are sicker than cats infected with either virus. Ishida and coworkers (1989) found that FeLV/FIV-infected cats were about a year younger at the time of clinical presentation than cats infected with FeLV or FIV alone. They also found that dually infected cats lived a shorter period of time following diagnosis. Grindem and associates (1989) also found that dually infected cats were sicker than cats infected with FIV alone, but they only studied a small group of animals. However, Shelton and coworkers (1989c) found that three-fourths of dually infected cats, two-thirds of FeLV-infected cats, and five-sixth of FIV-infected pet cats were sick at the time the infection was diagnosed. Pedersen and coworkers (1990) infected asymptomatic FeLV carrier cats with FIV and followed the subsequent course of disease. FeLV-infected cats that were given FIV developed a severe primary form of FIV infection 6–8 weeks later and about one-half of them died over a 2 week period. Following recovery from the primary stage of FIV infection, dually infected cats had inverted T4/T8 lymphocyte ratios and were significantly more leukopenic than cats infected with either FeLV or FIV alone. One of these surviving cats died 6 months later of a severe bowel infection.

Although FeLV and FIV infections appear to occur independently of each other, there was a strong correlation between FeSFV and FIV infections. Seventy-four percent of a group of FeSFV-infected cats in one FIV study group tested positive for FIV infection (Yamamoto et al., 1989). This was compared to a 37% FIV infection rate among a group of FeSFV negative cats from the same cohort. The linkage between FeSFV and FIV infection is probably related to the common mode of transmission for these two viruses. Feline immunodeficiency virus and FeSFV infections occur mainly in free-roaming cats, and bites have been implicated as a major route of infection for both viruses (Pedersen, 1987; Yamamoto et al., 1988b, 1989). The high incidence of FeSFV infection in FIV-infected cats greatly complicates attempts to isolate FIV.

### Mode of transmission

Feline immunodeficiency virus can be recovered in the blood, serum, plasma, cerebrospinal fluid, and saliva of experimentally or naturally infected cats (Yamamoto et al., 1988b, 1989). Although horizontal transmission can occur by contact alone (Pedersen et al., 1987), it is relatively inefficient when compared to the transmission of other feline pathogens (Yamamoto et al., 1988b, 1989). Only one of 15 susceptible cats that were housed in common rooms with infected animals became seropositive over a 3 year period (Pedersen, unpublished observation, 1989). Although horizontal infection appeared to occur in the original cattery where FIV was isolated (Pedersen et al., 1987), this may have been due to the owner's use of the same needles for treating sick animals and not from direct cat-to-cat contact (Pedersen, unpublished observation, 1989). Shelton and associates (1989c) found no evidence of infection among 31 feline housemates of infected cats. Venereal transmission from infected toms to non-infected females and from infected females to non-infected toms does not occur to any extent (Pedersen, unpublished observation, 1989). Likewise, in utero transmission and neonatal transmission through colostrum, milk, and maternal grooming are apparently uncommon (Yamamoto et al., 1988b). Parenteral inoculation of susceptible cats with blood, plasma, or infectious tissue culture fluids originating from infected animals will readily transmit the infection (Yamamoto et al., 1988b).

Bites appear to be one of the most efficient modes of transmission. A single experimentally administered bite from a naturally or experimentally infected cat will transmit the infection to susceptible animals (Yamamoto et al., 1989). Biting is infrequent among cats that are kept strictly indoors in stable groups. Cats kept strictly indoors express their territorial aggression by non-violent means, while the same cats will ferociously defend their territories when allowed to roam outdoors. This may also explain why male cats are more likely to be infected.

## Pathogenesis

FIV infection occurs in two stages; a transient primary illness occurring several weeks after infection and a terminal secondary stage that occurs years afterward (Barlough et al., 1990; Yamamoto et al., 1988b). In these regards, FIV infection is similar to HIV infection of man. The primary phase of the infection is characterized by varying degrees of fever, neutropenia (often associated with a mild to moderate leukopenia), and generalized lymphadenopathy. This primary transient disease is reminiscent of the primary stage of FeLV infection (Pedersen et al., 1977). Diarrhea and depression are additional signs in more severely affected animals. The fever and neutropenia persist for a few days to several weeks before disappearing. The generalized lymphadenopathy, which can be pronounced, persists for 2–9 months before subsiding. Mortality during the initial stage of infection is low, ranging from 5 to 20% at the worst. Death is usually due to a peculiar and florid type of necrotizing and pyogranulomatous vasculitis that is centered around the cecum and mesenteric lymph nodes (Yamamoto et al., 1988b). Lymph node changes are associated with pronounced follicular hyperplasia with a less marked increase in paracortical zones (Yamamoto et al., 1988b). The follicles are dysplastic in appearance, asymmetrical, and often intrude into the paracortex. Lymph node changes in FIV-infected cats resemble those described for cats in nature with peculiar types of lymphadenopathy (Moore et al., 1986).

Following the disappearance of fever, leukopenia, and generalized lymphadenopathy, experimentally infected cats go into a long period of clinical normalcy (Yamamoto et al., 1988b). The virus can be readily reisolated from the blood from all of the infected cats, and the carrier state is lifelong. The length of time between the primary phase of disease and the terminal secondary stage has not yet been determined. Specific-pathogen-free cats that were experimentally infected with FIV are still clinically normal after 3 years, but several animals have developed abnormalities in their T4/T8 lymphocyte ratios beginning 1–2 years after infection (Barlough et al., 1990). Shelton and coworkers (1989c) found that the median age of FIV-infected cats in nature was 4 years, while the median age of sick FIV-infected cats was 10 years. This would also suggest that the period between infection and terminal disease may be several years. Mortality among the index Petaluma cattery dramatically increased 2–5 years after the first infected animal was introduced into the household (Sparger and Pedersen, unpublished observation, 1989), again suggesting that the incubation period for the secondary stage of FIV infection can be as long as 5 years.

The ultimate proportion of FIV-infected cats that will go on to the final, or AIDS, stage of disease is also unknown at this time. Limited data from a single large household of FIV-infected cats show the mortality among a group of healthy appearing FIV-infected cats to be 15–20% per year (Sparger and Pedersen, unpublished observation, 1989). This is much lower than the 50% per year mortality for FeLV-infected cats (Pedersen et al., 1977).

## CLINICAL FEATURES

A number of distinct and intertwined disease syndromes are observed in FIV-infected cats, and these various syndromes are not unlike those seen in HIV infection of man (Hopper et al., 1989; Hosie et al., 1989; Ishida et al., 1989; Yamamoto et al., 1989). Signs referable to an AIDS-like syndrome occur in one-half or more of the cases. About one-third of FIV-infected cats present with vague chronic or intermittent signs of weight loss, inappetence, fever, lymphadenopathy, anemia, leukopenia, or behavioral changes. Disease syndromes of other types may also be seen as the predominant feature of infection in smaller proportions of infected cats. These syndromes may be neurologic (5%), immunologic (5%), hematologic (5%), or neoplastic (10%). Some cats may have combinations of these various manifestations.

About one-half of the cats with AIDS-like disease present with chronic progressive infections of the mouth, including the gingiva, periodontal tissues, cheeks, oral fauces, or tongue (Gruffydd-Jones et al., 1989; Hopper et al., 1989; Hosie et al., 1989; Ishida et al., 1989; Knowles et al., 1989; Shelton et al., 1989c; Swinney et al., 1989; Yamamoto et al., 1989). Such lesions may be present for years before the diagnosis is finally made. Although chronic oral cavity infections are a common feature of FIV infection, not every cat with mouth disease is FIV-infected. In the United States, about one-fourth or less of the cats with severe mouth infections are FIV-infected. In a study in the United Kingdom, 75% of a group of cats with severe stomatitis were FIV-infected (Knowles et al., 1989).

About one-fourth of the ill FIV-infected cats with AIDS-like disease present chronic upper respiratory infections involving the lungs (chronic bronchitis, bronchiolitis, pneumonitis), nasal passages (rhinitis) and conjunctival membranes of the eyes (conjunctivitis) (Bennett et al., 1989; Hosie et al., 1989; Hopper et al., 1989; Ishida et al., 1989; Pedersen et al., 1987; Swinney et al., 1988; Yamamoto et al., 1989). Respiratory signs can occur by themselves or in association with infections in other areas of the body.

About 15% of FIV-infected cats with AIDS-like disease present with chronic infections of the skin or external ear canals (Ishida et al., 1988, 1989; Pedersen et al., 1987; Yamamoto et al., 1989). Bacterial skin lesions are usually caused by Staphylococcus. Generalized mite infestations (demodectic and notoedric mange) have also tended to be concentrated in cats with FIV infection (Chalmers et al.,

1989; Ishida et al., 1989). Chronic abscesses have been observed in FIV-infected cats by several groups (Grindem et al., 1989; Ishida et al., 1989; Shelton et al., 1989c).

Chronic enteritis, usually manifested by loose or diarrheic stools and some degree of weight loss, is the main clinical complaint in about 10% of the animals with immunodeficiency (Belford et al., 1989; Hopper et al., 1989; Gruffydd-Jones et al., 1989; Ishida et al., 1988, 1989; Pedersen et al., 1987; Swinney et al., 1989; Yamamoto et al., 1989). Bowel disease is probably more common than this; many cat owners do not examine their cat's stools and are unaware of any problems. Chronic bacterial infections of the upper or lower urinary tract are seen in a small proportion of FIV-infected cats (Grindem et al., 1989).

About one-third of all FIV-infected cats are brought to veterinarians for vague signs of illness such as recurrent fevers of undetermined origin, leukopenia, lymphadenopathy, anemia, unthriftiness, inappetence, weight loss, or non-specified changes in normal behavior (Belford et al., 1989; Hopper et al., 1989; Gruffydd-Jones et al., 1989; Ishida et al., 1989; Swinney et al., 1989; Yamamoto et al., 1989). The lymphadenopathy seen in these cats resembles that previously described by Moore and coworkers (1986). If the cat is not showing any obvious signs of chronic secondary or opportunistic infections, the diagnosis of FIV infection can be missed. Therefore, cats with vague signs of illness should be routinely tested for FIV infection.

A number of infections of an opportunistic nature have been seen in FIV-infected cats in the AIDS phase of illness. The most common among these have been feline calicivirus infection (Knowles et al., 1989), poxvirus infection (Brown et al., 1989), toxoplasmosis (Witt et al., 1989), cryptococcoses and candidiasis (Ishida et al., 1989), generalized demodectic (Chalmers et al., 1989; Swinney et al., 1989) and notoedric mange (Ishida et al., 1989), mycobacteriosis (Ishida et al., 1989; Swinney et al., 1989), and haemobartonellosis (Belford et al., 1989; Grindem et al., 1989; Hopper et al., 1989; Ishida et al., 1988a). Feline infectious peritonitis, which is often linked with FeLV infection, does not appear to be associated with FIV infection (Ishida et al., 1989).

About 5% of clinically ill FIV-infected cats will have neurological abnormalities as the predominant clinical feature (Shelton et al., 1989c; Swinney et al., 1989; Yamamoto et al., 1989). Neurological signs can also be an accompanying feature of a more generalized AIDS-like syndrome in a similar proportion of cats (Harbour et al., 1988; Pedersen et al., 1987; Shelton et al., 1989c). Neurological signs can be a direct effect of the virus on brain cells (commonly), or a manifestation of some other opportunistic infection (uncommonly). Because most FIV-related lesions are in the cerebral cortex, clinical signs are more behavioral than motor. Dementia, twitching movements of the face and tongue, psychotic behavior (hiding, rage, over-aggression), loss of toilet training, and compulsive roaming have all been recognized in FIV-infected cats (Belford et al., 1989; Harbour et al., 1988; Shelton et al., 1989c; Yamamoto et al., 1989). Convulsions, nystagmus, ataxia, intention tremors, are also observed in some FIV-infected cats.

Renal disease of an unspecified type has been observed as a complicating feature of FIV infection in some cats (Belford et al., 1989; Ishida et al., 1989). Whether this merely reflects the tendency of FIV-diseased cats to be of advanced age (renal disease is common in old cats) or whether there is a definite cause and effect relationship remains to be established. Cystitis of bacterial or unknown origin has been seen in some FIV-infected cats (Gruffydd-Jones et al., 1989; Shelton et al., 1989a,c; Yamamoto et al., 1989).

Inflammatory disease of the eye, in particular the anterior uveal tract, has been seen in several FIV-infected cats from the field (Gruffyd-Jones et al., 1989). Some eye lesions are caused by other agents, in particular *Toxoplasma gondii.* In other cases, no obvious agent can be identified.

Several types of immune mediated diseases may be associated in some way with FIV infection in cats (Pedersen, unpublished observations, 1989). A proportion of anemic FIV-infected cats have a Coomb's positive anemia. Such anemias are common with haemobartonellosis, and because *Haemobartonella felis* is not easy to identify in the blood of some chronically infected animals, it is not always possible to ascribe the anemia solely to immunologic mechanisms when no organisms are seen. The author has treated several cats with immune-mediated thrombocytopenia and/or arthritis. Arthritis has also been observed in several FIV-infected cats by Hopper and associates (1989).

Hematologic abnormalities are common in ill FIV-infected cats (Belford et al., 1989; Grindem et al., 1989; Gruffydd-Jones et al., 1989; Harbour et al., 1988; Hopper et al., 1989; Ishida et al., 1988, 1989; Shelton et al., 1989a,c; Swinney et al., 1989; Yamamoto et al., 1989). The main abnormalities are leukopenia and anemia. The leukopenia can be due to an absolute granulocytopenia, an absolute lymphopenia, or both. The anemias are usually non-responsive in nature. Examination of bone marrow often shows either marrow hyperplasia or marrow dysplasia. Maturation arrests, particularly in the red blood cells series, are common. Monocytosis and lymphocytosis have been observed in a proportion of FIV-infected cats (Hopper et al., 1989). Hypergammaglobulinemia occurs in about one-third, and elevated levels of serum IgG in about one-half, of all FIV-infected cats presenting with clinical signs of illness (Hopper et al., 1989).

There is mounting evidence that FIV-infected cats have a higher incidence of certain types of cancers. It is not yet certain how FIV is associated with these cancers, i.e., is it oncogenic like FeLV, does it increase cancer incidence by decreasing tumor immunosurveillance mechanisms, or does it allow other cancer causing agents to be activated? Cancers that appear to be FIV-associated are of several types: (1) lymphoid tumors (lymphosarcoma), (2) myeloid tumors (myelogenous leukemia, myeloproliferative disease), and (3) miscellaneous solid carcinomas and sarcomas.

Lymphosarcomas have been observed in a number of FeLV negative, FIV-infected cats (Belford et al., 1989; Gruffyd-Jones et al., 1988; Hopper et al., 1989; Ishida et al., 1989; Sabine et al., 1988; Shelton et al., 1989b, 1990; Yamamoto et al., 1989). The most convincing study on the relationship between FIV infection and lymphosarcoma has been presented by Shelton and coworkers (1990). They found that the relative risks for developing leukemia/lymphoma were 5.6, 62.1 and 77.3 times greater in cats infected with FIV, FeLV, and FeLV/FIV, respectively. Lymphoid tumors tended to occur in FeLV-infected cats with a mean age of 3.8 years, and in FIV-infected cats with a mean age of 8.7 years (Shelton et al., 1990). Lymphoid tumors in FIV-infected cats have been usually associated with the head and neck (nasopharyngeal lymphomas). Lymphoid tumors in the nasal passages appear to arise out of surrounding plasmacytic-lymphocytic inflammation and to be of the B-cell type.

Myeloproliferative disorders have also been seen in some FeLV negative, FIV-infected cats that presented with severe anemias and leukopenias (Belford et al., 1989; Ishida et al., 1989; Pedersen, unpublished observation, 1989; Yamamoto et al., 1989). A myeloproliferative disorder has been induced in a specific-pathogen-free cat experimentally infected with just FIV for several months (Pedersen et al., 1987; Yamamoto et al., 1988), suggesting that FIV may be directly oncogenic. It is interesting to note that myeloid neoplasms and myelodysplasias (preleukemias) are common in cats, and only 70% of them can be directly linked to FeLV infection (Blue et al., 1988). It appears, therefore, that FIV might be another retrovirus cause of myeloid leukemias and myelodysplasias in cats.

FIV infection has also been diagnosed in some older cats with squamous cell and mammary gland carcinomas (Hopper et al., 1989; Ishida et al., 1989; Kraegel, unpublished observation, 1989). The rate of FIV infection among cats with squamous cell carcinomas of the mouth and skin at the School of Veterinary Medicine, University of California, Davis, has been around 10–20%, which appears higher than chance. However, cats with squamous cell carcinomas tend to be older, more often male, and inevitably outdoor roaming, all of which are risk factors for FIV infection as well. More studies are needed before FIV can be considered a cofactor of solid tumors of cats such as squamous cell carcinomas.

Shelton and coworkers (1990) observed feline sarcoma virus induced fibrosarcomas in two cats that were co-infected with both FeLV and FIV, which seemed unusual. Ishida and coworkers (1989) described FIV-infected cats with FeLV negative multicentric sarcomas. Hopper and coworkers (1989) reported a seemingly high incidence of various rare types of tumors in FIV-infected cats. Much more research needs to be done before it can be said with certainty that any of these unusual tumors of cats are etiologically related to FIV infection.

### Clinicopathologic features

FIV infection is currently diagnosed by detecting antibodies in the blood. Since cats do not recover from FIV infection, there is a direct correlation between the presence of antibodies and virus infection (Yamamoto et al., 1989). Antibodies can be detected by an indirect fluorescent antibody (IFA) assay using FIV-infected T-lymphocyte enriched peripheral blood mononuclear or Crandell feline kidney cells as a substrate, or by ELISA or Western blotting using gradient-purified tissue culture grown virus as a source of antigen (Pedersen et al., 1987; O'Connor et al., 1989; Yamamoto et al., 1988). Antibodies usually appear within 2–4 weeks of experimental infection and remain at detectable levels more or less for the rest of the animal's life (Yamamoto et al., 1988; O'Connor et al., 1989). However, a small proportion of experimentally infected cats may not demonstrate antibodies for up to a year following infection (Yamamoto et al., 1988).

The ELISA test suffers from a low percentage of false positives, perhaps in the order of 2% or less. False positive reactions are particularly troublesome in low-risk groups of cats, such as purebred catteries where testing is often required as a condition for sale. In such environments, the incidence of false positive serological reactions may actually exceed the true incidence of the infection. Such cats are heavily vaccinated and often have serum antibodies against cat cell antigens. Cat cell and tissue culture antigens often contaminate antigen preparations used for most ELISAs, because the virus is propagated in cat cell cultures. The Western blot and IFA tests are not quite as sensitive as ELISA, but may be more specific. However, care must be taken in reading weak bands of reaction in the 25 and 70 kDa regions of the immunoblot strips. Many cats have low levels of antibodies that react against non-viral proteins that band in these regions. The indirect immunofluorescent antibody test is also not entirely fool-proof, because the titer of antibodies in many cat sera is very low and the test is often read at the limits of its sensitivity. If FIV-infected T-lymphocytes are used as the substrate, a non-specific reaction can occur if the sera contain anti-lymphocyte antibodies.

A small proportion of cats never have detectable levels of antibody in their blood, yet have recoverable virus in their peripheral blood lymphocytes (Harbour et al., 1988; Hopper et al., 1988, 1989; Torten and Pedersen, unpublished observation, 1989). These cats may be analogous to the sexual partners of AIDS patients who have genomic virus in their body by the polymerase chain reaction (PCR) or virus isolation for years prior to seroconversion (Imagawa et al., 1989; Pezzella et al., 1989). Tests that detect viral antigen in the blood, similar to those used in FeLV testing, are being researched at this time (Yamamoto and Hansen, unpublished information, 1989). The level of antigen in the blood of FIV-infected cats is so low, however, that the specificity of antigen detection then becomes a problem. It appears that virus culture and PCR are the only tests that are presently sensitive enough to detect most of these seronegative animals.

Cats with FIV infection may show abnormalities in their hemograms that can alert clinicians to its presence. About one-half to two-thirds of clinically ill cats will show some degree of leukopenia and/or anemia (Yamamoto et al., 1989). The leukopenia in the initial stage of the experimentally induced infection is usually due to an absolute neutropenia (Yamamoto et al., 1988b). Leukopenia in naturally infected cats in the AIDS phase of illness can be associated with neutropenia and/or lymphopenia (Yamamoto et al., 1989). The anemia is of the depression or regenerative type, and bone marrow aspirates range from hyperplastic, to dysplastic, to aplastic, or to neoplastic.

## Infection and immunity

Antibodies to the 24, 41, and 50 kDa virion proteins are the first to appear in the serum following experimental infection, followed shortly by antibodies to the 10, 15, 31, and 62 kDa proteins (Yamamoto et al., 1988b; O'Connor et al., 1989). Antibodies to the major envelope protein, gp110/130, appear rather early in the course of infection and tend to remain high throughout the subsequent disease course (O'Connor et al., 1989). Unfortunately, gp120 antibodies are usually not measurable by ELISA or Western blotting. The envelope proteins are easily sheared from the virions during the purification of the ELISA and Western blot antigen. Envelope antibodies are most easily visualized by RIP-PAGE assay (O'Connor et al., 1989; Steinman et al., 1989). Virus neutralizing antibodies have not yet been studied in the FIV system.

Feline immunodeficiency virus is relatively easy to isolate from the blood during the initial and terminal stages of the disease. Isolation during the interim period of normalcy is more difficult. The easiest tissues for isolation are the bone marrow and the peripheral blood mononuclear cells. The viral genome is most prevalent by PCR in the bone marrow, followed by the mesenteric lymph nodes and the blood (Pedersen et al., 1989). The virus can be readily recovered from peritoneal macrophages, where it is present as a latent infection (Brunner and Pedersen, 1989).

## Treatment and prevention

Most FIV-infected cats in the AIDS phase of illness are treated symptomatically and supportively. Secondary and opportunistic infections often respond well to treatment in the early stages of infection, but become more and more refractory to treatment with time. This probably reflects the steady deterioration of the immune system that is occurring in the face of therapy. Specific anti-viral drugs, such as azidothymidine, have been used successfully in HIV-infected AIDS patients (Fischl et al., 1987). They have not been studied extensively in FIV-infected cats. Corticosteroid therapy may be helpful in controlling immunologic diseases in cats without AIDS-like complications.

The disease can best be prevented by keeping cats out of high risk environments excluding high risk practices. Basically, cats should be neutered, kept indoors whenever possible, and not exposed to new homeless, feral, abandoned, or stray cats without those cats being first tested for the virus.

## Public health considerations

There is no evidence that would link FIV infection to any human disease, and most especially AIDS. The virus is antigenically and genetically distinct from HIV, and appears to be highly species adapted (Egberink et al., 1989; O'Connor et al., 1989; Olmsted et al., 1989; Pedersen et al., 1987; Steinman et al., 1989; Talbot et al., 1989; Yamamoto et al., 1988b). Species adaptation is characteristic of all retroviruses, including lentiviruses, and although there is some evidence that retroviruses do cross species, this adaptation occurs over eons of time. Once retroviruses adapt themselves to a new host, they become species specific. There is no evidence that a lentivirus infection of one species of animal readily transmits itself back and forth to another. Limited studies have failed to identify FIV antibodies in people that have had intimate contact with FIV-infected cats and people that have been bitten by infected animals or inadvertently or accidentally injected themselves with virus-containing material (Yamamoto et al., 1989).

## FIV infection as an animal model for human AIDS

An ideal animal model for HIV infection of man should be caused by a genetically similar virus, it should cause as nearly identical disease as possible, the temporal evolution (pathogenesis) of the resulting disease should be similar, and the model should be easily accessible to all researchers. Feline immunodeficiency virus infection of cats meets all of these criteria. Several areas where FIV infection might be particularly useful as an animal model include: (1) cofactor studies; (2) the role of macrophages as lentivirus reservoirs; (3) vaccine strategies; and (4) drug testing in vitro and in vivo.

The role of incidental infectious diseases as cofactors for human AIDS is an important area of study. Of particular interest is whether immune stimulation caused by other diseases will accelerate the course of HIV infection from the asymptomatic to the AIDS stage of illness (Lane and Fauci, 1985; Quinn et al., 1987; Rosenberg and Fauci, 1989; Zagury et al., 1986). It has recently been shown that FeLV infection will greatly potentiate the severity and time course of both the primary and secondary stages of FIV infection (Pedersen et al., 1989). Specific-pathogen-free (SPF) cats with pre-existing persistent asymptomatic FeLV infections developed an extremely severe primary illness when subsequently infected with FIV. Dually infected cats that survived the initial stage of FIV infection tended to be more anemic than control cats infected with either virus alone, and their T4/T8 lymphocyte ratios were chronically inverted. Co-infection of asymptomatic FeLV carrier cats with FIV did not increase the levels of FeLV-p27 (major core protein) antigen present in their blood over that seen in cats infected with FeLV alone. The amount of proviral FIV DNA was greatly increased, however, in dually infected cats compared to cats that were infected just with FIV. There was a greater expression of FIV DNA in lymphoid tissues, where the genome was normally detected, and in non-lymphoid tissues where FIV DNA was not usually found. These findings indicated that it was the FIV infection that was potentiated by the asymptomatic FeLV infection, and not *vice versa.* It is interesting to note that HTLV-I infection of man will potentiate the severity of HIV-1 infection (Bartholomew et al., 1987), and that the less pathogenic HIV-2 infection will also potentiate AIDS caused by the more pathogenic HIV-1 infection (de Thé, 1987).

The immunopathogenesis of HIV infection could be studied using the FIV model system. Feline immunodeficiency virus and HIV differ considerably in genetic make-up (Olmsted et al., 1989; Talbot et al., 1989), yet both cause virtually identical diseases. It would be interesting, therefore, to see which of the conserved regions between HIV, SIV and FIV might be responsible for their immunological effects. At a more mechanistic level, it should also be possible to follow FIV-infected cats for long periods of time and to study events that precede the demise of their immune systems. Studies of the immune system of the cat have been previously restricted because of the limited numbers of reagents. Recently, however, monoclonal antibodies to panB, MHC-I and II antigens, CD4, and CD8 cell surface antigens have become available (Moore, Rideout, Levy and Pedersen, unpublished observations, 1989; Klotz and Cooper, 1986; Ackley et al., 1989).

The role of macrophages as reservoirs for HIV and for its immunopathogenicity is a topic of interest in human AIDS research (Narayan et al., 1987; Pauza, 1988; Roy and Wainberg, 1988). Preliminary experiments indicate that the FIV model can be used for such studies (Brunner and Pedersen, 1989). Peritoneal macrophages harvested from normal SPF cats could be infected with FIV in vitro. Following an initial stage of virus replication, the infection becomes latent. Virus can be recovered from latently infected macrophages by phorbol myristate acetate treatment and cocultivation with T-lymphocyte rich peripheral blood mononuclear cells.

The simian immunodeficiency virus (SIV) model is currently the main animal system for vaccine research. However, primates are difficult to obtain in large numbers, expensive to keep, and difficult to handle. With the development of appropriate genetic probes and publication of the entire viral genome (Olmsted et al., 1989; Talbot et al., 1989), it is now possible to research many of the same vaccine strategies in cats.

The reverse transcriptase is biologically identical to that of HIV and SIV (North et al., 1989). This means that FIV could be used instead of HIV for the development and assay of anti-lentivirus drugs. The ready availability of cats with naturally acquired FIV infection and AIDS-like diseases also opens the way for in vivo testing of promising anti-viral drugs.

## References

Ackley, C.D., Hoover, E.A. and Cooper, M.D. (1990) Identification of a CD4 homologue in the cat. *Tissue Antigens* 35, 92–98.

Barlough, J.E., Ackler, C.D., George, J.W., Levy, N., Acevedo, R., Moore, P., Rideout, B., Cooper, M.D. and Pedersen, N.C. (1990) Acquired immune dysfunction in cats with experimental induced feline immunodeficiency virus infection: comparison of short-term and long-term infections. *J. AIDS* (in press).

Bartholomew, C., Blattner, W. and Cleghorn, F. (1987) Progression to AIDS in homosexual men co-infected with HIV and HTLV-I in Trinidad. *Lancet* ii, 1469.

Belford, C.J., Miller, R.I., Mitchell, G., Rahaley, R.S. and Menrath, V.H. (1989) Evidence of feline immunodeficiency virus in Queensland cats: preliminary observations. *Aust. Vet. Practit.* 19, 4–6.

Bennett, M., McCracken, C., Lutz, H., Gaskell, C.J., Gaskell, R.M., Brown, A. and Knowles, J.O. (1989) Prevalence of antibody to feline immunodeficiency virus in some cat populations. *Vet. Rec.* 124, 397–398.

Blue, J.T., French, T.W. and Kranz, J.S. (1988) Non-lymphoid hematopoietic neoplasia in cats: a retrospective study of 60 cases. *Cornell Vet.* 78, 21–42.

Brown, A., Bennett, M. and Gaskell, C.J. (1989) Fatal poxvirus infection in association with FIV infection. *Vet. Rec.* 124, 19–20.

Brunner, D. and Pedersen, N.C. (1989) Infection of peritoneal macrophages in vitro and in vivo with feline immunodeficiency virus. *J. Virol.* 63, 5483–5488.

Chalmers, S., Schick, R.O. and Jeffers, J. (1989) Demodicosis in two cats seropositive for feline immunodeficiency virus. *J. Am. Vet. Med. Ass.* 194, 256–257.

de Thé, G. (1988) HIV-1 and HIV-2 epidemiology and disease association in Ivory Coast. In: *Proc. 2nd Colloque des Cent Gardes, Retroviruses of Human A.I.D.S. and Related Retrovirus Diseases,* Marnes-La-Coquette, Paris, October 28–30, 1987, pp. 51–54.

Egberink, H.E., Ederveen, J., Montelaro, R.C., Pedersen, N.C., Horzinek, M.C. and Koolen, M.J.M. (1990) Intracellular proteins of feline immunodeficiency virus (FIV) and their antigenic relationship to equine infectious anemia virus (EIAV). *J. Gen. Virol.* 71, 739–743.

Fischl, M.A., Richman, D.D., Grieco, M.H. et al. (1987) The efficacy of azidothymidine (AZT) in the treatment of patients with AIDS and AIDS-related complex: a double-blind, placebo controlled trial. *N. Engl. J. Med.* 317, 185–191.

Grindem, C.B., Corbett, W.T., Ammermann, B.E. and Tomkins, M.T. (1989) Seroepidemiologic survey of feline immunodeficiency virus infection in cats of Wake County, North Carolina. *J. Am. Vet. Med. Ass.* 194, 226–228.

Gruffyd-Jones, T.J., Hopper, C.D., Harbour, D.A. and Lutz, H. (1988) Serological evidence of feline immunodeficiency virus infection in UK cats from 1975–76. *Vet. Rec.* 123, 569–570.

Harbour, D.A., Williams, P.D., Gruffydd-Jones, T.J., Burbridge, J. and Pearson, G.R. (1988) Isolation of a T-lymphotropic lentivirus from a persistently leucopenic domestic cat. *Vet. Rec.* 122, 84–86.

Hopper, C., Sparkes, A., Gruffydd-Jones, T.J. and Harbour, D.A. (1988) Feline T-lymphotropic virus infection (letter). *Vet. Rec.* 122, 590.

Hopper, C.D., Sparkes, A.H., Gruffyd-Jones, T.J., Crispin, S.M., Harbour, D.A. and Stokes, C.R. (1989) Clinical and laboratory findings in cats infected with feline immunodeficiency virus. *Vet. Rec.* 125, 341–346.

Hosie, M.J., Robertson, C. and Jarrett, O. (1989) Prevalence of feline leukemia virus and antibodies to feline immunodeficiency virus in cats in the United Kingdom. *Vet. Rec.* 128, 293–297.

Imagawa, D.T., Lee, M.H., Wolinsky, S.M., Sano, K., Morales, F., Kwok, S., Sninsky, J.J., Nishanian, P.G., Giorgi, J., Fahey, J.L., Dudley, J., Visscher, B.R. and Detels, R. (1989) Human immunodeficiency virus type 1 infection in homosexual men who remain seronegative for prolonged periods. *N. Engl. J. Med.* 320, 1458–1462.

Ishida, T., Washizu, T., Toriyabe, K. and Motoyoshi, S. (1988) Detection of a feline T lymphotropic lentivirus (FTLV) infection in Japanese domestic cats. *Jpn. J. Vet. Sci.* 50, 39–44.

Ishida, T., Washizu, T., Toriyabe, K., Motoyoshi, S. and Pedersen, N.C. (1989) Feline immunodeficiency virus (FIV) infection in Japan. *J. Am. Vet. Med. Ass.* 194, 221–225.

Klotz, F.W., and Cooper, M.D. (1986) A feline thymocyte antigen defined by a monoclonal antibody (FT2) identifies a subpopulation of non-helper cells capable of specific cytotoxicity. *J. Immunol.* 136, 2510–2514.

Knowles, J.O., Gaskell, R.M., Gaskell, C.J., Harvey, C.E. and Lutz, H. (1989) Prevalence of feline calicivirus, feline leukaemia virus and antibodies to FIV in cats with chronic stomatitis. *Vet. Rec.* 124, 336–338.

Lane, H.C. and Fauci, A.S. (1985) Immunologic abnormalities in the acquired immunodeficiency syndrome. *Annu. Rev. Immunol.* 3, 477–500.

Lutz, H., Egberink, H., Arnold, P., Winkler, G., Wolfensberger, C., Jarrett, O., Parodi, A.L., Pedersen, N.C. and Horzinek, M.C. (1988) Felines T-lymphotropes Lentivirus (FTLV): Experimentelle Infektion und Vorkommen in einigen Ländern Europas. *Kleintierpraxis* 33, 445–492.

Moore, F.M., Emerson, W.E., Cotter, S.M. and DeLellis, R.A. (1986) Distinctive peripheral lymph node hyperplasia of young cats. *Vet. Pathol.* 23, 386–391.

Narayan, O., Clemments, J., Kennedy-Stoskopf, S., Sheffer, D. and Royal, W. (1987) Mechanisms of escape of visna lentiviruses from immunological control. *Contrib. Microbiol. Immunol.* 8, 60–79.

North, T.W., North, G.L.T. and Pedersen, N.C. (1989) Feline immunodeficiency virus, a model for reverse transcriptase-targeted chemotherapy for acquired immune deficiency syndrome. *Antimicrobial Agents Chemother.* 33, 915–919.

O'Connor, T.P. Jr., Tanguay, S., Steinman, R., Smith, R., Barr, M.C., Yamamoto, J.K., Pedersen, N.C., Andersen, P.R. and Tonelli, Q.J. (1989) Development and evaluation of immunoassay for detection of antibodies to feline T-lymphotropic lentivirus (feline immunodeficiency virus). *J. Clin. Microbiol.* 27, 474–479.

Olmsted, R.A., Barnes, A.K., Yamamoto, J.K., Hirsch, V.M., Purcell, R.H. and Johnson, P.R. (1989) Molecular cloning of feline immunodeficiency virus. *Proc. Natl. Acad. Sci. U.S.A.* 86, 2448–2452.

Pauza, C.D. (1988) HIV persistence in monocytes leads to pathogenesis and AIDS. *Cell. Immunol.* 112, 414–424.

Pedersen, N.C. (1987) Feline syncytium-forming virus infection. In: J. Holzworth (Ed.), *Diseases of the Cat.* W.B. Saunders Co., Philadelphia, PA pp. 268–278.

Pedersen, N.C., Theilen, G.H., Keane, M.A., Fairbanks, L., Mason, T., Orser, B., Chen, C. and Allison, C. (1977) Studies on naturally transmitted feline leukemia virus infection. *Am. J. Vet. Res.* 38, 1523–1531.

Pedersen, N.C., Ho, E., Brown, M.L. and Yamamoto, J.K. (1987) Isolation of a T lymphotropic virus from domestic cats with an immunodeficiency-like syndrome. *Science* 235, 790–793.

Pedersen, N.C., Torten, M., Rideout, B., Sparger, E., Tonachini, T., Luciw, P., Ackley, C., Levy, N. and Yamamoto, J. (1990) Feline leukemia virus infection as a potentiating cofactor for the primary and secondary stages of experimentally induced feline immunodeficiency virus infection. *J. Virol.* 64, 598–606.

Pezzella, M., Mannella, E., Mirolo, M. et al. (1989) HIV genome in peripheral blood mononuclear cells of seronegative regular sexual partners of HIV-infected subjects. *J. Med. Virol.* 28, 209–214.

Quinn, T.C., Piot, P., McCormick, J.B., Feinsod, F.M., Taelman, H., Kapita, B., Stevens, W. and Fauci, A.S. (1987) Serologic and immunologic studies in patients with AIDS in North America and Africa. The potential role of infectious agents as cofactors in human immunodeficiency virus infection. *J. Am. Med. Ass.* 257, 2617–2621.

Rosenberg, Z.F. and Fauci, A.S. (1989) Immunopathogenic mechanisms of HIV infection. *Clin. Immunol. Immunopathol.* 50, 5149–5156.

Roy, S. and Wainberg, M.A. (1988) Role of the mononuclear phagocyte in the development of the acquired immunodeficiency syndrome (AIDS). *J. Leukocyte Biol.* 43, 91–97.

Sabine, M., Michelsen, J., Thomas, F. and Zheng, M. (1988) Feline AIDS. *Aust. Vet. Practit.* 18, 105–107.

Shelton, G.H., Abkowitz, J.L., Linenberger, M.L., Russell, R.G. and Grant, C.K. (1989a) Chronic leukopenia associated with feline immunodeficiency virus infection in a cat. *J. Am. Vet. Med. Ass.* 194, 253–255.

Shelton, G.H., McKim, K.D., Cooley, P.L., Dice, P.F., Russell, R.G. and Grant, C.K. (1989b) Feline leukemia virus and feline immunodeficiency virus infections in a cat with lymphoma. *J. Am. Vet. Med. Ass.* 194, 249–252.

Shelton, G.H., Waltier, R.M., Connor, S.C. and Grant, C.K. (1989c) Prevalence of feline immunodeficiency virus infections in pet cats. *J. Am. Anim. Hosp. Ass.* 25, 7–12.

Shelton, G.H., Grant, C.K., Cotter, S.M., Gardner, M.B., Hardy, W.D. Jr. and DiGiacomo, R.F. (1990) Feline immunodeficiency virus (FIV) and feline leukemia virus (FeLV) infections and their relationships to lymphoid malignancies in cats: a retrospective study (1968–1988). *J. AIDS* 3, 623–630.

Steinman, R., Dombrowski, J., O'Connor, T., Tonelli, Q., Montelaro, R., Lawrence, K., Seymour, C., Goodness, J., Pedersen, N. and Andersen, P.R. (1990) Biochemical and immunological characterization of the major structural proteins of feline immunodeficiency virus. *J. Gen. Virol.* 71, 701–706.

Swinney, G.R., Pauli, J.V., Jones, B.R. and Wilks, C.R. (1989) Feline T-lymphotropic virus (FTLV) (feline immunodeficiency virus infection) in cats in New Zealand. *N.Z. Vet. J.* 37, 41–43.

Talbot, R.L., Sparger, E.E., Lovelace, K.M., Fitch, W.M., Pedersen, N.C., Luciw, P.A. and Elder, J.H. (1989) Nucleotide sequence and genomic organization of feline immunodeficiency virus. *Proc. Natl. Acad. Sci. U.S.A.* 86, 5743–5747.

van der Riet, F. de St. J., Sayed, A.R., Hess, A., Hazell, R.W. and Pedersen, N.C. (1988) Serologic evidence for feline immunodeficiency virus infection in Southern Africa. *Small Anim. Vet. Med.* 1, 122.

Witt, C.J., Moench, T.R., Gittelsohn, A.M., Bishop, B.D. and Childs, J.E. (1989) Epidemiologic observations on feline immunodeficiency virus and *Toxoplasma gondii* coinfection in cats in Baltimore, MD. *J. Am. Vet. Med. Ass.* 194, 229–233.

Yamamoto, J.K., Pedersen, N.C., Ho, E.W., Okuda, T. and Theilen, G.H. (1988a) Feline immunodeficiency syndrome-A comparison between feline T-lymphotropic lentivirus and feline leukemia virus. *Leukemia* 2 (Suppl.), 204S–215S.

Yamamoto, J.K., Sparger, E., Ho, E.W., Andersen, P.R., O'Connor, P., Mandell, C.P., Lowenstine, L., Munn, R. and Pedersen, N.C. (1988b) The pathogenesis of experimentally induced feline immunodeficiency virus (FIV) infection in cats. *Am. J. Vet. Res.* 49, 1246–1258.

Yamamoto, J.K., Hansen, H., Ho, E.W., Morishita, T.Y., Okuda, T., Sawa, T.R., Nakamura, R.M., Kau, W.P. and Pedersen, N.C. (1989) Epidemiologic and clinical aspects of feline immunodeficiency virus infection in cats from the continental United States and Canada and possible mode of transmission. *J. Am. Vet. Med. Ass.* 194, 213–220.

Zagury, D., Bernard, J., Leonard, R., Cheynier, R., Feldman, M., Sarin, P.S. and Gallo, R.C. (1986) Long term cultures of HTLV-III-infected cells: a model of cytopathology of T-cell depletion in AIDS. *Science* 231, 850–853.

*Eds. H. Schellekens and M.C. Horzinek*
*Animal Models in AIDS*



# 19

# Feline immunodeficiency virus (FIV): a model for antiviral chemotherapy

MARCK KOOLEN and HERMAN EGBERINK

Institute of Virology, Department of Infectious Diseases and Immunology, School of Veterinary Medicine, State University of Utrecht, 3584 CL Utrecht, The Netherlands

**Summary**

Feline immunodeficiency virus (FIV) was used as a model to study the effect of antiretroviral chemotherapeutics on an immunosuppressive lentivirus infection in vitro and in vivo. The antiviral activity of different nucleoside analogues with known anti-HIV activity was tested on FIV-infected feline thymocytes. Subsequently, the prophylactic and therapeutic effect of the compound 9-(2-phosphonomethoxyethyl)adenine (PMEA) on FIV infection was studied in vivo.

PMEA caused a dose-dependent suppression of FIV replication and virus-specific antibody production. Diseased animals with clinical signs of opportunistic infections recovered after treatment with PMEA. Thus, FIV infection in cats is a suitable model to study the efficacy of antiretroviral compounds on immunosuppressive lentivirus infections.

## FIV as a model for antiviral chemotherapy studies

Feline immunodeficiency virus (FIV) is a recently identified lentivirus (E-type retrovirus) which is widespread in the feline population (Pedersen et al., 1987). In cats the infection is characterized by a primary transient illness of several weeks or even years during which virus can be demonstrated (Yamamoto et al., 1988; Harbour et al., 1988). Subsequently, clinical abnormalities may develop consisting of behavioral changes, anorexia, weight loss, stomatitis, gingivitis, rhinitis, diarrhea, pustular dermatitis, anemia and generalized lymphadenopathy (Hardy, 1988). Ultimately, FIV-infected cats may die of opportunistic infections.

Feline immunodeficiency virus replicates in feline peripheral blood mononuclear cells, thymocytes and splenocytes stimulated with concanavalin A (conA; 5 $\mu g/ml$) and maintained on recombinant human interleukin-2 (IL-2; 100 U/ml). Besides in cells of the lymphoid and myeloid lineage, FIV can also infect and replicate in primary feline brain cell cultures. Astrocytes can be infected in vitro as has been demonstrated by double immunofluorescence staining using

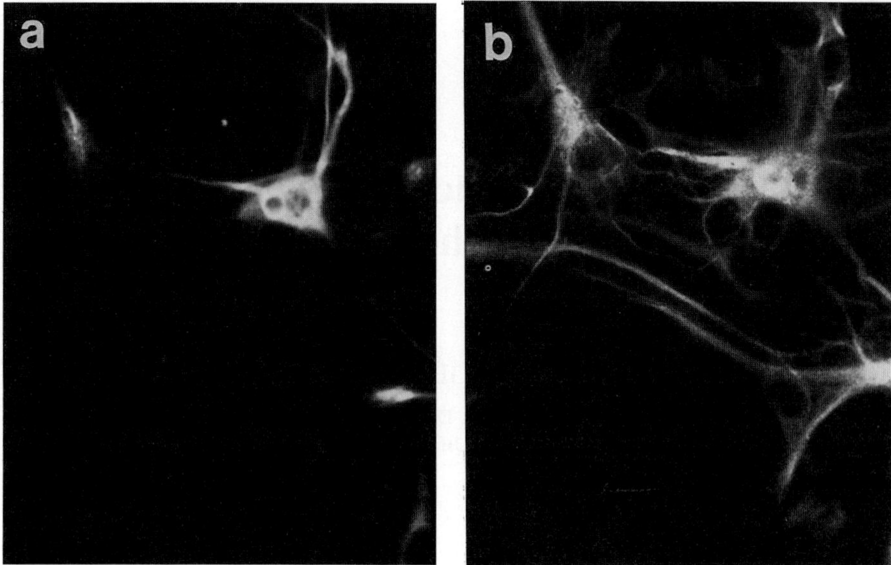


Fig. 1. Double immunofluorescence studies performed on primary feline brain tissue cultures infected with FIV. FIV antigen and astrocytes were stained with (a) polyclonal cat anti-FIV and (b) rabbit anti-glial fibrillary acidic protein antibodies.

specific antibodies to FIV antigens and to glial fibrillary acidic protein, a specific marker of astrocytes (Fig. 1).

With respect to cell tropism and outcome of disease, FIV infection of cats parallels the life threatening disease acquired immunodeficiency syndrome (AIDS) in many aspects (Ishida et al., this volume). Steps taken toward developing new efficacious treatments against this fatal disease have been focused on the crucial steps of the replication cycle of the virus. One of the major issues is the reverse transcriptase protein. Zidovudine (3′-azido-2′,3′-dideoxythymidine; AZT) and other nucleoside analogues operate at the level of the synthesis of DNA from viral RNA. This reaction is catalyzed by the enzyme reverse transcriptase. Despite toxic side effects and evidence that AZT resistance is developing among strains of human immunodeficiency virus type 1 (HIV-1), lives of AIDS patients are extended. Many other drugs that work on the same principle as AZT are being tested and may soon be available to treat AIDS patients. However, the development of drug-resistant strains after approximately 6 months of use is somewhat troubling. Molecular cloning studies of the reverse transcriptase gene revealed that many amino acids are changed but these changes cannot be linked to the enzymatic activity of the polypeptide. Cross-resistance to AZT is limited to 3′-azido-2′,3′-dideoxyuridine, a closely related nucleoside. AZT-resistant HIV strains appear not to be resistant to other reverse transcriptase inhibitors. Treatment of AIDS patients by using a regime of an alternating drug therapy offers hope that resistance can be eluded. Therefore, the demand for efficacious, specific and less toxic drugs becomes stronger. Up to now the development and testing of potential antiretroviral compounds of HIV has been postponed due to the lack of an ideal animal model. The FIV infection model in cats meets the major criteria of such a model; an immunosuppressive lentivirus that with respect to the pathogenesis causes a disease with many parallels to AIDS in man and is easily accessible to all researchers (Pedersen, this volume; Ishida et al., this volume).

The nucleoside analogues, AZT, PMEA (9-(phosphonomethoxy-ethyl)adenine) and FddClUrd (3′-fluoro-2′,3′-dideoxy-5-chlorouridine) with known anti-HIV activity in vitro (Balzarini et al., 1989) were tested for their potential to inhibit FIV replication in feline thymocytes in vitro. Cells were stimulated with concanavalin A (5 $\mu$g/ml) and maintained on recombinant interleukin-2. One hour prior to infection cells ($1 \times 10^6$ cells/ml) were incubated with different concentrations of the drugs. Cells were either infected with the Utrecht isolate FIV-113 or mock-infected. After 4 and 6 days of culturing in the presence of the drugs, culture medium supernatants were harvested and assayed for the presence of reverse transcriptase activity. The 50% effective dose ($ED_{50}$), defined as the concentration of compound that reduced the reverse transcriptase activity by 50% as compared to untreated control cultures, was determined. In addition, the 50% cytotoxic dose ($CD_{50}$), corresponding to the concentration of compound that reduced the number of viable mock-infected cells by 50%, was determined by the trypan blue exclusion method. Of the compounds listed in Table 1, AZT emerged as the most potent and selective inhibitor of FIV replication in feline thymocytes ($ED_{50}$: 0.05 $\mu$M), followed by PMEA ($ED_{50}$: 0.60 $\mu$M) and FddClUrd ($ED_{50}$: 4 $\mu$M). These data are in agreement with previously reported values for AZT and PMEA in HIV-infected MT-4 cells and Moloney murine sarcoma virus (MSV)-induced transformation of murine C3H embryo fibroblasts (Balzarini et al., 1989). The $CD_{50}$ values of all three compounds tested were 2.5–200 times greater than the $ED_{50}$ values.

## Effect of PMEA on FIV infection in vivo

The half-life of PMEA in vivo was determined in 4 month old kittens. Subsequently, the prophylactic and therapeutic effects of the drug on FIV infection were studied during 35 days. PMEA was administered intramuscularly twice a day at 12 h-intervals. Although full details have been published elsewhere

TABLE 1
Inhibitory effects of PMEA, AZT and FddClUrd on FIV replication in feline thymocytes

| Compound | $ED_{50}$ ($\mu$M) | $CD_{50}$ ($\mu$M) |
|---|---|---|
| PMEA | 0.60 | 80 |
| AZT | 0.05 | 120 |
| FddClUrd | 4.00 | $\geqslant$10 |

(Egberink et al., 1990) PMEA caused a dose-dependent suppression of FIV replication and virus-specific antibody production. Seropositive field cats with signs of opportunistic infection showed a marked clinical improvement during PMEA therapy (5 mg/kg/day). One cat showed a recurrence of symptoms 1 month after discontinuing therapy; again clinical improvement was observed when the same regime of PMEA treatment was applied. Four out of five cats are still healthy 10 months after therapy. However, virus could be isolated and antibody titers were not affected.

Opportunistic infections in cats are frequently associated with herpes- and calicivirus infections. As has been demonstrated (De Clercq et al., 1989) PMEA exhibits a dual antiviral activity, which may therefore broaden its therapeutic usefulness in controlling opportunistic infections.

In conclusion, feline immunodeficiency virus infection in cats is an excellent model to test the efficacy of selective anti-human immunodeficiency virus agents.

## Acknowledgements

We thank Drs. Jan Balzarini and Erik De Clercq for providing the necessary quantities of PMEA and FddClUrd and for their kind help and valuable discussions of these results. M.K. was supported by the TNO Primate Center, Rijswijk.

## References

Balzarini, J., Naesens, L., Herdewijn, P., Rosenberg, I., Holy, A., Pauwels, R., Baba, M., Johns, D.G. and De Clercq, E. (1989) Marked in vivo antiretrovirus activity of 9-(2-phosphonylmethoxyethyl)adenine, a selective anti-human immunodeficiency virus agent. *Proc. Natl. Acad. Sci. U.S.A.* 86, 332–336.

De Clercq, E., Holy, A. and Rosenberg, I. (1989) Efficacy of phosphonylmethoxyalkyl derivatives of adenine in experimental herpes simplex virus and vaccinia virus infections in vivo. *Antimicrobial Agents Chemother.* 33, 185–191.

Egberink, H., Borst, M., Niphuis, H., Balzarini, J., Neu, H., Schellekens, H., De Clercq, E., Horzinek, M. and Koolen, M. (1990) Suppression of feline immunodeficiency virus infection in vivo by 9-(2-phosphonomethoxyethyl)adenine. *Proc. Natl. Acad. Sci. U.S.A.* 87, 3087–3091.

Harbour, D.A., Williams, P.D., Gruffydd-Jones, T.J., Burbridge, J. and Pearson, G.R. (1988) Isolation of a T-lymphotropic lentivirus from a persistently leucopenic domestic cat. *Vet. Rec.* 122, 84–86.

Hardy, W.D. (1988) *J. Am. Anim. Hosp. Ass.* 24, 241–243.

Pedersen, N.C., Ho, E.W., Brown, M.L. and Yamamoto, J.K. (1987) Isolation of a T-lymphotropic virus from domestic cats with an immunodeficiency-like syndrome. *Science* 235, 790–793.

Yamamoto, J.K., Sparger, E., Ho, E.W., Andersen, P.R., O'Connor, P., Mandell, C.P., Lowenstine, L., Munn, R. and Pedersen, N.C. (1988) The pathogenesis of experimentally induced feline immunodeficiency virus (FIV) infection in cats. *Am. J. Vet. Res.* 49, 1246–1258.

*Eds. H. Schellekens and M.C. Horzinek*
*Animal Models in AIDS*



# 20

# Clinical and immunologic staging of feline immunodeficiency virus (FIV) infection

TAKUO ISHIDA, AKIKO TANIGUCHI, AKIHIRO KONNO, TSUKIMI WASHIZU and ISAMU TOMODA

Department of Clinical Pathology, Nippon Veterinary and Zootechnical College, 1-7-1 Kyonan-cho, Musashino, Tokyo 180, Japan

**Summary**

In order to elucidate the relationship between disease progress and immunologic alterations in feline immunodeficiency virus (FIV) infection, a classification of naturally infected cats into clinical stage groups was attempted on the basis of their clinical signs. As working criteria for clinical staging, those for human immunodeficiency virus (HIV) infection were used with some modifications based on clinical observations in naturally and experimentally infected cats. Of the five distinct stages described for HIV infection, the acute phase, asymptomatic carrier (AC), AIDS related complex (ARC), and acquired immunodeficiency syndrome (AIDS) were recognized in FIV infection. Naturally infected cats classified as AC, ARC, or AIDS were evaluated for concanavalin A (conA)-induced lymphocyte blastogenic activities using the glucose consumption assay. There was a significant decrease in lymphocyte responsiveness even in the AC phase. The loss of response became marked as the disease progressed to ARC and AIDS, with almost complete loss of mitogen response in the AIDS phase. In addition to the loss of lymphocyte function, the AIDS in FIV infection was characterized by marked emaciation, lymphopenia, anemia or pancytopenia, and post-mortem evidence of opportunistic infections and lymph node dysplasia.

## Introduction

Feline immunodeficiency virus (FIV), isolated from cats in 1986 by Pedersen and coworkers (1987), is a lentivirus with similar characteristics to human immunodeficiency virus (HIV), which causes acquired immunodeficiency syndrome (AIDS) in man (Barre-Sinoussi et al., 1983; Popovic et al., 1984). This feline virus is associated with a number of chronic disorders in cats, and the virus can be isolated from terminally ill cats showing AIDS-like diseases (Pedersen et al., 1987; Ishida et al., 1988, 1989). The close association of FIV with chronic disease problems has also been suggested by the observation that the infection is far more frequent in cats with chronic disorders than in clinically healthy cats

(Ishida et al., 1989; Yamamoto et al., 1989). The terminal AIDS-like stage has a great similarity to the human counterpart because opportunistic infections and neoplasms are common findings in such cats infected with FIV (Ishida et al., 1989).

Because of this clinical and virologic similarity to HIV infection and AIDS (Piot et al., 1984; Bowen et al., 1985; Niedt and Schinella, 1985), a similar pathogenesis of virus-induced T-lymphocyte deficiency (King, 1986; Lifson et al., 1986) has been considered (Yamamoto et al., 1989). In veterinary medicine, however, the lack of appropriate reagents to detect feline T-lymphocyte subpopulations has limited the use of immunologic evaluation of FIV infected cats.

The purpose of the present study is to document the presence of immunodeficiency and to investigate the relationship between disease progress and immunologic alterations occurring in infected cats. We have employed the lymphocyte blastogenesis test on peripheral blood lymphocytes which has been used for some time in small animal medicine (Cockerell et al., 1976; Cockerell and Hoover, 1977; Hebebrand et al., 1977). The FIV infected cats were first classified into one of the clinical stages using working criteria modified from those of HIV infection (CDC, 1986; Ishida and Tomoda, 1990), and the lymphocyte stimulation indices were compared between clinical stages and with those of healthy uninfected cats.

## Materials and methods

### Clinical staging

Working criteria for the clinical staging of FIV infection were developed on the basis of clinical observations and clinicopathologic findings in both naturally and experimentally infected cats with reference to the criteria for HIV infection staging (CDC, 1986; Ishida and Tomoda, 1990). The clinical findings were based on records of 700 FIV-infected animals showing various diseases (Ishida et al., 1989; Ishida and Tomoda, 1990). Classification mainly depended on the presence or absence of clinical signs characteristic of each stage.

### Animals

Five specific pathogen free (SPF) domestic short hair cats (two females and three males) were experimentally infected with FIV. They were 5–7 months of age, and feline leukemia virus (FeLV) p27 and FIV antibody negative. Twenty-seven naturally infected cats (seven females and 20 males), with positive FIV antibody titers, were used for the lymphocyte blastogenesis study. Their ages ranged between 2 and 11 years. Nine clinically healthy cats (three females and six males) free from FIV and FeLV infections, 2–3 years of age, were also used as uninfected controls. The infected cats were classified into stages using the working criteria described above. Another group of 12 FIV infected cats was obtained through veterinary hospitals and a local animal pound, and kept for clinical observations. They received symptomatic therapy as needed, and were observed for life.

### Experimental infection

An FIV isolate, Petaluma strain, was provided by Dr. N.C. Pedersen, University of California at Davis, and was propagated in interleukin-2 (rIL-2: Cetus Corporation, CA, U.S.A.) stimulated SPF cat peripheral blood lymphocyte culture (Pedersen et al., 1987; Ishida et al., 1988). The culture supernatant showing maximum cytopathic effect (CPE) was harvested and stored at $-80°$ C. A 1 ml aliquot was inoculated subcutaneously into the SPF cats.

### Serology

The rIL-2 stimulated FIV infected cat lymphocytes were used as the antigen for indirect immunofluorescence (IFA) (Pedersen et al., 1987; Ishida et al., 1988). Serum samples were tested for FIV antibody at a 1:10 dilution. Positive sera were then tested for confirmation by Western blot assay using electrophoresed FIV proteins (Pedersen et al., 1987; Ishida et al., 1988). The test for FeLV p27 viral antigen was carried out by a commercial enzyme-linked immunosorbent assay (ELISA) kit using monoclonal antibodies to this protein (Leukassay F: Pitmann-Moore, NJ, U.S.A.).

### Lymphocyte isolation

Heparinized peripheral blood was diluted 1:2 with Hanks' balanced salt solution (HBSS). Diluted blood (3–6 ml) was layered over 3 ml of Ficoll-Hypaque (SG: 1.077, Sigma, MO, U.S.A.), and was centrifuged at $250 \times g$ for 30 min. Mononuclear cells at the interface were harvested and washed three times with HBSS. The cell concentration was adjusted to $1 \times 10^6$ cells/ml in RPMI 1640 medium. The medium contained 10% fetal calf serum, 2 mM L-glutamine, 100 U/ml penicillin, and 100 $\mu$g/ml streptomycin. The cell suspension enriched with lymphocytes (> 95%) was cultured in triplicate with or without concanavalin A (conA) mitogen at 25 $\mu$g/ml under 5% $CO_2$ at 37°C for 120 h (Taniguchi et al., 1990).

### Lymphocyte blastogenic assay

The blastogenic activities of cultures were monitored by glucose consumption (Decock et al., 1980; Taniguchi et al., 1990). Supernatants of mitogen stimulated and control cultures were harvested and centrifuged at $500 \times g$ for 5 min. The glucose concentration (mg/dl) of the supernatant was determined by the glucose oxidase method employing spectrophotometry (AMCO, Tokyo, Japan). The stimulation index (SI) of each culture was calculated by the following formula;

$$\mathrm{SI}\ (\%) = \frac{\text{control culture glucose} - \text{stimulated culture glucose}}{\text{control culture glucose}} \times 100$$

## Results

### Experimental infection

All inoculated animals showed antibody to FIV p24 at 4–7 weeks post inoculation (p.i.) by Western blot immunoassay. One male cat (No. 1) showed lymphadenopathy in the submandibular and popliteal nodes starting 8 weeks p.i., and the rest showed it starting 10 weeks p.i. Cat 1 showed recurrent mild diarrhea associated with mild fever for 4 months, and hematologic examination revealed cyclic neutropenia. Cats 2 and 3 showed mild fever plus upper respiratory signs for 1 month. Cats 4 and 5 had repeated episodes of diarrhea of 1 week's duration over a 2 month period. Lymphadenopathy and other signs persisted for 7 months and 3 months, in No. 1 and the others, respectively. All animals were then asymptomatic with no abnormal hematologic findings, but were FIV antibody positive for 1 year.

### Clinical staging criteria

The case records of 700 FIV antibody positive cats were analyzed with reference to the clinical staging criteria for HIV infection (CDC, 1986; Ishida and Tomoda, 1990). The five clinical stages of FIV infection considered included acute phase, asymptomatic carrier (AC), persistent generalized lymphadenopathy (PGL), AIDS related complex (ARC) and AIDS (CDC, 1986). Clinical signs produced in experimental inoculation of SPF cats with a FIV isolate were also considered in establishing criteria for the early stages. The signs in the acute phase included lymphadenopathy, transient neutropenia, acute diarrhea and mild upper respiratory signs.

The mean ages for frequent clinical signs in 700 cases are presented in Table 1. These signs are classified into at least two groups according to the age of presentation: those seen in younger animals ($< 4.5$) and those seen in older animals ($> 5.0$). While enteritis, fever, lymphadenopathy and leukopenia tend to be detected in younger animals, chronic illnesses such as bacterial skin disease, upper respiratory disease, anemia, stomatitis and emaciation are seen in older animals, which may represent more advanced disease stages.

We first searched for acute phase FIV positive cases meeting the criteria based on experimental infection and field observations, including lymphadenopathy plus any of the acute phase signs, $< 2$ years of age, and FeLV negative. In the

TABLE 1
Mean age of FIV-infected cats with various clinical signs or clinicopathologic abnormalities

| Clinical signs | Age | SD |
|---|---|---|
| Enteritis | 4.0 | 2.3 |
| Fever of undetermined origin | 4.3 | 2.9 |
| Lymphadenopathy | 4.4 | 1.9 |
| Leukopenia | 4.5 | 3.3 |
| Chronic bacterial infection | 5.0 | 2.9 |
| Chronic upper respiratory disease | 5.0 | 3.2 |
| Chronic skin disease | 5.1 | 3.0 |
| Anemia | 6.1 | 3.2 |
| Stomatitis/gingivitis | 6.2 | 3.2 |
| Emaciation | 6.5 | 3.3 |

700 cases studied, there were 41 cases (5.9%) meeting the criteria, and thus they were considered to be in the acute phase.

In HIV infected individuals, the acute phase is followed by an asymptomatic period of variable duration (Reichert et al., 1983; CDC, 1986). In experimental FIV infection, the same transition has been documented. There were 74 (10.6%) healthy infected cats in the group studied here, which were considered to be asymptomatic carriers (AC). Consistent positive virus isolation from these cats also supports that they were infected carrier animals.

The mean age of those carriers was $4.2 \pm 3.2$ years as opposed to $5.3 \pm 3.1$ years in chronically ill cats, which suggests that the clinically healthy period may be followed by development of chronic illnesses. The asymptomatic carrier phase is followed by PGL in HIV infection, in which the patient is healthy except for lymphadenopathy. Although there were quite a few cats showing generalized lymphadenopathy comparable to the human PGL, all showed concurrent clinical sign(s), which made it impossible to classify these cats as PGL.

The ARC following PGL in HIV infection is characterized by fatigue, lymphadenopathy, night sweats, oral cavity disease, skin disease, and/or enteric disorders (CDC, 1986). In our cats, 537 out of 700 cases showed some chronic problems such as lymphadenopathy, stomatitis/gingivitis, skin disease, upper respiratory disease, and/or chronic enteric disease without marked emaciation. They were considered to be in the stage similar to human ARC.

In order to further prove the usefulness of this classification, we have selected FIV infected cats on the basis of the above working criteria of feline ARC, and a long-term clinical observation was performed. As shown in Table 2, all nine cats showed progression of disease and died within 8 months. They had anemia or pancytopenia and marked weight loss, and necropsy revealed lymphoid depletion and evidence of opportunistic infections suggestive of AIDS in all but one case. One out of nine cases died of bacterial pyothorax, but evidence of AIDS was not found post mortem.

On the basis of the above observations and the criteria for human AIDS (Reichert et al., 1983; CDC, 1986), we searched for FIV infected cats (FeLV

TABLE 2
Clinical observations on FIV infected cats classified as ARC

| Case | Age (years) | Time to death (months) | Necropsy diagnosis |
|---|---|---|---|
| 1328 | – [a] | 3 | AIDS [b] |
| 1397 | 7 | 3 | AIDS |
| 1461 | 3 | 6 | AIDS |
| 1573 | – | 2 | AIDS |
| 1575 | 5 | 4 | AIDS |
| 1579 | – | 5 | AIDS |
| 1609 | – | 3 | AIDS |
| 1616 | 6 | 8 | AIDS |
| 1628 | – | 7 | ARC (pyothorax) |

[a] unknown.
[b] based on the presence of lymphoid depletion, opportunistic infection or malignant neoplasm without other causes of immunodeficiency.

negative) with severe emaciation, anemia, and chronic diseases. Chronic renal failure and other readily diagnosed diseases which might give rise to immunologic disturbance were excluded. There were 48 (6.9%) such cats in our 700 and 36 (75%) of them had died within 6 months after FIV testing.

Three other FIV positive cats meeting these criteria were kept for observation, and they all died with severe wasting within 1 month (Table 3). Post-mortem revealed opportunistic infections as well as depletion in the lymph node which has been documented in human AIDS (Reichert et al., 1983).

Next, the clinical staging of 27 FIV antibody positive cats for the lymphocyte study was attempted using the working criteria described from above (Table 4). There were 13 clinically healthy cats, and they were considered AC. Of the 14 clinically ill cats, two had severe emaciation, anemia and opportunistic infections, and thus they were classified as AIDS. The remaining 12 cats showed moderate weight loss, lymphadenopathy, and some chronic diseases, and they were considered to be in the ARC phase. The distribution of clinical signs in each of the symptomatic cats is presented in Table 5. No cats were classified as pure PGL, since other clinical signs always accompanied the lymphadenopathy.

TABLE 3
Clinical observations on FIV infected cats previously diagnosed as AIDS

| Case | Age (years) | Time to death (months) | Necropsy diagnosis |
|---|---|---|---|
| 1167 | 6 | 1 | AIDS [a] |
| 1265 | 4 | 1 | AIDS |
| 1745 | 6 | 1 | AIDS |

[a] based on the presence of lymphoid depletion, opportunistic infection or malignant neoplasm without other causes of immunodeficiency.

TABLE 4
Clinical staging and disease manifestations of FIV infected cats

| Stage | Clinical signs or disease | Duration |
|---|---|---|
| Acute phase | Cyclic neutropenia, fever, lymphadenopathy | Weeks to months |
| Asymptomatic carrier (AC) | None | Years |
| Persistent generalized lymphadenopathy (PGL) | Generalized lymphadenopathy | Months? |
| AIDS-related complex (ARC) | Weight loss, chronic diarrhea, chronic upper respiratory disease, chronic stomatitis/gingivitis, chronic skin infections, lymphadenopathy | Months to 1 year |
| AIDS | ARC signs plus: emaciation, anemia or pancytopenia; Opportunistic infection and/or malignancy | Months |

TABLE 5
Clinical staging and disease manifestations of symptomatic FIV infected cats used for the blastogenesis study

| Case | Clinical stage | Stomatitis | Weight loss | Anemia | LAP | Other signs |
|---|---|---|---|---|---|---|
| 1 | ARC | + | + | − | + | |
| 2 | ARC | + | + | − | + | |
| 3 | ARC | + + | + | − | + + | |
| 4 | ARC | − | + | − | + | CURD |
| 5 | ARC | + | + | − | + | |
| 6 | ARC | + | + | − | + | |
| 7 | ARC | + | + | − | + | |
| 8 | ARC | − | + | + + | + | |
| 9 | ARC | + | + | − | + | |
| 10 | ARC | + + | + | − | + | |
| 11 | ARC | − | + | − | + | CURD |
| 12 | ARC | + + | + | − | + | |
| 13 | AIDS | + + | + + + | + + | − | OI, hepatitis |
| 14 | AIDS | + + | + + + | + + | − | OI, pneumonia |

+, present; + +, severe; + + +, very severe; −, absent.
LAP, lymphadenopathy; CURD, chronic upper respiratory disease; OI, opportunistic infection.

### Lymphocyte count

Peripheral blood total leukocyte counts in FIV infected cats were in the normal range except for the one case of AIDS (mean ± SD: AC, 17,560 ± 8377, ARC, 15,685 ± 5675, AIDS, 8785 ± 4221). While the lymphocyte counts of cats in the AC and ARC phases were normal, the AIDS group showed a significant

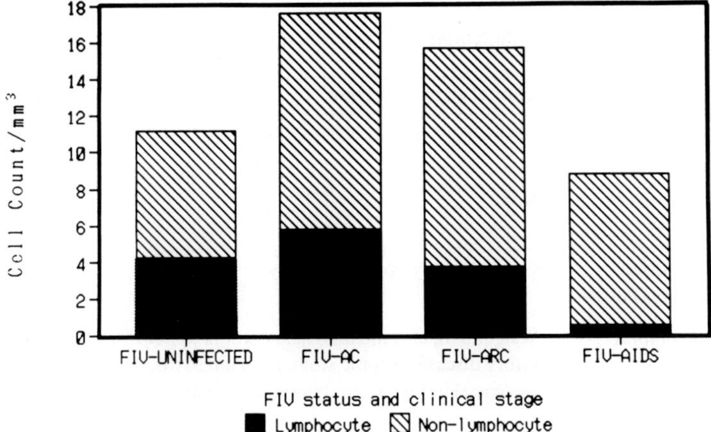


Fig. 1. The total leukocyte and lymphocyte count in peripheral blood of cats of different disease categories.

decrease ($P < 0.01$) as compared with ARC cats (mean ± SD: AC, 5774 ± 2896, ARC, 3705 ± 1266, AIDS, 528 ± 419) (Fig. 1).

### Lymphocyte blastogenic assay

ConA induced lymphocyte blastogenesis activity was measured by glucose consumption in the culture medium. The mean ± SD SIs of FIV infected cats were 51.2 ± 8.4, 22.4 ± 13.0, and 5.2 ± 4.9, in AC, ARC, and AIDS, respectively. These SI figures were all significantly lower ($P < 0.01$) than that of uninfected controls (mean ± SD 82.0 ± 10.7). There were significant differences between the AC and ARC ($P < 0.01$), and ARC and AIDS groups ($P < 0.05$) (Fig. 2). When the infected cats were classified into three groups according to their age, no

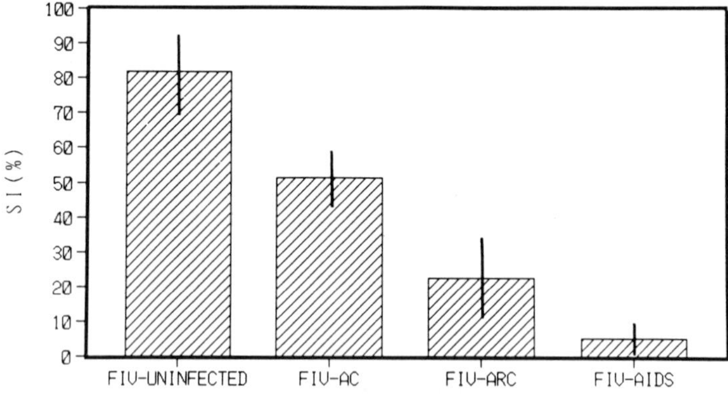


Fig. 2. Stimulation indices (SI) of peripheral blood lymphocytes with conA induced blastogenesis as determined by the glucose consumption assay.

significant difference was demonstrated between the groups. The mean ± SD SI values for each age groups were: < 5 years (n = 11), 43.1 ± 14.0, 6–8 years (n = 5), 40.24 ± 16.6; > 9 years (n = 5), 48.6 ± 17.5. No significant difference was observed between infected males and females: male, 34.2 ± 20.6; female, 44.5 ± 9.8.

## Discussion

The retrospective analysis of clinical records as well as clinical observations in naturally and experimentally infected cats suggested the possibility of clinically staging FIV infection into distinct stages comparable to those in HIV infection (Table 4).

Experimental inoculation of SPF cats with an FIV isolate has produced clinical syndromes considered as the acute phase. The acute phase may last several weeks to months on the basis of experimental infection. This may vary with the dose of the inoculum and/or the severity of the individual reaction. The lack of an appropriate virus infectivity assay limits the critical evaluation of this hypothesis.

In experimentally infected cats, the acute phase is followed by the asymptomatic phase, except in some animals that die with acute illnesses (Yamamoto et al., 1988). Since it was possible to isolate the virus in all asymptomatic FIV antibody positive cats in our previous study (Ishida et al., 1989), it is appropriate to designate this stage as the asymptomatic carrier (AC) phase. Although the length of the AC phase has not been determined, it may be variable, judging from the wide variation in age seen in the asymptomatic cats employed in this study (4–10 years of age). We have also seen an 18 year old healthy carrier as a clinical case.

In HIV infection, the AC phase is followed by the PGL phase characterized by lymphadenopathy without any evidence of clinical illness. In the present study, however, all the cats showing PGL or local lymphadenopathy were classified as ARC because of accompanying chronic clinical illnesses. We have encountered some PGL-like FIV infected cats on a few occasions, but have not performed any immunologic evaluations so far. Some cats may actually develop PGL prior to the ARC phase, but many are likely to be presented to veterinary hospitals after they develop additional signs such as chronic stomatitis/gingivitis or chronic upper respiratory disease, and are thus diagnosed as ARC.

Once ARC is established, the clinical diseases are likely to progress to AIDS within 1 year as evidenced by our observation. In AIDS, opportunistic infections or malignancies are common findings (CDC, 1986; Ishida et al., 1988, 1989), and these conditions may cause the death of the patient within a short period of time.

The present study has demonstrated that each putative clinical stage has a distinctly decreased level of lymphocyte response against conA stimulation. A good correlation between progress of clinical diseases and immunologic alterations may prove these criteria useful for clinical evaluation of patients.

It was striking that the decrease in lymphocyte blastogenic response paralleled the progression of the disease process. The approximately 50% decrease in the blastogenic response in asymptomatic FIV carriers is a very important finding. Our previous survey showed that these carriers comprise as much as 12% of the healthy cat population (Ishida et al., 1989). Although the apparent lack of clinical signs may prevent their presentation to veterinary clinics, it is speculated that a large number of such undetected carriers suffer from subclinical progression of the immunodeficiency.

The glucose consumption test (Decock et al., 1980), which measures the degree of lymphocyte stimulation in culture, is a simple way of determining cellular activation in culture without employing radioactive material. It has been shown to correlate with [$^3$H]thymidine uptake in the lymphocyte blastogenesis assay. Although it was not possible to evaluate the test results with age and sex matched SPF control animals in this study, the decrease in lymphocyte responsiveness in FIV infected cats was unrelated to age or sex, and may therefore be disease or stage specific. In the clinical observation of naturally infected cases, the ARC is apparently followed by the development of AIDS and death within 1 year. The conA response of lymphocytes clearly indicates a severe depression of lymphocyte function which may be related to T cell depletion. In the two clinical cases of AIDS in this study, however, the post-mortem evidence of opportunistic infections as well as the lymph node pathology with subcortical lymphocyte depletion may suggest the presence of T cell immunodeficiency in these cases.

The staging system backed up with the lymphocyte stimulation test will provide useful information leading to an accurate prognosis of the infected cats. Knowledge of the immunologic responsiveness characteristic of each stage may help the clinical management of the patients. Furthermore, repeated testing for the mitogen response may provide valuable information in monitoring the progress of immunodeficiency. On the other hand, the clear distinction between each stage, in terms of clinical signs and immunologic parameters, and the great similarity to the human disease make this FIV cat system an excellent animal model for HIV infection.

## References

Barre-Sinoussi, F., Chermann, J.C., Rey, F., Nugeyre, M.T., Chamaret, S., Gruest, J., Dauguet, C. and Axler-Blin, C. (1983) Isolation of T-lymphotropic retrovirus from a patient at risk for acquired immunodeficiency syndrome (AIDS). *Science* 220, 868–871.

Bowen, D.L., Lane, H.C. and Fauci, A.S. (1985) Immunopathogenesis of the acquired immunodeficiency syndrome. *Ann. Intern. Med.* 103, 704–709.

Centers for Disease Control (1986) *Morbidity and Mortality Weekly Report* 35, 334.

Cockerell, G.L., Hoover, E.A., Krakowka, S., Olsen, R.G. and Yohn, D.S. (1976) Lymphocyte mitogen reactivity and enumeration of circulating B- and T-cells during feline leukemia virus infection in the cat. *J. Natl. Cancer Inst.* 57, 1095–1099.

Cockerell, G.L. and Hoover, E.A. (1977) Inhibition of normal lymphocyte mitogen reactivity by serum from feline leukemia virus-infected cats. *Cancer Res.* 37, 3985–3989.

Decock, W., Decree, J., Vanwauwe, J. and Verhaegen, H. (1980) Measurement of mitogen stimulation of lymphocytes with a glucose consumption test. *J. Immunol. Methods* 33, 127–131.

Hebebrand, L.C., Mathes, L.E. and Olsen, R.G. (1977) Inhibition of concanavalin A stimulation of feline lymphocytes by inactivated feline leukemia virus. *Cancer Res.* 37, 4532–4533.

Ishida, T., Washizu, T., Toriyabe, K. and Motoyoshi, S. (1988) Detection of feline T-lymphotropic lentivirus (FTLV) infection in Japanese domestic cats. *Jpn. J. Vet. Sci.* 50, 39–44.

Ishida, T., Washizu, T., Toriyabe, K., Motoyoshi, S., Tomoda, I. and Pedersen, N.C. (1989) Feline immunodeficiency virus infection in cats of Japan. *J. Am. Vet. Med. Ass.* 194, 221–225.

Ishida, T. and Tomoda, I. (1990) Clinical staging of feline immunodeficiency virus infection. *Jpn. J. Vet. Sci.* 52, 657–660.

King, N.W. (1986) Simian models of acquired immunodeficiency syndrome (review). *Vet. Pathol.* 23, 345–353.

Lifson, J.D., Reyes, G.R., McGrath, M.S., Stein, H.S. and Engleman, E.G. (1986) AIDS retrovirus induced cytopathology: giant cell formation and involvement of CD4 antigen. *Science* 232, 1123–1127.

Niedt, G.W. and Schinella, R.A. (1985) Acquired immunodeficiency syndrome. *Arch. Pathol. Lab. Med.* 109, 727–734.

Pedersen, N.C., Ho, E.W., Brown, M.L. and Yamamoto, J.K. (1987) Isolation of a T lymphotropic virus from domestic cats with an immunodeficiency-like syndrome. *Science* 235, 790–793.

Piot, P., Quinn, T.C., Taelman, H., Feinsod, F.M., Mbendi, N., Mazebo, P., Ndangi, K., Steven, W., Kalambayi, K., Mitchell, S., Bridts, C. and McCormick, J.B. (1984) Acquired immunodeficiency syndrome in a heterosexual population in Zaire. *Lancet* i, 65–69.

Popovic, M., Sarngadharan, M.G., Read, E. and Gallo, R.C. (1984) Detection, isolation and continuous production of cytopathic retroviruses from patients with AIDS and pre-AIDS. *Science* 224, 497–500.

Reichert, C.M., O'Leary, T.J., Levens, D.L., Simrell, C.R. and Machaer, A.M. (1983) Autopsy pathology of AIDS. *Am. J. Pathol.* 112, 357–382.

Taniguchi, A., Ishida, T., Konno, A., Washizu, T. and Tomoda, I. (1990) Altered mitogen response of peripheral blood lymphocytes in different stages of feline immunodeficiency virus infection. *Jpn. J. Vet. Sci.* 52, 525–530.

Yamamoto, J.K., Hansen, H., Ho, E.W., Morishita, T.Y., Okuda, T., Sawa, T.R., Nakamura, R.M. and Pedersen, N.C. (1989) Epidemiologic and clinical aspects of feline immunodeficiency virus infection in cats from the continental United States and Canada and possible mode of transmission. *J. Am. Vet. Med. Ass.* 194, 213–220.

Yamamoto, J.K., Sparger, E., Ho, E.W., Andersen, P.R., Connor, T.P., Mandell, C.P., Lowenstine, L., Munn, R. and Pedersen, N.C. (1988) Pathogenesis of experimentally induced feline immunodeficiency virus infection in cats. *Am. J. Vet. Res.* 49, 1246–1258.

*Eds. H. Schellekens and M.C. Horzinek*
*Animal Models in AIDS*



# 21

# Clinical symptoms and humoral antibody response in cats experimentally infected with FIV and FeLV

M. FRANCHINI, A. DITTMER, B. KOTTWITZ, R. LEHMANN and H. LUTZ

Department of Veterinary Medicine, University of Zurich, CH-8057 Zurich, Switzerland

## Introduction

The most important viral pathogen in the domestic cat is feline leukemia virus (FeLV), which occurs in high prevalence around the world. The biology, the epidemiology, the pathogenic potential of FeLV and the immune reaction of cats to this virus have been the subject of intensive studies for more than 20 years. The discovery of a feline lentivirus by Pedersen et al. (1987), which is now designated feline immunodeficiency virus (FIV), marked the beginning of another era of research conducted internationally.

FIV is a major cause of a chronic immunodeficiency-like syndrome in cats. In field cats FIV infection is associated with chronic stomatitis and gingivitis, infections of the respiratory tract, diarrhea, weight loss and other diseases caused by secondary infections (Yamamoto et al., 1989). FIV is now known to occur in the U.S.A. (Yamamoto et al., 1989), Japan (Ishida et al., 1988) and in many countries of Europe (Lutz et al., 1988a).

Experimental FIV infection of specific-pathogen-free (SPF) cats has been shown to cause transient fever, lymphadenopathy and neutropenia (Pedersen et al., 1987; Yamamoto et al., 1988a; Lutz et al., 1988a). Besides these manifestations, which are seen in the early phase of the infection, no major additional symptoms were observed during the first 30 months of experimental FIV infection (Pedersen, personal communication, 1989; Lutz, 1989). The absence of clinical symptoms in SPF cats infected with FIV may be attributed to the lack of additional infectious agents when cats are housed under SPF conditions. In the present study we investigated the clinical outcome of combined experimental infection with FeLV and FIV (part 1). To specifically test the humoral immune response, cats with the combined infection, cats infected with FIV alone and non-infected controls were immunized with a synthetic peptide and the antibody response was measured (part 2).

## Material and methods

### Experimental design

Five 12 week old cats were infected oronasally with $1.2 \times 10^6$ ffu FeLV A; at 1 year of age the FeLV-infected and five age-matched SPF cats were infected intraperitoneally with 2 ml of FIV-infected lymphocyte cell culture supernatant. A third group of four SPF cats served as controls. Nine months later all cats were immunized subcutaneously with 1 mg of (T,G)AL (Trainin et al., 1983) in 0.5 ml of phosphate-buffered saline and 0.5 ml of Freund's complete adjuvant.

### Cats

SPF cats were kindly provided by Ciba-Geigy AG, Basel, Switzerland.

### Viruses

FeLV subtype A, Glasgow was kindly provided by Dr. Os Jarrett. The Petaluma strain of FIV (kindly provided by Dr. Niels Pedersen) was maintained in feline lymphocyte cultures in the presence of recombinant interleukin-2 (IL-2, a generous gift of Dr. M.H. Schreier, Sandoz AG, Basel) under conditions described earlier (Lutz et al., 1988b). The lymphocyte cultures were established from cats negative for feline syncytia forming virus (FeSFV).

### Detection of FeLV and FIV infection

FeLV infection was detected by demonstration of FeLV p27 in the serum (Lutz et al., 1983). FIV infection was detected by virus isolation from lymphocytes and the demonstration of serum antibodies to FIV. For virus isolation lymphocytes were purified from cat blood in LeucoSep tubes (Assaf Pharmaceutical Industries Ltd., Mevasseret-Zion, Israel) over Ficoll-Paque gradients (Pharmacia LKB Biotechnology Inc., Piscataway, NJ, U.S.A.) and stimulated in RPMI 1640 medium (Gibco) with concanavalin A and IL-2 as described above. Presence of onco- or lentivirus in the cell culture fluid was determined by assaying reverse transcriptase (RT) in the presence of $Mg^{2+}$ (FIV) or $Mn^{2+}$ (FeLV).

Antibodies to FIV were detected by immunofluorescence assay (IFA) and Western blot (Lutz et al., 1988a), and by a commercial ELISA (Idexx Corp., Portland, ME, U.S.A.)

### Synthetic peptide and measurement of antibodies

Poly(L-tyr,L-glu)-poly-DL-ala-poly-L-lys (=(T,G)AL, Sigma No. 3649) was used to immunize the cats. Antibodies to (T,G)AL were measured by ELISA using 0.2 $\mu$g antigen per well for coating. The sera were diluted 1:400. A rabbit

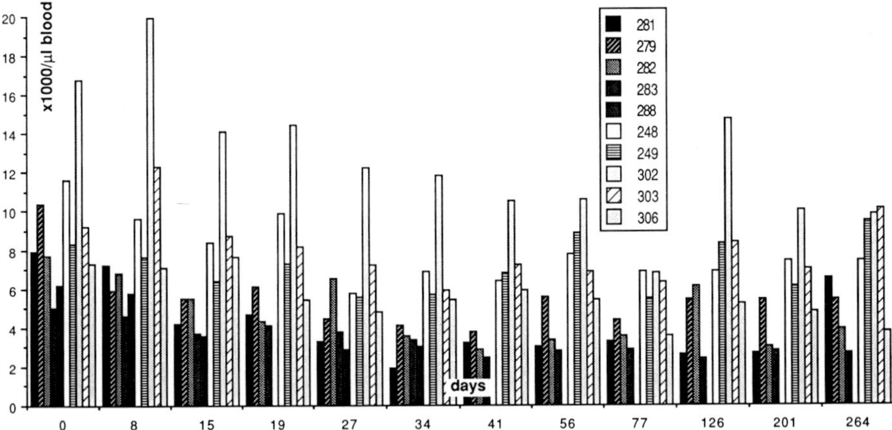


Fig. 1. Leukocyte counts in cats with combined FeLV/FIV infection and sole FIV infection. Cats viremic with FeLV (Nos. 281, 279, 282, 283, 288) and five age-matched SPF cats (Nos. 248, 249, 302, 303, 306) were infected with FIV by intraperitoneal injection of cell culture supernatant. Leukocyte counts were determined for up to 37 weeks. While the leukocyte counts at the time of FIV infection were not statistically different between the two groups, they were significantly lower in the FeLV/FIV cats after day 8 p.i. and later ($P < 0.05$, Mann-Whitney test).

anti-cat IgG peroxidase conjugate (Dako, Copenhagen, Denmark) and ABTS (Lutz et al., 1983) were used as revealing systems.

## Results

### Part 1

*Clinical symptoms*

All cats remained healthy except one of the FeLV/FIV-infected cats (No. 288) which developed severe anemia and neutropenia and had to be killed 34 days after FIV inoculation. In the five FeLV/FIV cats a distinct drop in leukocyte counts was observed by week 2 post inoculation (p.i.) with the lowest values in week 8 p.i. No systematic decrease in leukocyte counts was found in the FIV-infected cats (Fig. 1).

*Course of infection*

All cats—with the exception of cat 288—seroconverted 2–5 weeks after FIV inoculation (Table 1). FIV was generally isolated 1–2 weeks prior to seroconversion. Cat 288 (FeLV/FIV-infected) did not seroconvert, although FIV was isolated three times within 2 weeks. FIV-RT in the cell culture supernatant could easily be distinguished from FeLV-RT using $Mg^{2+}$ instead of $Mn^{2+}$ (data not shown).

TABLE 1
Isolation of FIV and serology during the first 42 days after experimental FIV infection

| Cat no. | Pre infection | Post infection (days) | | | | | |
|---|---|---|---|---|---|---|---|
| | | 8 | 15 | 19 | 27 | 34 | 41 |
| *FeLV positive cats* | | | | | | | |
| 279 | VI – | nd | + | + | + | + | + |
| | AB – | – | – | + | + | + | + |
| 283 | VI – | nd | nd | + | + | + | + |
| | AB – | – | – | – | – | + | + |
| 282 | VI – | nd | + | + | + | + | + |
| | AB – | – | – | – | + | + | + |
| 281 | VI – | nd | + | + | + | + | + |
| | AB – | – | – | + | + | + | + |
| 288 | VI – | nd | + | + | + | nd | |
| | AB – | – | nd | – | – | – | |
| | | | | | | (killed) | |
| *FeLV negative cats* | | | | | | | |
| 306 | VI – | nd | + | + | + | + | nd |
| | AB – | – | – | – | + | + | + |
| 303 | VI – | nd | – | + | + | + | + |
| | AB – | – | – | + | + | + | + |
| 302 | VI – | nd | + | nd | + | + | + |
| | AB – | – | – | – | + | + | + |
| 248 | VI – | nd | + | + | + | + | + |
| | AB – | – | – | + | + | + | + |
| 249 | VI – | nd | + | nd | + | + | + |
| | AB – | – | – | + | + | + | + |

VI: virus isolation; AB: antibody (immunofluorescence/Western blot or ELISA).

### Part 2, humoral immune response to (T,G)AL

No difference in the humoral immune response to (T,G)AL was seen between the FIV-infected cats and the controls. The FeLV/FIV cats however responded to immunization with distinctly lower antibody titers than the FIV-infected cats and the controls (Fig. 2)

## Discussion

The finding that experimental infection with FIV did not result in clinical disease confirms our previous observations (Lutz et al., 1988a). The combined FeLV/FIV infection resulted in mild (in one case severe) leukopenia and anemia. It appeared that the drop in blood cell counts was associated with FIV infection. However, this effect may have been induced by FeLV alone. As no FeLV-infected control group was available, no firm conclusion can be drawn in this respect.

All cats became infected with FIV as confirmed by virus isolation in the

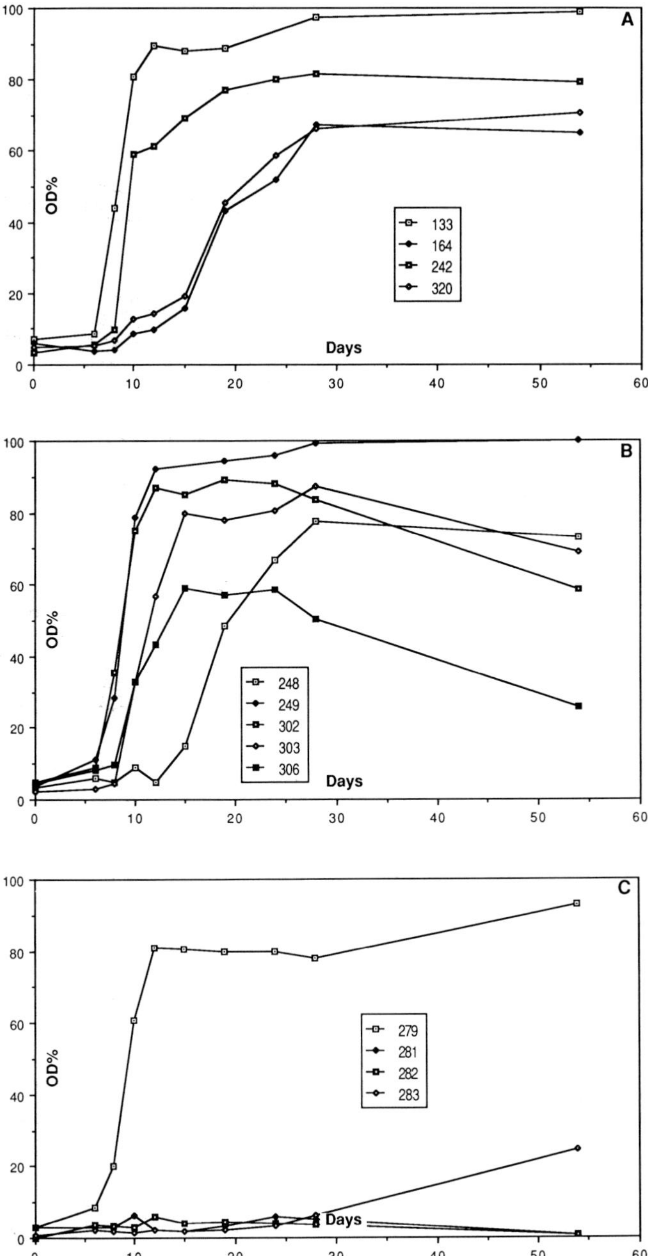


Fig. 2. Humoral immune response to (T,G)AL. Cats with combined FeLV/FIV infection (Fig. 2a, cats 279, 281, 282, 283), with sole FIV infection (Fig. 2b, cats 248, 249, 302, 303, 306) and control cats (Fig. 2c, cats 133, 164, 242, 320) were immunized with 1 mg of (T,G)AL in 0.5 ml of phosphate-buffered saline and 0.5 ml of Freund's complete adjuvant. While the immune reaction of the FIV-infected animals was similar to that of the controls, no antibodies were detected in three of four FeLV/FIV-infected cats up to day 28.

second week p.i. The observation that the FeLV-infected cats seroconverted to FIV later than the non-FeLV-infected animals may be explained by immune suppression due to FeLV infection. Severe immune suppression may also explain that in cat 288 no antibodies to FIV were detected, although the animal was clearly infected with FIV as judged by repeated virus isolation. FeLV and FIV infection do occur simultaneously in the field (Yamamoto et al., 1988, 1989; Shelton et al., 1989; Kölbl and Schuller, 1989). Whether FeLV and FIV infection are etiologically linked cannot be decided at this time. While Yamamoto et al. (1988, 1989) and Shelton et al. (1989) did not find a correlation between the two infections, according to Kölbl and Schuller (1989) they may be linked. Our observation that one out of five FeLV-infected cats did not seroconvert to FIV after experimental infection may be significant. Cats immunosuppressed by FeLV or by other agents may not or only poorly respond with the formation of FIV antibody. It has also been reported by Hopper and colleagues (1988) that a number of cats may be infected with FIV and yet have no detectable antibody to the virus. Therefore, the determination of viral antibody may not be a completely dependable method of testing for FIV infection. If our assumption holds true that a certain number of FIV-infected cats are not detected by testing for viral antibody, the prevalence of FIV infection in the field—especially among sick cats—may have been underestimated. The question whether FeLV and FIV may be linked, therefore, needs further investigation.

From the identical humoral immune response to (T,G)AL in the FIV-infected and the control cats it was concluded that FIV—at least in the first months of infection—may not be strongly immune suppressive. The strong immune suppression found in FeLV/FIV-infected cats may therefore be attributed to FeLV rather than FIV. This would be in agreement with the data of Trainin et al. (1983) who also observed a strongly depressed humoral immune response to (T,G)AL in FeLV-viremic cats.

## Acknowledgements

This study was supported by Grant 3.633.87 from the Swiss National Science Foundation and by donations from cat clubs (FIFE, Katzenclub Ostschweiz, Katzenclub Zürileu). The cats were provided by Ciba-Geigy AG, Basel, the IL-2 by Dr. M.H. Schreier, Sandoz AG, Basel and the cat food by Effems AG. The authors thank Dr. Niels Pedersen and Dr. Os Jarrett for providing FIV and FeLV, respectively, and Dr. B. von Beust for helping with the preparation of the manuscript.

## References

Hopper, C., Sparkes, A., Gruffyd-Jones, T.J. and Harbour, D.A. (1988) Feline T-lymphotropic virus infection. *Vet. Rec.* 122, 590.

Ishida, T., Washizu, T., Toriyabe, K. and Motoyoshi, S. (1988) Detection of feline T-lymphotropic lentivirus (FTLV) infection in Japanese domestic cats. *Jpn. J. Vet. Sci.* 50, 39–44.

Kölbl, S. and Schuller, W. (1989) Serologische Untersuchungen zum Vorkommen des Felinen Immundefizienzvirus (FIV) bei Katzen in Oesterreich. *Wien. Tierärztl. Mschr.* 76, 185–189.

Lutz, H. (1989) Feline retroviruses *Vet. Microbiol.* (in press).

Lutz, H., Pedersen, N.C., Durbin, R. and Theilen, G.H. (1983) Monoclonal antibodies to three epitopic regions of feline leukemia virus p27 and their use in enzyme linked immunosorbent assay of p27. *J. Immunol. Methods* 56, 208–221.

Lutz, H., Egberink, H., Arnold, P., Winkler, G., Wolfensberger, C., Jarrett, O., Parodi, A.L., Pedersen, N.C. and Horzinek, M.C. (1988a) Felines T-lymphotropes Lentivirus (FTLV): Vorkommen in einigen Ländern Europas. *Kleintierpraxis* 33, 445–452.

Lutz, H., Arnold, P., Hübscher, U., Egberink, H., Pedersen, N.C. and Horzinek, M.C. (1988b) Specifity assessment of feline T-lymphotropic lentivirus serology. *J. Vet. Med. B* 35, 773–778.

Pedersen, N.C., Ho, E.W., Brown, M.L. and Yamamoto, J.K. (1987) Isolation of a T-lymphotropic virus from domestic cats with an immunodeficiency-like syndrome. *Science* 235, 790–793.

Shelton, G.H., Waltier, R.M., Connor, S.C. and Grant, C.K. (1989a) Prevalence of feline immunodeficiency virus and feline leukemia virus infections in pet cats. *J. Am. Anim. Hosp. Ass.* 25, 7–12.

Shelton, G.H., McKim, K.D., Cooley, P.L., Dice, P.F., Russell, R.G. and Grant, C.K. (1989b) Feline leukemia virus and feline immunodeficiency virus infections in a cat with lymphoma. *J. Am. Vet. Med. Ass.* 194, 249–252.

Trainin, Z., Wernicke, D., Ungar-Waron, H. and Essex, M. (1983) Suppression of the humoral antibody response in natural retrovirus infection. *Science* 220, 858–859.

Yamamoto, J.K., Sparger, E., Ho, E.W., Andersen, P.R., O'Connor, T.P., Mandell, C.P., Lowenstine, L., Munn, R. and Pedersen, N.C. (1988a) Pathogenesis of experimentally induced feline immunodeficiency virus infection in cats. *Am. J. Vet. Res.* 49, 1246–1258.

Yamamoto, J.K., Pedersen, N.C., Ho, E.W., Okuda, T. and Theilen, G.H. (1988b) Feline immunodeficiency syndrome—A comparison between feline T-lymphotropic lentivirus and feline leukemia virus. *Leukemia* 2, 204–215.

Yamamoto, J.K., Hansen, H., Ho, E.W., Morishita, T.Y., Okuda, T., Sawa, T.R., Nakamura, R.M. and Pedersen, N.C. (1989) Epidemiologic and clinical aspects of feline immunodeficiency virus infection in cats from the continental United States and Canada and possible mode of transmission. *J. Am. Vet. Med. Ass.* 194, 213–220.

Ishida, T., Washizu, T., Toriyabe, K. and Motoyoshi, S. (1988) Detection of feline T-lymphotropic lentivirus (FTLV) infection in Japanese domestic cats. Jpn. J. Vet. Sci. 50, 39-44.

Kölbl, S. and Schuller, W. (1989) Serologische Untersuchungen zum Vorkommen des Felinen Immunschwächevirus (FIV) bei Katzen in Österreich. Wien. Tierärztl. Mschr. 76, 169-172.

[illegible] (in press).

[illegible]

[illegible] 225-236.

[illegible]

[illegible]

*Eds. H. Schellekens and M.C. Horzinek*
*Animal Models in AIDS*



# 22

# Co-infection of cats with feline immunodeficiency virus (FIV) and feline leukemia virus (FeLV) enhances the severity of FIV infection and affects the distribution of FIV DNA in various tissues

MICHAEL TORTEN [1] *, BRUCE A. RIDEOUT [1], P.A. LUCIW [2], E.E. SPARGER [1] and NIELS C. PEDERSEN [1]

[1] Department of Veterinary Medicine, School of Veterinary Medicine and [2] Department of Medical Pathology, School of Medicine, University of California, Davis, CA 95616, U.S.A.

**Summary**

A study was conducted to determine whether a pre-existing asymptomatic feline leukemia virus (FeLV) infection would act as a cofactor to increase the severity of the acute primary and chronic secondary stages of feline immunodeficiency virus (FIV) infection in otherwise specific-pathogen-free (SPF) cats. Pre-existing FeLV infection, even though largely asymptomatic, greatly potentiated the severity of a primary FIV infection. FIV-infected cats with pre-existing FeLV infections developed severe depression, anorexia, fever, diarrhea, dehydration, weight loss, and leukopenia 4–6 weeks after infection and were moribund within 2 weeks, while cats infected only with FIV developed much milder gross and hematologic abnormalities. Though more widespread and severe, pathologic findings in dually infected cats that died were similar to those observed in cats dying from primary FIV infection alone.

Co-infection of asymptomatic FeLV carrier cats with FIV did not increase the levels of FeLV p27 antigen present in their blood over that seen in a similar group of cats infected with FeLV alone. The amount of proviral FIV DNA was greatly enhanced in dually infected cats over cats infected just with FIV. Not only was there a greater quantity of FIV DNA in lymphoid tissues, where the genome can normally be detected in all FIV-infected cats, but viral DNA was also found in non-lymphoid tissues that usually do not contain detectable levels of FIV DNA.

Dually infected cats that recovered from the primary stage of FIV infection remained more leukopenic than cats infected with either FIV or FeLV alone. It was concluded, therefore, that a

* On leave from the Israel Institute for Biological Research, P.O. Box 19, Nes Ziona, Israel and Department of Medical Microbiology, Faculty of Medical Sciences, Tel Aviv University, Tel Aviv, Israel.

pre-existing asymptomatic FeLV infection enhanced replication and spread of FIV in the body and increased the severity of both transient primary and chronic secondary stages of FIV infection. This study demonstrated the usefulness of the FIV model for investigating the role of incidental infectious diseases as cofactors for immunodeficiency diseases caused by lentiviruses.

## Introduction

Feline immunodeficiency virus (FIV) is a T-cell tropic cytopathic lentivirus associated with the feline acquired immunodeficiency syndrome (FAIDS), (Pedersen et al., 1987, 1989; Yamamoto et al., 1988). In a recent study performed in our laboratory we found that experimental co-infection of specific-pathogen-free (SPF) cats with FIV and feline leukemia virus (FeLV) led to fulminating clinical FAIDS involving multiple organ pathology and death. Experimental infection of SPF cats with FIV alone led basically only to transient lymphadenopathy and latent asymptomatic infection. The purpose of the present study was to investigate the potential influence of FeLV as a cofactor affecting the severity of disease as well as the distribution and quantity of FIV DNA in various tissues. If a viral cofactor does indeed affect spread of FIV in tissues, its influence could aid in understanding the clinical progression of disease. FAIDS could thus serve as a model for understanding the suggested role of cofactors in the distribution and expression of HIV in AIDS patients (Fauci, 1988; Rosenberg and Fauci, 1989). FeLV was chosen as a candidate for analysis of cofactor activity since: (1) it is widespread among cats (Hardy, 1980); (2) it causes a depression of the immune system and is tumorigenic (Anderson et al., 1971; Perryman et al., 1972); (3) it affects lymphatic as well as other tissues (Hoover et al., 1987); and (4) it has been incriminated as causing immunodeficiency disease by interacting with other viruses (Neil and Onions, 1988). In addition several strains of FeLV have been sequenced and could be used for studying co-interactions on molecular basis (Berry et al., 1988; Laprevotte et al., 1984; Overbaugh et al., 1988; Stewart et al., 1986). Recent elucidation of the complete sequence of FIV (Talbott et al., 1989) enabled us to use polymerase chain reaction (PCR) amplification for detection and identification of specific proviral sequences in various body tissues. Sequences in the *gag* region were chosen for PCR amplification because they are highly conserved and are quite different from any known FeLV sequence that may interfere with the specificity of FIV identification.

## Materials and methods

### Experimental animals and infection

SPF domestic cats were obtained from the breeding colony of the Feline Retrovirus Research Laboratory, University of California at Davis. Animals were housed in facilities of the Animal Resource Services, University of California at Davis. A total of 30 cats were selected for the study. Twenty cats had been experimentally infected with FeLV and were chronic asymptomatic viremic carriers for 4–6 months. The infecting FeLV strain was CT600 as previously described (Pedersen et al., 1985, 1986). Seven cats were age, litter, and sex matched FeLV recovered animals that had been non-viremic for the same period of time. Three cats were never exposed to FeLV or any other pathogen. Ten FeLV viremic carriers and the seven recovered non-viremic cats were infected with FIV. FIV infection was induced by inoculation of each cat intravenously with 0.5 ml of whole heparinized blood collected from a chronic FIV carrier cat. The donor cat was chosen because it showed signs of persistent leukopenia and had an inverted CD4 + /CD8 + T-cell ratio.

### Naturally FIV-infected cats

Cats with naturally acquired FIV infection, that were FeLV negative and suffered from terminal AIDS-like disease, were seen in the Veterinary Medical Teaching Hospital, School of Veterinary Medicine, University of California at Davis. Tissues were taken at the time of necropsy.

### Complete blood counts

Complete blood counts (CBCs) included electronic total white blood cell (WBC) and red blood cell (RBC) counts, microhematocrit, total blood platelet count by hematocytometer, and WBC differential from Wright-Leishman stained blood smears.

### FeLV antigen and FIV antibody tests

The presence of the 27,000 Da major core protein of FeLV was measured in serum by an antigen capture ELISA (Lutz et al., 1983). FeLV p27, used for preparation of a standard ELISA curve, was purified by immunoaffinity column chromatography by procedures previously described (Pedersen et al., 1986), except that mouse monoclonal antibodies to FeLV p27 were used for antigen capture. Antibodies to FIV were measured by an indirect immunofluorescence assay using Crandell feline kidney cells chronically infected with the Petaluma strain of FIV as a substrate (Yamamoto et al., 1989).

### Gross and microscopic pathology

Cats were killed with an overdose of intravenous barbiturate when they failed to respond to routine symptomatic supportive therapy (fluid and electrolyte replacement, systemic antibiotics) and it became apparent that their disease course would probably be terminal without extreme therapeutic measures. Tissues were fixed in Carson's fixative and processed routinely for histopathology. Fixed tissue sections were stained with hematoxylin and eosin. Special stains, when necessary, consisted of Brown and Brenn, Fite's acid fast, periodic acid-Schiff, and Gomori's methenamine silver.

### Synthesis and labeling of oligonucleotides

Oligonucleotides were synthesized in a gene assembler using $\beta$-cyanomethyl phosphoramidite chemistry on a support matrix of Monobeads optimized for 0.2 $\mu$M synthesis scale (Pharmacia LKB Biotechnology Inc.). The sequences of the oligonucleotides to be used as primers in the PCR and as probes for Southern blots were chosen from FIV sequence data representing specific locations in the *gag* region between base pairs 929 and 1394. Sequencing was obtained from a cloned virus grown on Crandell feline kidney cell line (CRFK) (Miller et al., 1985). The oligonucleotides were purified by elution from a polyacrylamide gel as previously described (Berger et al., 1987; Maniatis et al., 1982). Radioactive labeling of the 5′ end of the oligonucleotide probes were done using 20 pmol of probe, 20 units of T4 polynucleotide kinase and 100 $\mu$Ci of [$^{32}$P]ATP at 5000 Ci/mmol in a total volume of 30 $\mu$l. Unincorporated [$^{32}$P]ATP was removed by passage over Sephadex G-50 by a spun column procedure (Berger et al., 1987).

### Preparation of samples for PCR amplification

DNA was prepared from various frozen tissues taken at post-mortem from cats infected with FIV, FIV and FeLV, or FeLV alone, as well as from non-infected (control) cats. The tissue samples, weighing 200–1200 mg, were cut into small pieces, added to 3 ml Tris-HCl, EDTA, NaCl buffer (TEN) and passed through a Dounce homogenizer. After homogenization 3 ml of TEN containing 1% SDS and 200 $\mu$g/ml proteinase K were added (final volume $\pm$ 7.0 ml). Digestion continued for 24 h at 50°C. Following primary digestion and light vortexing, proteinase K and SDS were added to final concentrations of 300 $\mu$g/ml and 2%, respectively. Digestion was continued for an additional 16 h followed by boiling for 10 min to stop the kinase activity. DNA was isolated by two repetitive cycles of phenol-chloroform extraction followed by precipitation in cold ethanol as previously described (Berger et al., 1987; Maniatis et al., 1982). 1 $\mu$l of DNA containing 200 ng of DNA was used for PCR amplification of each of the tissue samples.

DNA from FIV-infected and non-infected control CRFK cells was prepared as previously described (Berger et al., 1987; Maniatis et al., 1982). DNA from an FeLV-infected feline lung cell line and non-infected control cells was prepared in the same manner.

Samples of peripheral blood lymphocytes (PBL) were processed for PCR amplification by a method that does not require DNA extraction. Whole blood (5 ml) in EDTA was collected. After separation of the PBL by Ficoll-Hypaque gradients and washing three times in phosphate-buffered saline (PBS), the cells were dispersed in 1 ml of a solution containing 0.45% NP40, 0.45% Tween 20 and 100 $\mu$g/ml proteinase K. The cell lysates were frozen and thawed three times, incubated for 2 h at 50°C, followed by boiling for 10 min and centrifugation to remove debris. Of each preparation 20 μl was used for PCR amplification.

### Enzymatic amplification of proviral DNA sequences

Two sets of primer pairs were synthesized, representing two consecutive sequences in the GAG region. The first pair of primers (1 and 2) was intended to amplify a sequence of 327 base pairs (929–1255) while the second pair of primers (3 and 4) was designed to amplify the adjacent sequence of 159 base pairs (1236–1394). The above design enabled us to use primers 1 and 4 to also amplify a sequence of 466 base pairs representing amplification of both of the above sequences (929–1394). A sample of 200 ng of purified DNA from each of the samples to be tested was subjected to 30 cycles of PCR amplification (Mullis and Faloona, 1987).

Amplifications were performed in a DNA thermal cycler (Cetus, Perkin-Elmer, Norwalk, CT). Denaturation was at 94°C for 1 min, renaturation at 55°C for 1 min and elongation at 72°C for 1 min and 30 s. The enzyme used for amplification was a thermostable DNA polymerase (TAQ), as previously described (Saiki et al., 1988).

### Identification of amplified DNA products

Two specific probes were prepared along with each of the two sets of primers. Probe A represents base pairs 1108–1141 while probe B represents base pairs 1277–1306. The above design made it possible to test for specific amplification of the 466 long sequence with either of the two probes. 18 μl of each amplified sample was subjected to electrophoresis (at 97 V) in a gel consisting of 1.5% NuSieve GTG agarose and 1.5% agarose (FMC Bioproducts) in Tris, Borate, EDTA (TBE) buffer. Amplified DNA bands were visualized using ethidium bromide and compared for sequence length against a marker of $\Theta$ X 174 RF DNA *Hae*III digest (Biolabs, New England). After denaturation and neutralization of the DNA in the agarose gel, the PCR reaction products were transferred to a 0.2 μm nitrocellulose sheet for Southern blotting. Specific identification of oligonucleotide sequences with $^{32}$P-labeled probes (A or B) was done under conditions previously described (Berger et al., 1987; Maniatis et al., 1982). Prehybridization was done at 47°C for 2 h and the hybridization at 55°C for approximately 16 h.

## Results

All 17 cats injected with whole blood from an FIV positive cat developed an active FIV infection. Infection was demonstrated by: (1) persistent presence of anti-FIV antibodies; (2) presence of FIV DNA in tissues; and (3) clinical manifestations. All 20 cats infected with FeLV, whether alone or followed by

TABLE 1
Histopathologic data from cats that succumbed from FIV

| Dead/Alive<br>Infecting agent | 5/10<br>FeLV + FIV | | | | | 1/7<br>FIV |
|---|---|---|---|---|---|---|
| Time to death<br>Lesion | 42 days | 52 days | 52 days | 52 days | 56 days | 54 days |
| Typhlocolitis | | | | | | |
| Mural inflammation | + + + | + + + | + + + + | + + + | + + | − |
| Mucosal necrosis | + + + | + + + + | + + + + | − | − | − |
| Enteritis | − | − | − | − | − | + |
| Tonsillitis | + + + | + + + + | + + + + | − | − | + |
| with necrosis | + + + | + + + + | + + + + | − | − | − |
| Lymph node necrosis | − | + + + + | + + + + | + + + | + + + | − |
| Marrow left shift | + + + + | + + + + | ND | + + + + | + + + + | + + + |
| Gingivitis | − | − | + + + | − | − | + |
| Stomatitis | − | − | − | − | − | + |
| Nephritis | − | + | − | − | + + + | + + |

ND: not done; −: negative; +: minimal; + +: mild; + + +: moderately severe; + + + +: severe.

FIV, developed p27 antigenemia which remained essentially the same for both groups throughout the experiment.

Five out of 10 cats (50%) co-infected with FIV and FeLV died or had to be killed within 56 days of FIV infection. Table 1 presents the histopathologic findings in all cats that developed lethal FIV infection. All five cats developed severe leukopenia. The remainder of the co-infected cats developed a transient

```
929        PRIMER 1        948
CTACTGCTGC  TGCAGCTGAA  AATATGTATT  CTCAAATGGG  ATTAGACACT  AGGCCATCTA  TGAAAGAAGC
GATGACGACG  ACGTCGACTT  TTATACATAA  GAGTTTACCC  TAATCTGTGA  TCCGGTAGAT  ACTTTCTTCG

AGGTGGAAAA  GAGGAAGGCC  CTCCACAGGC  ATATCCTATT  CAAACAGTAA  ATGGAGTACC  ACAATATGTA
TCCACCTTTT  CTCCTTCCGG  GAGGTGTCCG  TATAGGATAA  GTTTGTCATT  TACCTCATGG  TGTTATACAT

                                              1108              PROBE A
GCACTTGACC  CAAAAATGGT  GTCCATTTTT  ATGGAAAAGG  CAAGAGAAGG  ACTAGGAGGT  GAGGAAGTTC
CGTGAACTGG  GTTTTTACCA  CAGGTAAAAA  TACCTTTTCC  GTTCTCTTCC  TGATCCTCCA  CTCCTTCAAG

   1141
AACTATGGTT  TACTGCCTTC  TCTGCAAATT  TAACACCTAC  TGACATGGCC  ACATTAATAA  TGGCCGCACC
TTGATACCAA  ATGACGGAAG  AGACGTTTAA  ATTGTGGATG  ACTGTACCGG  TGTAATTATT  ACCGGCGTGG

                                  1236       PRIMER 3    1255                         1277
AGGGTGCGCT  GCAGATAAAG  AAATATTGGA  TGAAAGCTTA  AAGCAACTGA  CAGCAGAATA  TGATCGCACA
TCCCACGCGA  CGTCTATTTC  TTTATAACCT  ACTTTCGAAT  TTCGTTGACT  GTCGTCTTAT  ACTAGCGTGT
                                             PRIMER 2
              PROBE B             1308
CATCCCCCTG  ATGCTCCCAG  ACCATTACCC  TATTTTACTG  CAGCAGAAAT  TATGGGTATA  GGATTAACTC
GTAGGGGGAC  TACGAGGGTC  TGGTAATGGG  ATAAAATGAC  GTCGTCTTTA  ATACCCATAT  CCTAATTGAG

                                 1325                    1394
AAGAACAACA  AGCAGAAGCA  AGATTTGCAC  CAGCTAGGAT  GCAGTG
TTCTTGTTGT  TCGTCTTCGT  TCTAAACGTG  GTCGATCCTA  CGTCAC
                                            PRIMER 4
```

Fig. 1. Oligonucleotide sequences from sequence data of the *gag* region used as primers and probes for amplification and identification of FIV DNA.

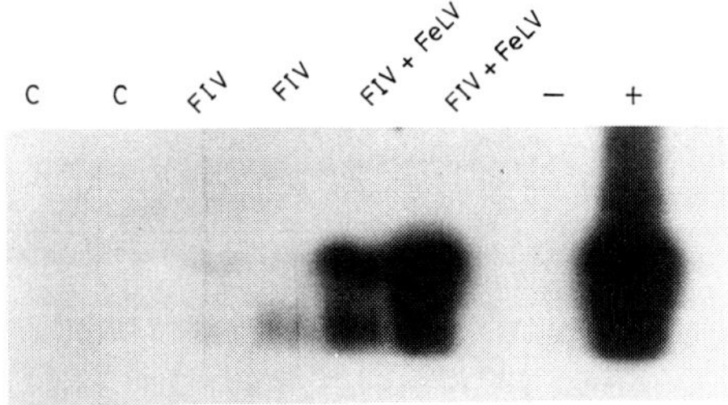


Fig. 2. Detection of FIV DNA in mesenteric lymph nodes of infected and non-infected cats. C: two non-infected cats; FIV: two cats infected with FIV alone; FIV + FeLV: two cats co-infected with FIV and FeLV.

lymphadenopathy with mild elevation of fever as did six of the seven cats which were infected with FIV alone. One cat infected with FIV alone died after 54 days and its histopathologic data are also presented in Table 1. None of the uninfected controls developed any infection while two out of the 10 cats infected with FeLV alone succumbed after more than 100 days with symptoms and lesions which differed from those observed in the FIV-infected cats.

Fig. 1 shows the FIV primers and probes used for the amplification and identification of specific sequences in the FIV *gag* region. When compared to sequences of known length, the primers were shown to amplify the expected three sequences of 327, 159 and 466 bp. As expected the 327 bp sequence was recognized by probe A but not by probe B; the 159 bp sequence was recognized by probe B but not by probe A; the 466 bp sequence was recognized by both probes A and B. Neither probe reacted with FeLV DNA. Fig. 2 shows that FIV

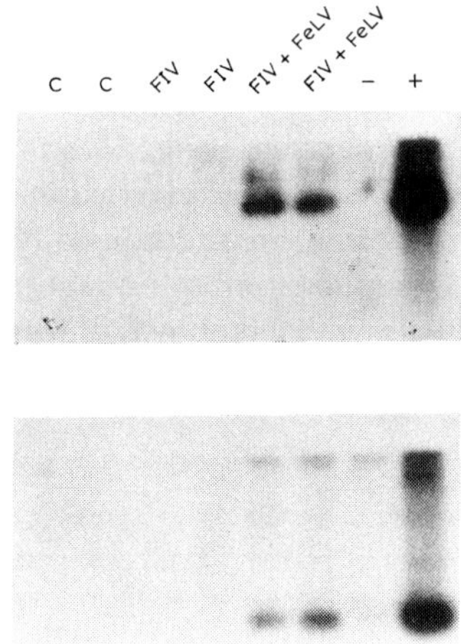


Fig. 3. Detection of FIV DNA (Top amplification by primers 1 and 2, bottom amplification by primers 3 and 4) in kidneys of infected and non-infected cats. C: two non-infected cats; FIV: two cats infected with FIV alone; FIV + FeLV: two cats co-infected with FIV and FeLV.

TABLE 2
Distribution of FIV proviral DNA in various tissues

| Cat No. | Infecting agent(s) | Mode of infection | Peripheral | Mesen-teric | Kid-ney | Liver | Brain |
|---|---|---|---|---|---|---|---|
| 1 | FIV | Experimental | + | + | − | − | − |
| 2 | FIV | Experimental | + | ND | − | ND | ND |
| 3 | FIV | Experimental | + | + | − | ND | ND |
| 4 | FIV | Experimental | + | + | − | − | − |
| 5 | FIV | Natural | + | + | − | − | − |
| 6 | FIV + FeLV | Experimental | + + | + + | + | + | + |
| 7 | FIV + FeLV | Experimental | + | + | + | + | − |
| 8 | FIV + FeLV | Experimental | + + | + + | + | ND | + |
| 9 | FIV + FeLV | Experimental | + + | + + | + | ND | + |
| 10 | FeLV | Experimental | − | − | − | − | − |
| 11 | FeLV | Experimental | − | − | − | − | − |
| 12 | None | None | − | − | − | − | − |
| 13 | None | None | − | − | − | − | − |

+: high but definite identification; + +: heavy band.

genomic DNA could be identified in mesenteric lymph nodes taken from cats infected either with FIV or with FIV and FeLV. Since the amount of tissue DNA amplified was the same in all samples (see Materials and methods), the data in Fig. 2 also indicate that the FIV genome is much more abundant in lymphatic tissue in cats infected with both FIV and FeLV than in cats infected with FIV alone. In addition, FIV genomic DNA could be identified only in kidneys of cats infected with both FIV and FeLV and not in kidneys of cats infected with FIV alone (Fig. 3). Similar data to those shown in Fig. 3 were obtained from other tissues and are summarized in Table 2.

The data in Table 2 reveal that infection with FIV alone caused involvement of only lymphatic tissue (peripheral blood lymphocytes, peripheral and mesenteric lymph nodes) which is in agreement with the clinical data of latency and transient lymphadenopathy (Pedersen et al., 1989; Yamamoto et al., 1988). On the other hand, co-infection of FIV and FeLV led to involvement of FIV in other tissues (kidney, liver, brain, cecum) in addition to lymphatic tissue. Thus, FeLV is a potent activator of FIV replication both quantitatively (i.e., more FIV DNA is seen in tissues of animals with combined infection) and qualitatively (i.e., co-infection affected the ability of FIV to disseminate to tissues of non-lymphatic origin).

## Discussion

The aim of this study was to evaluate an animal model that could aid in understanding in vivo molecular regulation of lentivirus activation from a latent or low level infection to a fulminating stage with pathologic manifestations involving many tissue systems. Our data show that co-infection of cats with FIV, a lentivirus, and FeLV, an unrelated oncornavirus, affects the distribution of FIV in various tissues. Also we have shown that lymphoid tissues of co-infected cats contain a higher number of FIV DNA copies than lymphoid tissues of cats infected with FIV alone. The implication of FeLV as an effector of qualitative and quantitative changes of FIV replication in co-infected cats should enable further study of the correlation between molecular events and the pathologic manifestations leading to progressive and terminal disease. Our study is also supported by sero-epidemiologic data that reveal a more rapid progressive FAIDS in cats which were co-infected with FeLV (Pedersen et al., 1989).

Studies in the FIV FAIDS system may provide insight into HIV and AIDS. Many postulates have been offered in an attempt to explain induction of HIV expression in infected individuals and its relation to the ensuing pathologic effects. One hypothesis suggested that concomitant viral infections such as CMV, EBV, hepatitis B or HSV could induce HIV expression in various cell types (Andiman et al., 1985; Fauci, 1988; Ho et al., 1987; Mosca et al., 1987; Nelson et al., 1988). This notion was supported by studies showing that regulatory genes of non-related DNA viruses transactivated expression directed by the HIV long terminal repeats (LTR) (Gendelman et al., 1986).

The progressive pathologic events of an immunodeficiency syndrome could be influenced by any of the following factors which could be evaluated in an in vivo cat model.

(1) Formation of FIV pseudotypes that are capable of entering cell types not normally infected in cats with FIV alone. Formation of highly infectious recombinant hybrid pseudotypes of gibbon ape leukemia virus *env* genes with *gag* and *pol* sequences of a Moloney leukemia virus, as previously described, is one example of what may occur in vivo (Wilson et al., 1989). Other examples have also been described (Cone and Mulligan, 1984; Miller et al., 1985).

(2) Alterations of target cell surface properties by pre-infection with another virus may enable FIV to enter cells which are otherwise non-permissive. Though the order of infection is unknown, co-infection of human brain cells with HIV and CMV in AIDS was previously recorded (Nelson et al., 1988).

(3) Co-infected cells may lose their ability to maintain and control a latent stage of FIV integration, which leads to a massive increase in FIV replication in these cells. Incriminating evidence that an increase in retroviral DNA density and hyperexpression could lead to cell pathology in human AIDS has already been described (Albert et al., 1989; Fenyo et al., 1988; Shaw et al., 1984).

(4) Specific and non-specific immunosuppression by an oncorna retrovirus such as FeLV may serve as a synergistic factor for increased sensitivity to FIV replication and expression. Recent findings of a similar nature have been described in human AIDS (Andiman et al., 1985).

Pathologic progression of AIDS, SAIDS and probably FAIDS which originally starts as a mild disease with latent or low level infection of lentivirus in T-lymphocytes and macrophages is dependent on invasion of non-lymphoid organs by either non-related microorganisms or lentiviruses or their pseudotypes. It is felt that treatment as well as prognosis is dependent upon the nature of the invasion of non-lymphatic organs.

## References

Albert, J., Bottiger, B., Biberfeld, G. and Fenyo, E.M. (1989) Replicative and cytopathic characteristics of HIV-2 and severity of infection. *Lancet* i, 852–853.

Anderson, L.J., Jarrett, W.F., Jarrett, O. and Laird, H.M. (1971) Feline leukemia-virus infection of kittens: mortality associated with atrophy of the thymus and lymphoid depletion. *J. Natl. Cancer Inst.* 47, 807–813.

Andiman, W.A., Eastman, R., Martin, K., Rubinsteen, A., Pahwa, S., Katz, B.Z., Pitt, J. and Miller, G. (1985) Opportunistic lymphoproliferation associated with Epstein-Barr viral DNA in infants and children with AIDS. *Lancet* ii, 1390–1393.

Berger, S.L. and Kimmel, A.R. (1987) In: J.N. Abelson and M.I. Simon (Eds.), *Methods in Enzymology, Vol. 152.* Academic Press, New York, NY.

Berry, B.T., Ghosh, A.K., Kumar, D.W., Spodick, D.A. and Roy-Burman, P. (1988) Structure and function of endogenous feline leukemia virus long terminal repeats and adjoining regions. *J. Virol.* 62, 3631–3641.

Cone, R.D. and Mulligan, R.C. (1984) High efficiency gene transfer into mammalian cells: Generation of helper-free recombinant retrovirus with broad mammalian host range. *Proc. Natl. Acad. Sci. U.S.A.* 81, 6349–6353.

Fauci, A.S. (1988) The human immunodeficiency virus: infectivity and mechanisms of pathogenesis. *Science* 239, 617–622.

Fenyo, E.M., Morfeldt-Mansson, L., Chiodi, F., Lind, B., Von Gegerfelt, A., Albert, J., Olafson, E. and Asjö, B. (1988) Distinct replicative and cytopathic characteristics of human immunodeficiency virus isolates. *J. Virol.* 62, 4414–4419.

Gendelman, H.E., Phelps, W., Feigenbaun, L., Ostrove, J.M., Adachi, A., Howley, P.M., Khoury, G., Ginsberg, H.S. and Martin, M.A. (1986) Transactivation of the human immunodeficiency virus long terminal repeat sequence by DNA viruses. *Proc. Natl. Acad. Sci. U.S.A.* 83, 9759–9763.

Hardy, W.D. (1980) Feline leukemia virus disease. In: W.D. Hardy, M. Essex and A.J. McCelland (Eds.), *Feline Leukemia Virus.* Elsevier/North Holland, Amsterdam.

Ho, D.D., Pomerantz, R.J. and Kaplan, J.C. (1987) Pathogenesis of infection with human immunodeficiency virus. *N. Engl. J. Med.* 317, 278–286.

Hoover, E.A., Mullins, J.I., Quackenbush, S.L. and Gasper, P.W. (1987) Experimental transmission and pathogenesis of immunodeficiency syndrome in cats. *Blood* 70, 1880–1892.

Laprevotte, I., Hampe, A., Sherr, C.J. and Gilbert, F. (1984) Nucleotide sequence of the *gag* and *gag-pol* junction of feline leukemia virus. *J. Virol.* 50, 884–894.

Lutz, H., Pedersen, N.C., Durbin, R. and Theilen, G.H. (1983) Monoclonal antibodies to three epitopic regions of feline leukemia virus p27 and their use in enzyme-linked immunosorbent assay of p27. *J. Immunol. Methods* 56, 209–220.

Maniatis, T., Fritsch, E.F. and Sambrook, J. (1982) *Molecular Cloning: A Laboratory Manual.* Cold Spring Harbor Laboratory, Cold Spring Harbor, NY.

Miller, A.D., Law, M.-F. and Verma, I.M. (1985) Generation of helper-free amphotropic retroviruses that transduce a dominant-acting, methotrexate-resistant dihydrofolate reductase gene. *Mol. Cell. Biol.* 5, 431–437.

Mosca, J.D., Bednarik, D.P., Raj, N.B.K., Rosen, C.A., Sodroski, J.G., Haseltine, W.A., and Pitha, P.M. (1987) Herpes simplex virus type-1 can reactivate transcription of latent human immunodeficiency virus. *Nature* 325, 67–70.

Mullis, K.B., and Faloona, F.A. (1987) Specific synthesis of DNA in vitro via a polymerase catalyzed chain reaction. In: R. Wu (Ed.), *Methods in Enzymology, Vol. 155.* Academic Press, New York, NY, pp. 335–350.

Neil, J.C., and Onions, D.E. (1985) Feline leukemia viruses: molecular biology and pathogenesis. *Anticancer Res.* 5, 49–64.

Nelson, J.A., Reynolds-Kohler, C., Oldstone, M.B.A. and Wiley, C.A., (1988) HIV and HCMV co-infect brain cells in patients with AIDS. *Virology* 165, 286–293.

Overbaugh, J., Donahue, P.R., Quackenbush, S.L., Hoover, E.A. and Mullins, J.I. (1988) Molecular cloning of a feline leukemia virus that induces fatal immunodeficiency in cats. *Science* 239, 906–910.

Pedersen, N.C., Johnson, L. and Ott, R.L. (1985) Evaluation of a commercial feline leukemia virus vaccine for immunogenicity and efficacy. *Feline Pract.* 15, 790–793.

Pedersen, N.C., Johnson, L. and Theilen, G.H. (1986) Possible immuno enhancement of persistent viremia by feline leukemia virus envelope glycoprotein in challenge-exposure situations where whole inactivated virus vaccines were protective. *Vet. Immunol. Immunopathol.* 11, 123–148.

Pedersen, N.C., Ho, E.W., Brown, M.L. and Yamamoto, J.K. (1987) Isolation of a T-lymphotropic virus from domestic cats with an immunodeficiency-like syndrome. *Science* 235, 790–793.

Pedersen, N.C., Yamamoto, J.K., Ishida, T. and Hansen, H. (1989) Feline immunodeficiency virus infection. *Vet. Immunol. Immunopathol.* 21, 111–129.

Perryman, L.E., Hoover, E.A. and Yohn, D.S. (1972) Immunologic reactivity of the cat: immunosuppression in experimental feline leukemia. *J. Natl. Cancer. Inst.* 49, 1357–1362.

Rozenberg, Z.F. and Fauci, A.S. (1989) Minireview: Induction of expression of HIV in latently or chronically infected cells. *AIDS Res. Human Retroviruses* 5, 1–4.

Saiki, R.K., Gelfand, D.H., Stoffel, S., Schart, S.J., Higuchi, R. and Horn, G.T. (1988) Primer-directed enzymatic amplification of DNA with a thermostable DNA polymerase. *Science* 239, 487–491.

Shaw, G.M., Hahn, B.H., Arya, S.K., Groopman, J.E., Gallo, R.C. and Wong-Staal, F. (1984) Molecular characterization of human T-cell leukemia (lymphotropic) virus type III in the acquired immune deficiency syndrome. *Science* 226, 1165–1171.

Stewart, M.A., Warnock, M., Wheeler, A., Wilkie, N., Mullins, J.I., Onions, D.E. and Neil, J.C. (1986) Nucleotide sequence of a feline leukemia virus subgroup A envelope gene and long terminal repeat and evidence for the recombinational origin of subgroup B viruses. *J. Virol.* 58, 825–834.

Talbott, R.L., Sparger, E.E., Lovelace, K.M., Pedersen, N.C., Luciw, P.A. and Elder, J.H. (1989) Nucleotide sequence and genomic organization of feline immunodeficiency virus (FIV). *Proc. Natl. Acad. Sci. U.S.A.* 86, 5743–5747.

Wilson, C., Reitz, M.S., Okayama, H. and Eiden, M.V. (1989) Formation of infectious hybrid virions with Gibbon-ape leukemia virus and human T-cell leukemia virus retroviral envelope glycoproteins and the *gag* and *pol* proteins of moloney murine leukemia virus. *J. Virol.* 63, 2374–2378.

Yamamoto, J.K., Sparger, E., Ho, E.W., Andersen, P.R., O'Connor, T.P., Mandell, C.P., Lowenstine, L., Nunn, R. and Pedersen, N.C. (1988) Pathogenesis of experimentally induced feline immunodeficiency virus in cats. *Am. J. Vet. Res.* 49, 1246–1258.

Yamamoto, J.K., Hansen, H., Ho, E.W., Morishita, T.Y., Okuda, T., Sawa, T.R., Nakamura, R.M. and Pedersen, N.C. (1989) Epidemiologic and clinical aspects of feline immunodeficiency virus infection in cats from the continental United States and Canada and possible mode of transmission. *J. Am. Vet. Med. Ass.* 194, 213–220.

# *Large animal models*

*Eds. H. Schellekens and M.C. Horzinek*
*Animal Models in AIDS*



# 23

# Immunologic management of equine infectious anemia virus: a model for AIDS vaccine development

RONALD C. MONTELARO [1] and CHARLES J. ISSEL [2]

Departments of [1] Biochemistry and [2] Veterinary Science and Veterinary Microbiology and Parasitology, Louisiana State University, Baton Rouge, LA 70803, U.S.A.

## Introduction

One of the most difficult challenges in contemporary acquired immunodeficiency syndrome (AIDS) research is the development of an effective vaccine for the prevention of human immunodeficiency virus (HIV) infections. There are numerous reasons to be pessimistic about the prospects of a successful vaccine in the foreseeable future. Despite significant efforts over the past 20 years, only very limited success has been realized in preventing oncovirus infections by a variety of immunization strategies; in general, prevention of disease has been more easily achieved than protection against infection. An AIDS vaccine that can prevent disease but not HIV infection would result in a population of inapparent carriers which poses an uncertain threat of spreading virus infection. Compared to oncoviruses, lentiviruses present a greater array of persistence mechanisms (discussed below) that can compound attempts at immunoprophylaxis or immunotherapy. Most relevant to vaccine development is the need to protect macrophages from infection and the necessity of overcoming the extensive genetic/antigenic variation intrinsic to lentiviruses.

Efforts to develop an effective HIV vaccine are also severely limited by the restricted access to suitable human populations for testing candidate vaccines. This latter complication creates a critical need for the development of appropriate animal models for evaluating lentivirus vaccine strategies. Finally, there exists a belief among some researchers that a vaccine cannot be developed against a viral infection that appears to be 100% fatal in humans and never controlled effectively in animals. Thus, a strong case can be made against having any hope for an AIDS vaccine or for setting vaccine efforts at a high priority in AIDS research. Early failures of HIV vaccines in chimpanzees seem to document the dire predictions of failure (Laskey, 1989).

There are, however, compelling reasons to be optimistic that an effective HIV vaccine can be developed in due time. These factors include the availability of novel adjuvants (ISCOMS, MDP, etc.), modes of antigen presentation (recombinant viruses, synthetic peptides) and immune modulators that were unavailable to previous retrovirus vaccine studies. In addition, in considering immunoprophylaxis, most of the virus persistence mechanisms and effects on immune functions are not real concerns if virus infection is indeed prevented initially. Finally, it is being recognized that certain lentivirus infections can be brought under immunologic management despite the array of persistence strategies employed by these viruses. Based on these factors, a strong argument can and should be made for the feasibility and high priority of vaccine development in AIDS research. Recent vaccine studies (Murphey-Corb et al., 1989; Desroisiers et al., 1989) in which rhesus macaques were protected by experimental immunizations from simian immunodeficiency virus infection and/or disease lend encouragement to this effort.

Thus, the purpose of this presentation is to review recent developments in the study of equine infectious anemia virus (EIAV), a lentivirus of practical importance both to veterinary medicine and as an animal model in AIDS research. Although EIAV initially served a central role in defining the nature and role of antigenic variation during a persistent lentivirus infection, more recent studies have focused on EIAV as a model for the natural immunologic management of a lentivirus infection and as a model for evaluating experimental vaccine strategies.

## Properties of EIAV infection of horses

### Clinical course of disease

The clinical responses of horses following natural or experimental infections by EIAV can be divided into characteristic stages (Issel and Coggins, 1979). Acute EIA, characterized by fever and hemorrhages, is typically associated with the first exposure to virus and appears to correlate with massive virus replication and the destruction of macrophages. The more classical symptoms of EIA (anemia, weight loss, edema, leukopenia, etc.) are observed later during recurring cycles of viremia and illness which appear at irregular intervals separated by weeks or months. This stage of disease is called chronic EIA. The frequency and severity of disease episodes decline with time, and the chronic stage of disease usually ends within the first year after infection and an average of six to eight clinical episodes. The exact progression of disease, however, depends on the infecting strain of EIAV and characteristics of the individual animal and its environment (general health, work load, etc). For example, some infections may result in extensive encephalopathy, while others may show no manifestations of this pathology.

During disease episodes, viremia levels can range from $10^2$ to $10^4$ tissue culture infectious doses ($TCID_{50}$) allowing easy recovery of virus from plasma incubated on cultured cells (Orrego et al., 1982). In contrast, plasma viremia levels are typically negligible during afebrile periods. It has been clearly demonstrated that EIA can be transmitted by whole blood transfer to naive animals from infected animals in the chronic stage of disease. These blood transfers can be mediated by man (hypodermic needles, scalpels, etc.) or by insect vectors (Issel et al., 1984; Foil et al., 1987). In fact, transmission has been accomplished by allowing a single horse fly (*Tabanus fuscicostatus*) to take a partial blood meal on an infected pony during an acute clinical period and to immediately finish its meal on a naive pony. This transfer of blood by this species has been estimated at 6 nl, and efficient transmission of EIAV from donors with plasma viremias of $10^6$ horse $ID_{50}$ per ml have been reported with this horse fly species. Mosquitoes or other biting insects are less efficient in transmitting EIAV between animals.

Following the chronic stage of disease, most infected horses enter an inapparent stage during which there is an absence of any clinical symptoms or detectable levels of plasma viremia. The animal continues to harbor EIAV, however, as evidenced by the fact that infection can be efficiently transmitted by experimental transfer of whole blood (250 ml) from inapparently infected to naive horses. In addition, it has been demonstrated that recrudescence of chronic EIA can be induced in some inapparently infected horses by administration of immunosuppressants (e.g., dexamethasone) or by stress, even in certain animals that have been free of febrile episodes for years (Kono et al., 1976). The ability to induce chronic EIA in inapparent carriers suggests an active immunologic management of virus replication that can be overcome by suppressing or stressing the immune system. The role of immune responses in mediating the management of EIAV infections has recently been clearly documented by experimental infections of horses that have genetic defects resulting in deficiencies in both humoral and cellular immune systems (Perryman et al., 1988). Infection of these immunodeficient horses with EIAV results in a progressive viremia and a rapid pathogenesis leading to death. This course of infection is in distinct contrast to the usual chronic EIA induced in experimental infections and demonstrates the necessary role of competent host immune responses in controlling EIAV replication and pathogenesis.

Thus, the periodic nature of EIAV offers a uniquely dynamic model for examining lentivirus persistence in the presence of apparently competent host immune responses. In addition, EIAV-infected horses represent the only lentivirus system in which the infected animal routinely establishes control of viral replication, presumably resulting from cumulative immune factors which affect control of EIAV replication, even in the face of rapid and extensive antigenic variations of the infecting virus. Thus, EIAV should provide important insights into potential strategies for lentivirus vaccine development.

## Mechanisms of EIAV persistence

EIAV, like other lentiviruses, employs an array of escape mechanisms to confound host defense systems and to establish a persistent infection. These escape mechanisms include proviral integration and possible latency in target cells (Rasty et al., 1990), extensive genomic and antigenic variations that can circumvent host defense systems (Montelaro et al., 1984; Payne et al., 1987a,b), and suppression of certain immune functions (Gerencer et al., 1989).

The role of antigenic variations in maintaining a persistent lentivirus infection has perhaps been demonstrated most clearly for EIAV. Extensive studies of EIAV populations during the course of chronic EIA indicate that the recurrent viremias and disease episodes can be attributed to the sequential evolution and replication of novel antigenic variants that can temporarily elude established host immune responses. Each clinical cycle is associated with a distinct predominant virus population, and the predominant virus strain can change in as little as 2 weeks. Moreover, there appears to be a wide spectrum of possible antigenic variants of EIAV which need to differ in their surface glycoproteins by only a few amino acids to produce distinct serotypes. Of the more than 30 EIAV isolates characterized to date, no two reveal identical antigenic properties. Thus, EIAV infections present host immune systems with a rapidly changing, unpredictable array of antigenic targets. Despite this challenge, the horse immune system is capable of eventually controlling virus replication (cf. section on vaccine development).

## Immunologic management of EIAV replication

### Immune responses to EIAV infection

To identify the immunologic factors mediating control of EIAV replication, it is necessary to characterize the nature and kinetics of both humoral and cellular immune responses from the time that a horse is infected, through the period of chronic disease, and to the eventual state of inapparent infection. Unfortunately, very little is known about cellular immune responses during EIAV infection, although procedures and reagents are currently being developed to analyze this critical component of the immune system. Analyses of humoral immune responses, however, have already yielded intriguing results (Rwambo et al., 1990). Fig. 1 (top panel) summarizes schematically the general kinetics of humoral immune responses during the course of experimental infections as determined in Western blot and ELISA assays. The initial antibodies detected following EIAV infection are directed against the major surface glycoprotein gp90. Antibodies to gp90 are typically detectable 7–10 days post infection and the levels of gp90-specific antibody continue to rise over the next few months post infection, regardless of the number of observable clinical episodes. The gp90-specific antibody titer eventually reaches a plateau, remaining the predominant antibody response through the course of infection. The second detectable antibody is directed against the major core protein of the virus, p26. The antibody is first observed 10–14 days post infection, however, its level reaches a plateau very rapidly, remaining at a level that is about 100-fold less than that observed for

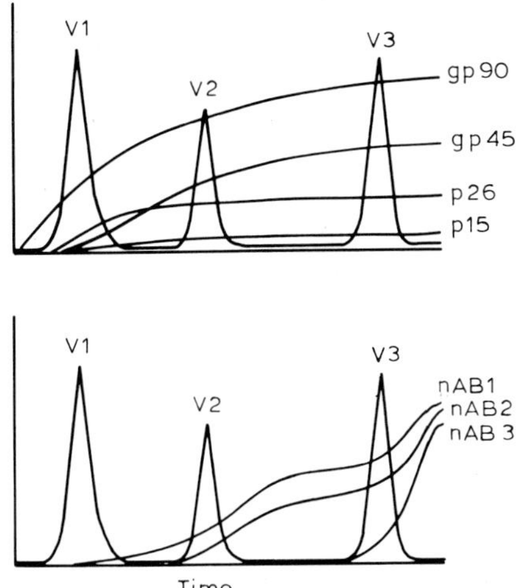


Fig. 1. Schematic representation of the kinetics of humoral immune responses during the course of experimental persistent infections. The top panel displays antibody responses to distinct viral antigens as determined by immunoblot and ELISA assays. The bottom panel demonstrates the temporal emergence of type-specific neutralizing antibodies as measured in in vitro neutralization assays. V1, V2, etc. indicate sequential viremias experienced during chronic EIA and nAB1, nAB2, etc. represent neutralizing antibodies specific for virus strains V1, V2, etc. respectively.

gp90. Interestingly, antibody to the EIAV transmembrane protein is not routinely detected until about 3–4 weeks post infection. These gp45-specific antibody levels rise slowly over the next few months eventually stabilizing at levels that are about one-half those observed for gp90. Only minor antibody levels are detected against the other viral core proteins p15, p11, and p9. The serum antibodies measured in these binding assays appear to be predominantly group-specific as the patterns of antibody reactivity remain essentially the same among a panel of antigenic variants of EIAV analyzed in parallel Western blot assays.

The results of these studies suggest that quantitative changes in EIAV-specific antibody responses typically occur within the first few months post infection and that relative antibody levels remain fairly consistent thereafter. However, these quantitative analyses do not provide any apparent identification of changing immune responses that can be correlated with control of virus replication.

A more qualitative and more discriminating analysis of humoral immune responses produced during persistent EIAV infections is provided by assaying neutralizing antibody responses during chronic EIA. A schematic of the most common pattern of neutralizing antibody responses is presented in Fig. 1 (lower panel). These data indicate that the initial control of EIAV replication is not necessarily mediated by neutralizing antibodies, at least not by those antibodies that can be measured in our in vitro assays. This observation suggests that the initial management of EIAV replication may be accomplished by non-specific immune responses (natural killer cells, etc.) or by cytotoxic T-lymphocytes. In this regard, Gerencer et al. (1989) have detected significant levels of ADCC at the beginning of an acute attack of disease, but cytotoxic activity was absent or very low during the chronic stage of disease. As the infection progresses, however, neutralizing antibody titers increase and the specificity of neutralization broadens significantly.

An interesting phenomenon that occurs during the evolution of type-specific neutralizing responses is their kinetics of appearance. Although neutralizing antibodies to the first virus isolate (V1) are not frequently detectable immediately after the first disease cycle, neutralizing antibodies to both V1 and V2 appear relatively rapidly after the second viremia and associated clinical episode. The rapidity of this neutralizing response after the second disease cycle suggests an immunologic priming during the initial viremia. The possible significance of these antibody kinetics in explaining the mechanisms of the eventual immunologic management of EIAV replication will be discussed below.

The broadening of antibody responses does not necessarily require the cyclic disease episodes characteristic of chronic EIA. Horses experimentally infected with *avirulent* strains of EIAV display no apparent clinical symptoms. Yet during the first year post infection, the specificity of neutralizing antibodies broadens as observed in horses with chronic EIA. These observations indicate that immune responses can evolve in the absence of apparent disease cycles and significant viremia levels, presumably due to the exposure of virus antigens during low level replication in the experimentally infected pony. The induction of these protective immune responses in the absence of high levels of virus replication may signal a role of cell mediated immune responses in addition to the increased neutralization capacities in managing EIAV replication.

Neutralizing antibodies are undoubtedly a narrow window to view the myriad immune responses generated in response to EIAV infection. Several non-neutralizing epitopes have been identified in EIAV gp90 and gp45, and T-lymphocytes from EIAV-infected horses can be stimulated in vitro with EIAV antigens (Hussain et al., 1987; Issel and Coggins, 1979). Thus non-neutralizing and cell mediated immune responses must also be examined in the immunologic management of EIAV infections. For example it will be critical to evaluate cellular immune responses to the EIAV core proteins during the course of experimental infections, as cytotoxic T-lymphocyte responses against the internal proteins of other viruses have proven to be an important factor in establishing a protective immune response.

### Possible mechanisms for immunologic management

How does the infected horse achieve an immunologic management of EIAV replication? It is possible that in response to the sequential production of EIAV variants during the chronic stage of infection, the immune system accumulates type-specific responses which eventually are able to control any possible variant that may be generated. This possibility, however, is unlikely for several reasons. First, there appears to be a very large number of EIAV variants that exist in nature. Thus it is improbable that an adequate array of type-specific responses could ever be generated to be effective against all possible variants of EIAV. Second, it is likely that different virus type specificities are present only very briefly in the infected horse before they are eliminated and further replication suppressed by immunosurveillance systems. The limited exposure of a type-specific antigenic determinant would probably limit the overall strength of the corresponding type-specific immune responses, especially in terms of the production of memory cells and antigen-specific T-cells. Thus, it appears that although EIAV type specificities can be immunodominant, their role in controlling virus replication is questionable. This model appears to be true for HIV gp120, where the immunodominant neutralizing epitope contained in a loop structure is type-specific (Javaherian et al., 1989).

The second model for achieving immunologic management of EIAV replication is a gradual "strengthening" of immune responses against antigenic determinants that are conserved but immunorecessive, i.e., they are relatively weak immunogens. These antigenic determinants would not be expected to induce strong humoral or cellular immune responses during the first exposure to the immune system, but because these determinants are conserved, they will be presented repeatedly at high concentrations to the immune system during the sequential viremias characteristic of chronic EIA. In the absence of obvious disease cycles, persistently infected animals may be chronically exposed to low levels of virus replication resulting in a continual exposure to these conserved antigenic determinants. This type of exposure would maximize anamnestic responses which could eventually result in strong responses even to relatively weak epitopes.

A definitive elucidation of the protective immune responses generated during persistent EIAV infections requires further detailed characterizations of humoral and cellular immune responses in infected horses and an extensive characterization of conserved and variable antigenic determinants, both immunodominant and immunorecessive. These studies, which are currently in progress, should provide important fundamental information that can be employed in the development of effective vaccine strategies for EIAV and for HIV.

## Vaccine development

### Immunization regimen

To address directly the feasibility of an EIAV vaccine, we have recently completed the evaluation of an inactivated whole virus vaccine for its ability to protect Shetland ponies against challenges with homologous and heterologous strains of EIAV (Issel et al., 1990). Table 1 summarizes the results of these studies.

The vaccine recipients consisted of groups of three ponies, each receiving from five to eight immunizations at 2 week intervals with gradient purified prototype (cell-adapted) EIAV inactivated with formalin and formulated in threonyl

TABLE 1

Efficacy of an inactivated EIAV whole virus vaccine in Shetland ponies [a]

| Vaccinate | | | Challenge | |
|---|---|---|---|---|
| Pony | Doses | LNI | Prototype VI/ΔLNI | PV VI/ΔLNI/HI |
| 717 | 8 | 2.5 | 0/0 | +/ND/ND |
| 722 | 8 | 4.5 | 0/0 | 0/0/+ |
| 730 | 8 | 3.5 | 0/0 | 0/0/+ |
| 732 | 7 | 2.5 | 0/0 | 0/0/+ |
| 733 | 7 | 2.5 | 0/0 | 0/0/+ |
| 734 | 7 | 3.5 | +/+ | 0/0/+ |
| 84 | 6 | 2.0 | 0/0 | 0/+/+ |
| 85 | 6 | 2.5 | 0/0 | +/+/+ |
| 86 | 6 | 2.5 | 0/+ | +/+/ND |
| 88 | 5 | 3.5 | 0/0 | 0/+/+ |
| 89 | 5 | 0.5 | 0/+ | 0/0/+ |
| 810 | 5 | 2.5 | 0/0 | 0/+/+ |

[a] Ponies were immunized with five to eight doses of formalin-inactivated prototype EIAV, monitored for antibody responses, and challenged sequentially with standard inocula of prototype EIAV (homologous challenge) at 2 weeks post immunization, and with the virulent PV strain of EIAV (heterologous challenge) at 3.5 months post immunization. The $\log_{10}$ neutralization index (LNI) of serum from all vaccinates was measured in in vitro assays against prototype or the PV strain of virus, and changes in LNI (ΔLNI) were monitored after challenges with prototype and PV-EIAV strains for evidence of virus infection. Other criteria for monitoring virus infection were the ability to succeed with virus isolations (VI) from plasma samples and the ability to transfer EIAV infection by whole blood transfers (250 ml) in horse inoculation (HI) assays.

muramyl dipeptide (MDP) adjuvant. Multiple immunizations were employed to ensure immune responses to immunorecessive as well as immunodominant EIAV antigenic determinants.

All ponies received their last immunization on the same day and were monitored for antibody responses and for possible infection from the inactivated vaccine stock. None of the vaccinates displayed signs of viral infection as measured by multiple attempts to recover virus from plasma samples (data not shown). These results indicate complete inactivation of the EIAV vaccine. Analyses of antibody responses by Western blots of EIAV revealed antibodies against all of the major EIAV proteins in a pattern of relative reactivities similar to that observed with serum from virus-infected ponies (data not shown). Analyses of neutralizing antibody in the serum of vaccine recipients (Table 1) demonstrated $\log_{10}$ neutralizing index (LNI) values of 2.0–4.5, except for a single pony (no. 89) that apparently failed to produce significant neutralizing antibody to the prototype EIAV.

### Homologous virus challenge

Two weeks after the last immunization, all of the immunized ponies were inoculated with $10^5$ $TCID_{50}$ of prototype EIAV, the same virus strain used to prepare the inactivated vaccine stock. This quantity of prototype EIAV represents about $10^3$ horse infectious doses (HID) and results in 100% infection of experimentally inoculated ponies. However, the prototype strain of virus has been adapted to growth in cell culture and does not usually cause disease in experimentally infected ponies. Thus, the prototype EIAV-challenged ponies were monitored for viral infection by repeated attempts to isolate virus from plasma and by monitoring for anamnestic antibody responses indicative of viral replication (Table 1). The results of these assays over a 3 month observation period indicated that nine of 12 ponies were protected against infection from the homologous live virus (prototype) challenge. Three ponies displayed anamnestic antibody responses (nos. 734, 86, and 89), while only a single pony (no. 734) was positive once in the plasma virus isolation assays. Thus, these data demonstrate that the inactivated whole virus vaccine was capable of providing a high degree of protection against a vigorous homologous virus challenge.

### Heterologous virus challenge

To examine further the extent of protection provided by the inactivated vaccine regimen, the same ponies after the 3 month observation period were subjected to a heterologous EIAV challenge consisting of about $10^6$ HID of the PV strain of virus. The PV-EIAV strain is a *virulent* biological clone of EIAV derived after backpassage of the prototype strain of EIAV in ponies and selected in vitro in the presence of convalescent polyclonal horse serum (Rwambo et al., 1990). The dose of PV-EIAV used in the challenge produces chronic EIA in 100% of infected ponies with recoverable plasma virus within 10 days and initial clinical symptoms within 2–3 weeks post infection.

Thus the challenged ponies were monitored for 6 months post challenge for recoverable virus, for anamnestic responses, and for clinical symptoms. Eight of the 11 ponies thus challenged remained without clinical signs of EIA during the observation period. One (no. 717) died 40 days after challenge and two (nos. 85, 86) had fever peaks with demonstrable plasma viremia within 3 weeks of challenge. However, all of the ponies were shown to have become infected after the heterologous challenge with PV-EIAV by one or more of the following criteria: recoverable plasma virus, anamnestic antibody responses, or whole blood transfers to naive ponies (Table 1). Thus, the vaccine appeared to provide protection against the development of EIA disease, but not against infection with a heterologous strain of virus. Protection against disease following PV strain challenge did not appear to be mediated by neutralizing antibody. Although sera from all 12 of the immunized ponies had neutralizing antibody to the prototype strain prior to their challenge with the PV strain, they had no detectable neutralizing activity against the PV strain. Four of the ponies failed to develop detectable plasma viremia or neutralizing antibody to the PV strain following PV strain challenge. This was suggestive evidence for protection against infection with the virulent challenge. These data further compel us to critically investigate all immune factors for protection against EIAV. Although preliminary data suggest that passively transferred serum with neutralizing activity confers a level of protection against avirulent and virulent strains of EIAV, factors other than neutralizing antibody appear to play important roles in recovery from initial febrile episodes in naive horses and in resistance to disease by the PV strain.

Taken together, the results of this initial vaccine trial suggest that an inactivated whole virus vaccine can provide protection against a relatively large challenge of homologous virus and against the development of disease after challenges with heterologous strains of virus. Further experiments are required to determine if the lack of protection against infection after heterologous challenge is due to the high levels of virus employed in the challenge inoculum or because of the absence of appropriate immune responses to inactivate heterologous virus strains.

## Discussion

In the preceding sections we have described aspects of the EIAV system which make it an important animal model for the immunologic management of lentivirus infections. The broadly protective immune responses produced during persistent EIAV infections demonstrate the capacity of the immune system to control lentivirus replication despite the battery of escape mechanisms employed by these viruses. The identification of these controlling immune factors can provide a defined goal for future immunoprophylactic or immunotherapeutic studies. A significant amount of time and effort will be required to identify the immune factors capable of controlling virus replication and to learn how to induce a protective immune status by a particular vaccine protocol.

The initial vaccine studies described here, however, support the idea that a vaccine can be developed for lentivirus infections. In this first attempt, we employed a relatively rigorous immunization protocol and virus challenge levels typically employed in classic virus vaccine development. Despite the stringent virus challenge, 75% of the immunized animals were protected from infection with the homologous strain of EIAV. This level of protection is similar to that observed recently in Rhesus macaques immunized with inactivated whole SIV and challenged with 10 ID of that virus (Murphey-Corb et al., 1989). Although we did not achieve protection against infection after massive challenges with heterologous EIAV strains, it is significant that the vaccine-induced immune responses were able to prevent or delay the development of clinical disease. It is possible that the vaccine protocol can prevent virus infection from lower challenge doses of heterologous EIAV. Further experiments to titer the level of protection against various levels of heterologous challenge are currently in progress.

Why are current EIAV and SIV vaccine trials succeeding where previous attempts have failed? The primary difference between previous studies and those reported here is in the nature of the vaccine preparation. We have chosen to use formalin-inactivated gradient purified virus preparations to insure that all potential virion immunogens are presented and to maximize the preservation of multimeric protein structures. In other vaccine trials, detergent solubilized SIV (Desrosiers et al., 1989) or purified or recombinant viral proteins (Laskey, 1989) have been employed as vaccine immunogens. Thus it is likely that these latter vaccines do not induce as broad a spectrum of immune responses compared to a whole virus vaccine. In support of this assertion is our observation that a vaccine composed of lectin-purified SIV glycoproteins protected only two of four rhesus macaques from a homologous challenge with 10 ID of SIV after immunization procedures parallel to those employed previously for the successful whole virus SIV vaccine (Murphey-Corb et al., 1990). Thus it appears somewhat premature to attempt subunit vaccines until whole virus vaccines are "perfected" and their critical protective immune factors clearly elucidated. It may then be feasible to constitute appropriate viral immunogens for a subunit vaccine. Until this time, more emphasis should be placed on methods of producing safe whole virus vaccines, such as the "virus like particles" (VLP) produced by baculovirus expression systems and the RNA-deficient virus particles produced by retroviruses with specific mutations in their *gag* proteins. These viral antigen preparations could be employed for immunoprophylaxis and immunotherapeutic procedures.

In summary, there appears to be an increasing body of data from animal lentivirus systems supporting the feasibility of AIDS vaccine development. However, success will depend on resourceful and vigorous investigations of all available animal lentivirus models, of different viral immunogen compositions and modes of presentation, and of novel adjuvant formulations. For this we shall need patience and perseverance in the crisis atmosphere of AIDS research.

## Acknowledgements

This research is supported by funds from the Louisiana Agricultural Center and by Public Health Service Grants AI2580 and CA49296 from the National Institute of Health.

## References

Desrosiers, R.C., Wyand, M.S., Kodama, T., Ringler, D.J., Arthur, L.O., Sehgal, P.K., Letvin, N.L., King, N.W. and Daniel, M.D. (1989) Vaccine protection against simian immunodeficiency virus infection. *Proc. Natl. Acad. Sci. U.S.A.* 86, 6353–6357.

Foil, L.D., Adams, W.V., McManus, J.M. and Issel, C.J. (1987) Bloodmeal residues on mouthparts of *Tabanus fuscicostatus* (Diptera: Tabanidae) and the potential for the mechanical transmission of pathogens. *J. Med. Entomol.* 24, 613–616.

Gerencer, M., Valpotic, I., Jukic, B., Tomaskovic, M. and Basic, I. (1989) Qualitative analyses of cellular immune functions in equine infectious anemia show homology with AIDS. *Arch. Virol.* 104, 249–257.

Hussain, K.A., Issel, C.J., Schnorr, K.L. and Montelaro, R.C. (1987) Antigenic analysis of equine infectious anemia virus (EIAV) variants using monoclonal antibodies: epitopes of glycoprotein 90 (gp90) of EIAV stimulate neutralizing antibodies. *J. Virol.* 61, 2956–2961.

Issel, C.J. and Coggins, L. (1979) Equine infectious anemia: current knowledge. *J. Am. Vet. Med. Ass.* 174, 727–733.

Issel, C.J. and Foil, L.D. (1984) Studies on equine infectious anemia virus transmission by insects. *J. Am. Vet. Med. Ass.* 184, 293–297.

Issel, C.J., McManus, J., Haguis, S., Adams, W.V. and Montelaro, R. (1990) Efficacy of an inactivated whole virus vaccine in protecting against homologous and heterologous EIAV challenges. Submitted for publication.

Jahaverian et al. (1989) *Proc. Natl. Acad. Sci. U.S.A.* 86, 6772.

Kono, Y., Hirasawa, K., Fukunaga, Y. and Taniguchi, T. (1976) Recrudescence of EIA by treatment with immunosuppressive drugs. *Natl. Inst. Anim. Health Q. (Tokyo)* 16, 8–15.

Laskey, L.A. (1989) Current status of the development of an AIDS vaccine. *CRC Crit. Rev. Immunol.* 9, 153–172.

Montelaro, R.C., Parekh, B., Orrego, A. and Issel, C.J. (1984) Antigenic variation during persistent infection by equine infectious anemia virus, a retrovirus. *J. Biol. Chem.* 259, 10539–10544.

Murphey-Corb, M., Martin, L., Davison-Fairburn, B., Montelaro, R., Miller, M., West, M., Okawa, S., Baskin, G., Zhang, J.Y., Putney, S.D., Allison, A.C. and Eppstein, D.A. (1989) A formalin inactivated whole simian immunodeficiency virus vaccine confers protection in macaques. *Science* 246, 1293–1297.

Murphey-Corb, M., Martin, L., Montelaro, R., West, M., Zhang, J.Y., Allison, A.C. and Eppstein, D.A. (1990) Evaluation of a subunit SIV vaccine in macaques. *AIDS* (in press).

Orrego, A., Issel, C.J., Montelaro, R.C. and Adams, W.V. Jr. (1982) Virulence and in vitro growth of a cell-adapted strain of equine infectious anemia virus after serial passage in ponies. *Am. J. Vet. Res.* 43, 1556–1560.

Payne, S.L., Fang, F.D., Lui, C.P., Dhruva, B., Rwambo, P., Issel, C.J. and Montelaro, R.C. (1987a) Antigenic variation and lentivirus persistence: variations in envelope gene sequences during EIAV infection resemble changes reported for sequential isolates of HIV. *Virology* 161, 321–331.

Payne, S.L., Salinovich, O., Montelaro, R.C., Issel, C.J. and Nauman, S.M. (1987b) Course and extent of variation of equine infectious anemia virus during parallel persistent infections. *J. Virol.* 61, 1266–1270.

Perryman, L., O'Rourke, K. and McGuire, T. (1988) Immune responses are required to terminate viremia in EIAV infection. *J. Virol.* 62, 3073–3076.

Rasty, S., Dhruva, B., Schiltz, L., Shih, D., Issel, C. and Montelaro, R. (1990) Proviral DNA integration and transcriptional patterns of EIAV during persistent and cytopathic infections. *J. Virol.* 64, 86–95.

Rwambo, P.M., Issel, C.J., Adams, W.V., Hussain, K.A., Miller, M. and Montelaro, R.C. (1990) Equine infectious anemia virus (EIAV): Humoral responses of recipient ponies and antigenic variation during persistent infection. *Arch. Virol.* (in press).

*Eds. H. Schellekens and M.C. Horzinek*
*Animal Models in AIDS*



# 24

# Contemporary developments in the biology of the bovine immunodeficiency-like virus *

MATTHEW A. GONDA, M. STEVEN OBERSTE, KEVIN J. GARVEY, LUKE A. PALLANSCH, JANE K. BATTLES, DOMINIQUE Y. PIFAT and KUNIO NAGASHIMA

Laboratory of Cell and Molecular Structure, Program Resources, Inc., National Cancer Institute-Frederick Cancer Research and Development Center, Frederick, MD 21702-1201, U.S.A.

## Introduction

The human immunodeficiency virus types 1 and 2 (HIV-1 and HIV-2) are members of the lentivirus subfamily of retroviruses (reviewed in Gonda et al., 1989) and the etiologic agents of the acquired immunodeficiency syndrome (AIDS) (Wong-Staal and Gallo, 1985a,b; Gallo and Wong-Staal, 1985). AIDS is characterized by a slow, progressively debilitating, degenerative disease of the immune and central nervous systems and is accompanied by cancers and opportunistic infections. At least in the case of HIV-1, the virus induces a long-term persistent infection, during which time the vast majority of infected individuals go on to develop AIDS and/or neurologic symptoms; most eventually die of AIDS-related complications. There is a critical need for an effective vaccine and, in its absence, the development of antiviral drugs to arrest the progression of HIV-related disease. The continuing growth of the HIV pandemic makes these discoveries all the more urgent (McGowan and Hoth, 1989; Haseltine, 1989).

Because HIV-1 and HIV-2 are lentiviruses, they have a number of virus counterparts in various animal species (Table 1). Lentiviruses are exogenous, non-oncogenic viruses that cause chronic, multisystemic diseases with insidious outcomes (Haase, 1986; Gonda et al., 1989). They are one of three subfamilies of retroviruses; the other two are the spumaviruses and the oncoviruses. While

---

* By acceptance of this article, the publisher or recipient acknowledges the right of the U.S. Government to retain a nonexclusive, royalty-free license in and to any copyright covering the article.

TABLE 1
Clinical manifestations of lentivirus infections in natural hosts

| Lentivirus | Disease description |
|---|---|
| Ovine visna, maedi, and progressive pneumonia virus | Progressive lethal pneumonia, chronic encephalomyelitis, spasticity, paralysis, lymphadenopathy, mastitis, generalized wasting, opportunistic infections |
| Caprine arthritis encephalitis virus | Generalized wasting, chronic leukoencephalomyelitis, progressive arthritis, osteoporosis, paralysis |
| Equine infectious anemia virus | Fever, persistent viremia, hemolytic anemia, lymphoproliferation, immune-complex glomerulonephritis, bone marrow depression, central nervous system lesions |
| Bovine immunodeficiency-like virus | Persistent lymphocytosis, lymphadenopathy, central nervous system lesions, weakness, emaciation |
| Feline immunodeficiency virus | Immunodeficiency-like syndrome, generalized lymphadenopathy, leukopenia, fever, anemia, emaciation, opportunistic infections |
| Simian immunodeficiency virus | Immunodeficiency, neuropathologic changes, wasting, opportunistic infections |
| Human immunodeficiency virus | Immunodeficency, lymphadenopathy, opportunistic infections, encephalopathy, emaciation, Kaposi's sarcoma and other cancers |

Adapted from Gonda (1988) with permission of the editors and Alan R. Liss, Inc.

lentiviruses have been recognized as novel animal pathogens for some time, the discovery that the HIVs are lentiviruses (Gonda et al., 1985, 1986) has given new importance to lentivirus studies. The search for a related animal lentivirus that may have given rise to HIV-1 led to the discovery and/or characterization of several new lentivirus agents, including the simian immunodeficiency viruses (SIVs) (Desrosiers et al., 1989), feline immunodeficiency virus (FIV) (Pedersen et al., 1987), and bovine immunodeficiency-like virus (BIV) (Van Der Maaten et al., 1972; Gonda et al., 1987; Braun et al., 1988; Garvey et al., 1990).

The lack of appropriate animal models susceptible to HIV infection for in vivo studies presents an obstacle to the testing of new leads in candidate AIDS drugs. Animal models became all the more important with the decision to liberalize the distribution of potentially beneficial antiretroviral drugs to HIV-infected individuals prior to the completion of validation studies. This policy, although humane, has resulted in reductions in the numbers of volunteers available for drug efficacy studies. The identification of and advancement in knowledge about animal models, which use animal retroviruses related to those that cause AIDS in humans (Table 1), is considered an important step in the development and testing of both novel vaccine strategies and therapeutic agents for AIDS; developments in lentivirus animal models may play a crucial role in understanding the pathogenesis of HIV (Gardner and Luciw, 1989). What follows is a historical perspective on the discovery, characterization, and salient features of the molecular biology of BIV and an overview of progress in the development of BIV as a model of lentivirus disease of relevance to HIV infection.

## Historical perspective

The intensive search, in the late 1960s, for an infectious agent that might be the cause of bovine lymphosarcoma was probably the motivating factor that led to the discovery of and subsequent research on several distinct classes of retroviruses in cattle. Of course, it was not until the finding of reverse transcriptase (RT) that this animal virus group became known as retroviruses. Four unique retrovirus isolates have been found in cattle (Malmquist et al., 1969; Miller et al., 1969; Van Der Maaten et al., 1972; York et al., 1989) and there is at least one representative bovine virus for each retrovirus subfamily (Oncovirinae, Lentivirinae, and Spumavirinae). These bovine isolates are briefly described below in order to highlight some of the distinctions between them.

Bovine leukemia virus (BLV), an oncovirus, was isolated from the peripheral leukocytes of cattle with lymphosarcoma (Miller et al., 1969). It is the best known and most studied bovine retrovirus and the cause of enzootic lymphosarcoma and associated persistent lymphocytosis (Burney et al., 1980). BLV is closely related to human T-cell leukemia viruses types 1 and 2 (HTLV-1 and HTLV-2); HTLV-1 is the etiologic agent of adult T-cell leukemia (Wong-Staal and Gallo, 1985b). Because of its relationship to the HTLVs, BLV is a useful model of infectious human cancers (Burny et al., 1987). Another recently described bovine oncovirus is structurally and immunologically related to the type D retroviruses, some of which cause immunodeficiencies in primates (Heidecker et al., 1987; Gardner and Luciw, 1989); this putative bovine type D virus is not known to be associated with any disease (York et al., 1989).

Bovine syncytial virus (BSV) is the only bovine representative of the spumavirus subfamily and was isolated, at about the same time as BLV, from both lymphosarcomatous and normal cattle (Malmquist et al., 1969). However, BSV has not been etiologically linked to any disease. It is a frequently encountered contaminant in primary cultures of bovine peripheral leukocytes.

Like BSV and BLV, the virus now known as BIV (Gonda et al., 1987) was discovered during the search by Van Der Maaten et al. (1972) for the cause of lymphosarcoma. These workers became interested in a novel bovine virus that induced syncytia in cultured cells (similar to BLV and BSV) and structurally resembled visna, maedi, and progressive pneumonia viruses (OPPV) of sheep; this virus was isolated in Louisiana from a Holstein herd with persistent lymphocytosis. Lymphoproliferative disease is also frequently seen in herds infected with BLV (Burny et al., 1980). The clinical signs of disease in animals infected with BIV included a generalized hyperplasia of lymph nodes, mild prolonged lymphocytosis, central nervous system lesions, weakness, and emaciation. When BIV was introduced into specific-pathogen-free calves, it induced a mild lymphocytosis and lymphadenopathy. There was no gross evidence of lymphosarcoma in animals from which BIV was isolated or in the experimentally infected calves. Since there was no conclusive evidence to support BIV's role in bovine lymphosarcoma, the virus was put into low-temperature storage.

Chronologically, BIV was the third unique lentivirus to be isolated. Neverthe-

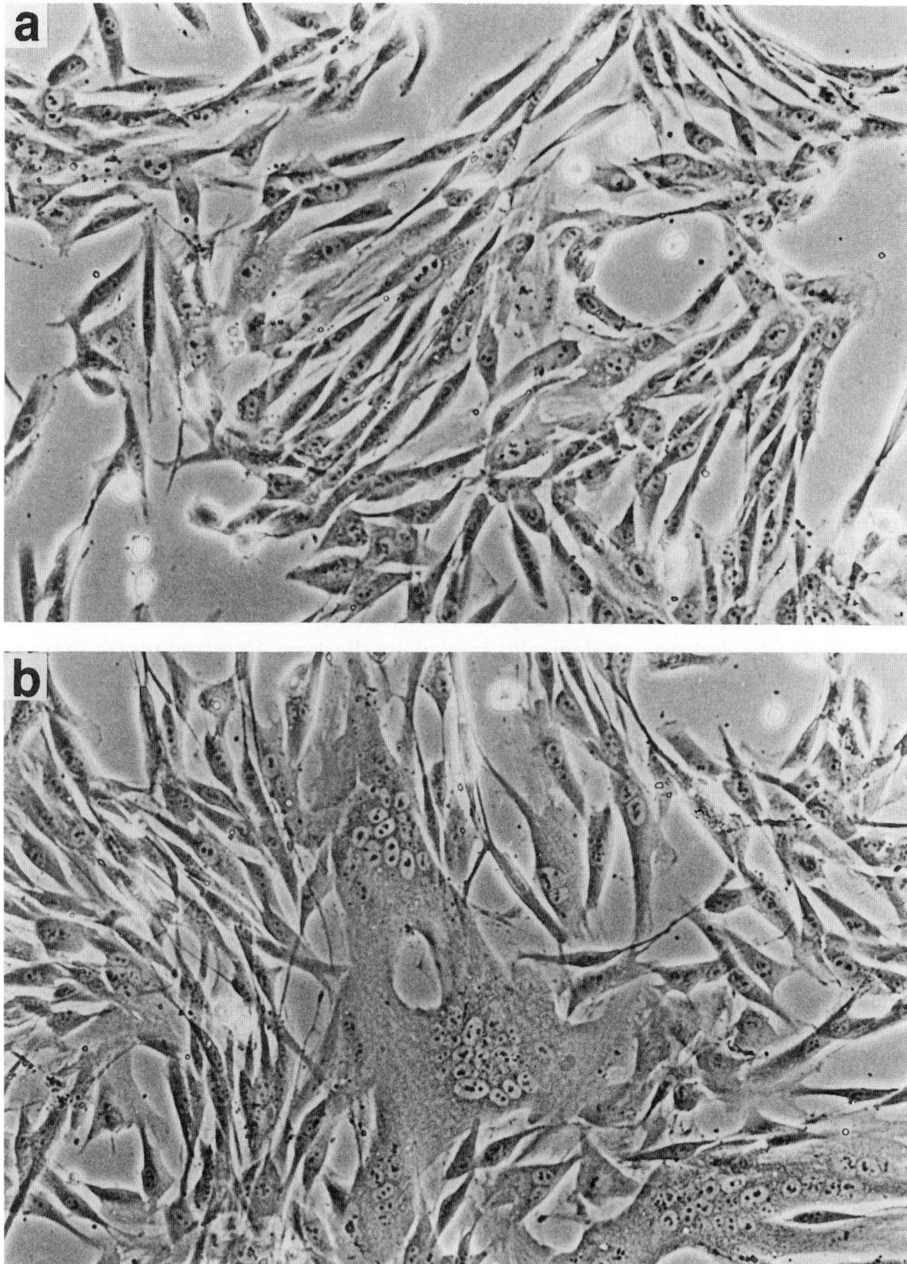


Fig. 1. Syncytia induction caused by BIV infection. (a) Uninfected control EREp cells. (b) EREp cells infected with cell-free BIV.

less, its importance went unappreciated and its biology unstudied for nearly a decade and a half after the initial discovery. Not until the emergence of the AIDS pandemic did researchers recognize that it shared morphologic, serologic, and genetic characteristics with the first human lentivirus, HIV (Gonda et al., 1987). Since that time, interest in the virus has been renewed and much progress has been made in characterizing BIV's molecular biology and in producing useful reagents for developing animal models of BIV infection and pathogenesis.

## In vitro characterization of BIV

BIV grows in a number of primary explants of bovine embryonic tissues, including brain, testis, spleen, lung, thymus, choroid plexus, and kidney (Gonda et al., 1987). Replication in bovine spleen and lung cells is preferred, as the virus grows to higher titers in these primary cells. The infection can be readily transmitted to uninfected cultures with cell-free supernatants, but the use of infected cells is the most efficient method. Infection of primary and established cell cultures leads to the formation of syncytia (Fig. 1), the release of virus particles as observed by electron microscopy, and an increase in supernatant RT activity (Gonda et al., 1987, 1990; Braun et al., 1988). Although BLV, BSV, and BIV all induce syncytia, each has distinctive in vitro cytopathologic characteristics that facilitate the identification of the agent (Gonda, unpublished data). In addition to cells that grow on a solid substrate, cell-free BIV stocks can effectively infect bovine leukocytes; however, the particular cell type(s) involved have not been sufficiently characterized to be identified definitively (Pifat et al., unpublished data).

The initial characterization of BIV was hampered by the lack of both an adequate cell culture system to sustain virus replication and methods for the large-scale production and purification of virus for experimental investigations. In an effort to establish persistently infected virus-producing cells, we have developed other established cell culture systems from several animal species that are capable of supporting BIV replication indefinitely (Gonda et al., 1990). Two of these cell lines originate from dog thymus (Cf2Th) and embryonic rabbit epithelium (EREp); these cells are more resistant than primary cell cultures to the cytopathic effects of the virus and can be passaged more than 20 times to produce virus for antigen, although there is a decline in antigen production on later passage. For this reason, we occasionally add uninfected cells to the persistently infected cultures to enhance the amount of virus production as necessary. These and primary bovine cell cultures have been used to mass-produce BIV stocks according to methods described for other retroviruses (Benton et al., 1978), with only slight modifications. Purified and concentrated BIV from large-scale production has been used to make BIV-specific polyclonal antisera, to analyze viral RT activity and viral structural proteins, and to develop various immunoassays (Gonda et al., 1987, 1990).

When studied under assay conditions optimal for HIV (Hoffman et al., 1985),

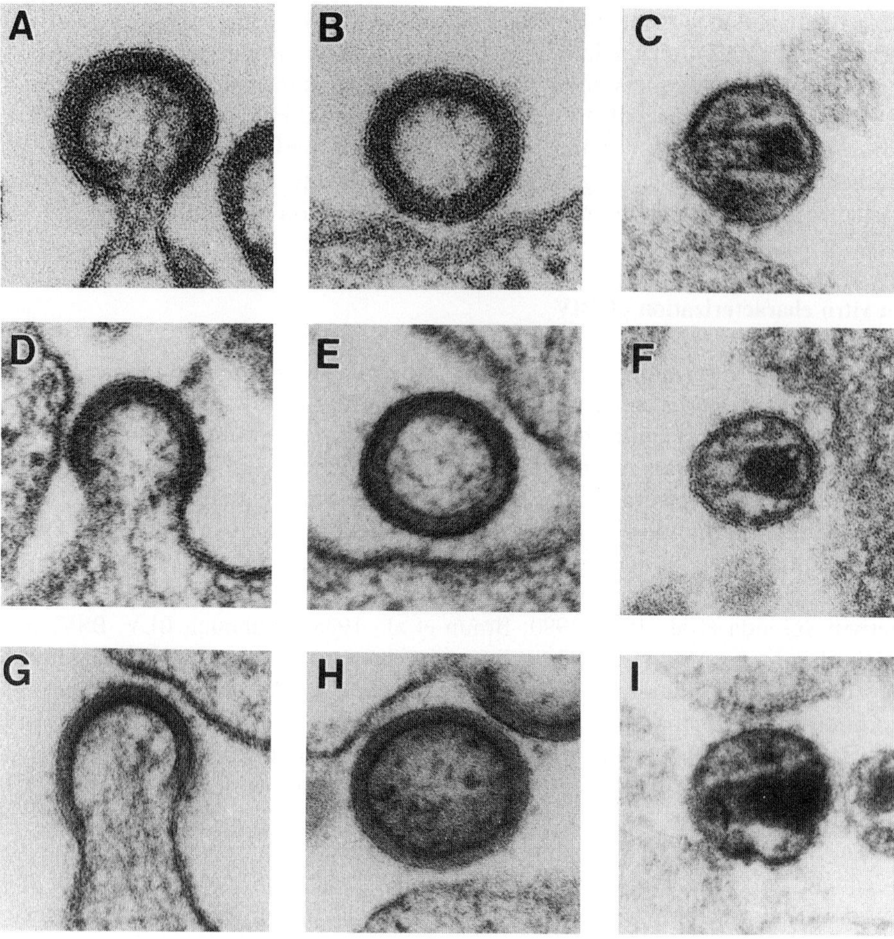


Fig. 2. Electron microscopy of the morphogenesis of BIV and several members of the lentivirus family for comparison. (A–C) HIV-1; (D–F) BIV; (G–I) OPPV; (A), (D), and (G) and (B), (E), and (H) are immature budding and extracellular forms, respectively, and (C), (F), and (I) are mature forms of HIV-1, BIV, and OPPV. (Reprinted from Gonda et al., 1989, with permission of the publisher).

the BIV RT in concentrated purified virions shows optimal activity using a poly(rA)-oligo ($dT_{12-18}$) template primer and has a significant preference for $Mg^{2+}$ cations as a cofactor (Gonda et al., 1987, 1990). Interestingly, the BIV RT is also active at low concentrations of $Mn^{2+}$ cation, although higher concentrations of $Mn^{2+}$ are inhibitory to the activity of BIV RT.

Transmission electron microscopy of BIV shows that its morphology and morphogenesis are typical of the lentivirus subfamily and are most similar to those reported for HIV (Gonda et al., 1985, 1989; Braun et al., 1988; Gelderblom et al., 1989). Fig. 2 shows the comparative ultrastructure of BIV, HIV, and OPPV. Particles of BIV initially form as a crescent beneath the plasma membrane; the electron-dense inner core is separated from the viral envelope by a semielectron-dense region (Fig. 2D). Virus particles are released from the cell after closure of the crescent by a budding process. Recently released, immature extracellular particles are round, with a doughnut-shaped core and an electron-lucent center (Fig. 2E). The core of the mature extracellular particle is condensed

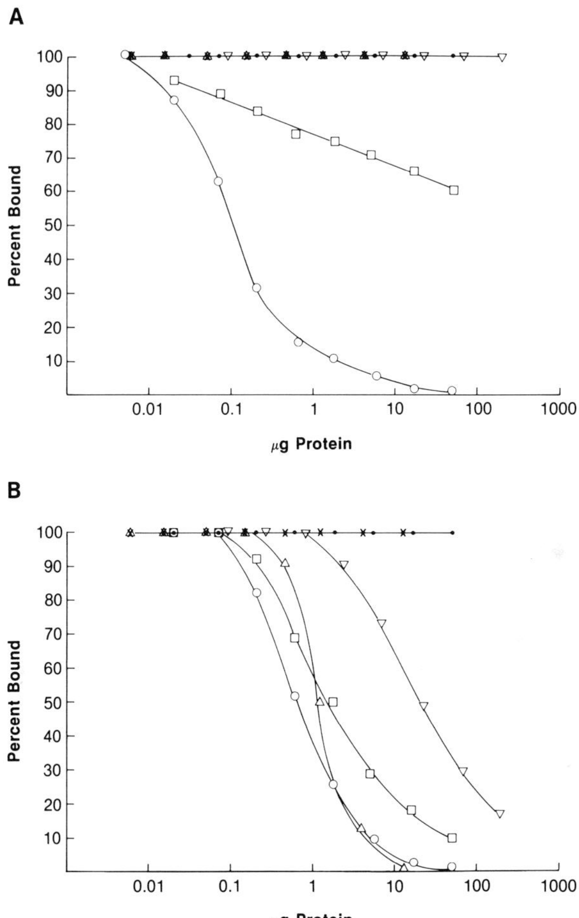


Fig. 3. Immunologic relatedness of major core proteins of retroviruses using a competitive radioimmunoassay for the major capsid protein (p24) of the *gag* gene of HIV-1. The viruses (or mock virus preparations) used to compete were HIV-1 (○), BIV (△), SIV (□), visna virus and caprine arthritis encephalitis virus (×), EIAV (▽), feline leukemia virus, BLV, HTLV-1, HTLV-2, and uninfected concentrated H9 cell supernatants (●). Sucrose gradient-purified viruses were disrupted in detergent and tested for their ability to compete for the binding of $^{125}$I-labeled HIV p24 at limiting dilutions of antiserum to BIV or HIV. (A) Homologous assay using $^{125}$I-labelled HIV p24 and anti-HIV polyclonal rabbit serum. (B) Heterologous assay using $^{125}$I-labeled HIV p24 and anti-BIV polyclonal rabbit antiserum. (Reprinted from Gonda et al., 1987, with permission of the editors and Macmillan Magazines Ltd.).

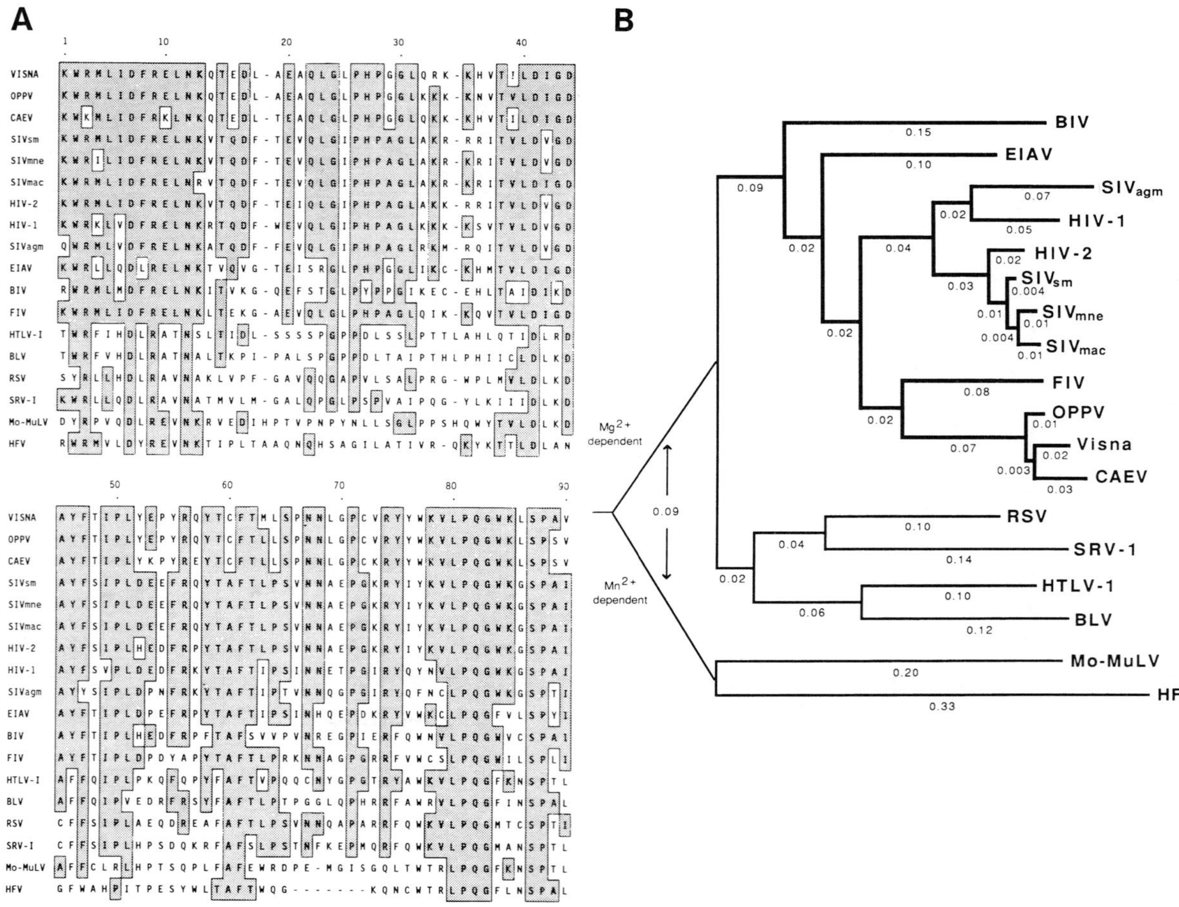
A
B
BIV
EIAV
SIVagm
HIV-1
HIV-2
SIVsm
SIVmne
SIVmac
FIV
OPPV
Visna
CAEV
RSV
SRV-1
HTLV-1
BLV
Mo-MuLV
HFV
Mg2+ dependent
Mn2+ dependent
0.09

(Fig. 2F); the condensation of the immature core presumably occurs following cleavage of *gag* precursors by the viral protease. The mature extracellular particles are 100–130 nm in diameter.

**Evolutionary relationship of BIV to other retroviruses**

Retroviruses are a genetically diverse group of protein-enveloped, high-molecular-weight, RNA-containing viruses that encode a unique enzyme, RT. RT is capable of catalyzing the flow of the virus's genetic information in the reverse direction (RNA → DNA) from that normally associated with cell processes (DNA → RNA); as a consequence, a replicative DNA intermediate called the provirus is created. Segments of the RT gene are the most conserved in the evolution of retroviruses and are useful markers for determining evolutionary relationships. Thus, RT not only plays a key role in the life cycle of the virus but also serves as a genetic hallmark to unify, as well as distinguish, members of this virus family. The *gag* genes of these viruses are also relatively conserved within retrovirus subfamilies and *gag* proteins have been used to demonstrate serologic relationships.

While it was obvious to us that BIV shared some biologic and structural properties with HIV and other lentiviruses, it remained unclear whether BIV was a unique lentivirus. To answer this question, we developed polyclonal antisera to BIV and several representative molecular clones of BIV that contained intact RT regions of the *pol* gene to assess its serologic and genetic relationship, respectively, to other retroviruses (Gonda et al., 1987).

Using polyclonal antisera to BIV and HIV, we initially observed gross cross-reactivity between BIV and HIV in immunofluorescence assays, and we localized the reactivity to the major capsid (CA) proteins, p26 and p24 of BIV and HIV, respectively, in Western blotting experiments. To further assess the relatedness of BIV, HIV, and other retrovirus *gag* proteins, we developed competitive radioimmunoassays using $^{125}$I-labeled HIV p24 CA antigen and polyvalent antisera to

Fig. 4. Evolutionary relationship of BIV. (A) Alignment of 90 consecutive amino acids in the conserved RT domain of *pol* genes from lentiviruses with those of other retroviruses. Retroviruses used are visna virus, OPPV, CAEV, $SIV_{sm}$, $SIV_{mne}$, $SIV_{mac}$, HIV-2, HIV-1, $SIV_{agm}$, EIAV, BIV, FIV, HTLV-1 (human T-cell leukemia virus), BLV, Rous sarcoma virus (RSV), simian AIDS retrovirus type 1 (SRV-1), Moloney leukemia virus (Mo-MuLV), and human foamy virus (HFV). The alignment shown is that generally found optimal with visna virus; slight improvements in the other pairwise alignment scores can be made by minor shifts in the placement of gaps. Shaded boxes are drawn around identical residues when seven or more lentiviruses share that residue. (B) Fitch-Margoliash phylogenetic tree of retroviral relationships based on the *pol* gene sequences shown in (A). Branch lengths are in units of $-\log M$, where M is the frequency of matching residues. The tree was rooted with HFV and Mo-MuLV as the outgroup taxons because they consistently had the lowest alignment scores and because their RTs preferentially use $Mn^{2+}$ cations as cofactor. The average percent standard deviation of the tree was 5.17. (Reprinted from Garvey et al., 1990, with permission of the editors and Academic Press, Inc.)

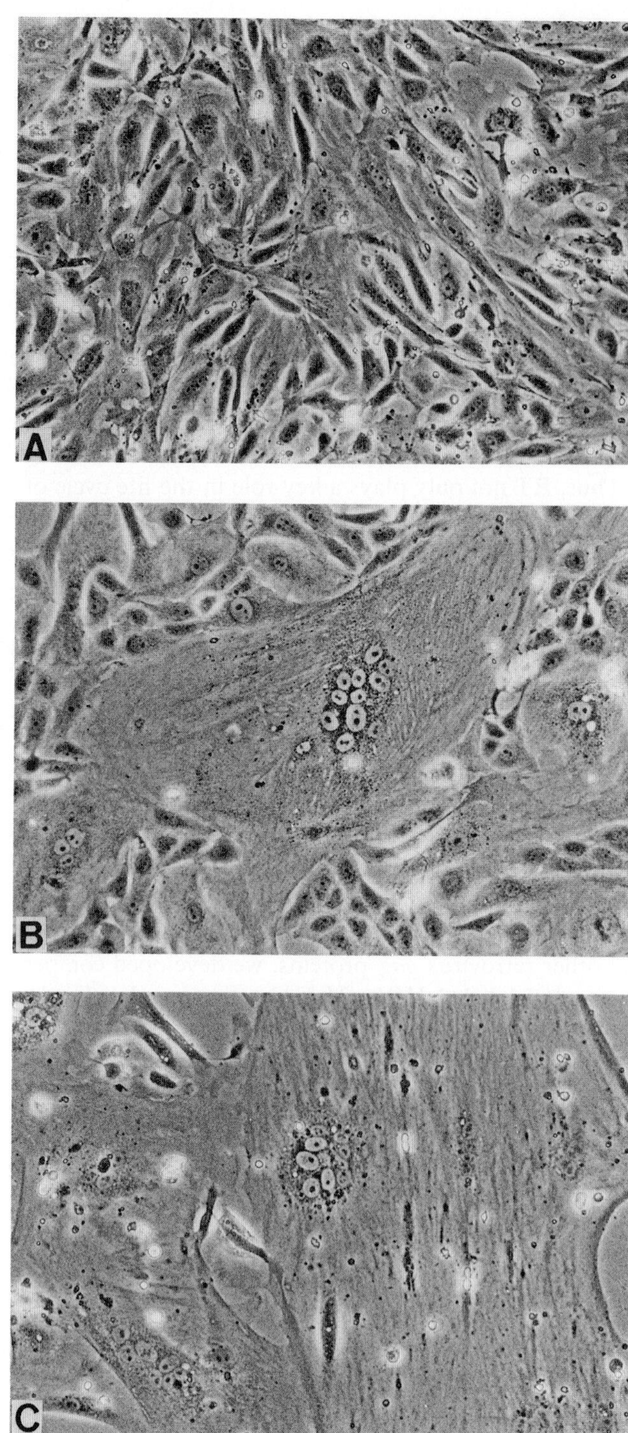
A
B
C

BIV and HIV (Fig. 3). In the homologous assay (using HIV antiserum), only SIV competed (partially) with HIV for HIV p24 CA antigen (Fig. 3A). In the heterologous assay (using BIV antiserum), BIV, HIV, equine infectious anemia virus (EIAV), and SIV all competed for HIV p24 CA antigen (Fig. 3B). These studies were the first to effectively extend the relationship between BIV and other lentiviruses beyond biologic and ultrastructural observations.

The phylogenetic relationship between BIV and other retroviruses has been quantified by aligning 90 consecutive amino acid residues deduced from the DNA sequence of the highly conserved RT domain of BIV to the sequences of the other retroviruses (Fig. 4A) (Garvey et al., 1990), as performed previously to demonstrate the ancestral relationship of HIV to the lentiviruses (Gonda et al., 1985, 1986, 1987, 1988, 1989). Pairwise comparisons between the amino acid residues in this region of RT indicate extensive sequence conservation between lentiviruses (50–53% or greater matching residues; no gaps); the sequence identity weakens when other retrovirus subfamily members are compared to the lentiviruses (38–42% or fewer matching residues; with gaps). It is obvious on inspecting this alignment that BIV clusters with the lentiviruses and is a unique entry.

A Fitch-Margoliash phylogenetic tree (Fig. 4B) was generated from the derived amino acid sequence shown in Fig. 4A. The tree was rooted with the retroviruses whose RTs preferentially use $Mn^{2+}$ cations as the outgroup taxons. Among the retroviruses whose RTs have a preference for $Mg^{2+}$ cations, there are two main branches, one that leads to the oncoviruses and one that leads to the lentiviruses. The branching order of the lentiviruses has BIV diverging first from an ancestor that gave rise to the lentiviruses. From calculations of the evolutionary distances on the tree, we find that BIV is positioned about equidistant from all of the other lentiviruses, although it may appear that BIV is more closely related to EIAV.

## Molecular cloning and characterization of functional proviruses

Biologic activity could not be demonstrated for the initial molecular clones of BIV (Gonda et al., 1987). Nevertheless, these non-functional proviral clones proved useful in establishing the uniqueness of BIV, and, more importantly, were used to develop highly specific DNA probes to screen recombinant libraries in search of functional proviruses with which to study the biology and pathogenesis of the virus. We obtained two distinct full-length, biologically active proviral clones (BIV 106 and 127), as well as numerous non-functional clones (Braun et

Fig. 5. Microinjection of BIV clones 106 and 127 into bovine embryonic spleen cells. (A) Mock-injected control cells. (B) Cells injected with BIV clone 106. (C) Cells injected with BIV clone 127. The photographs were taken 48 h after microinjection of the DNA into the nucleus. (Reprinted from Braun et al., 1988, with permission of the editors and Academic Press, Inc.).

al., 1988). These clones were derived from the DNA of cells carrying the infection from a single virus isolate. The biologic activity of the functional proviral clones was demonstrated by microinjecting the cloned proviral DNA into permissive cells (Braun et al., 1988). Cells microinjected with biologically active BIV provirus formed syncytia within 24–48 h (Fig. 5); RT activity was detectable in supernatants from these cultures within 2 weeks. Biologic activity was transmissible to other permissive bovine cell cultures by cell-free supernatants, thus confirming the generation of infectious virus from these proviral clones.

## Genome organization

The complete nucleotide sequence of the two infectious BIV proviral clones (BIV 106 and BIV 127) has been determined (Garvey et al., 1990). The sequences of the two functional clones diverge slightly, but the genomes are identical in genetic organization (Fig. 6). The overall topography for the BIV genome is 5′LTR-*gag-pol*-"central region"-*env*-3′LTR. In addition to the structural genes, *gag, pol,* and *env,* which are flanked on the 5′ and 3′ ends by the viral long terminal repeats (LTRs), BIV also contains five other open reading frames (ORFs) in the "central region" between and overlapping the *pol* and *env* genes. The central region is a hallmark of the lentiviruses and proteins encoded by this region are believed to play an important role in their pathogenesis (Haseltine, 1989).

Three of the central region ORFs, *vif, tat,* and *rev,* have been identified by comparing their deduced amino acid sequences with those of other lentiviruses. In addition, the positions of these ORFs are analogous to that of the non-structural/regulatory genes found in HIV (Fig. 6) and/or visna virus (not shown), suggesting that they may encode proteins with similar functions. BIV *vif* has little amino acid identity with other lentivirus *vif* proteins, but a local search of

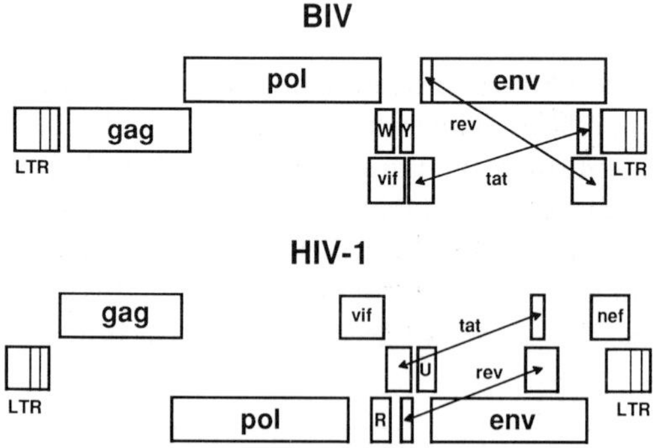


Fig. 6. Comparative genomic organization of BIV and HIV. The major structural ORFs (*gag, pol,* and *env*) are shown as well as those corresponding to the non-structural/regulatory genes (*vif, tat, rev, vpu, vpr,* W, and Y) found in either BIV or HIV.

amino acid similarity has delineated a conserved sequence motif, S-L-Q-X-L-A, where X is arginine, phenylalanine, or tyrosine (Oberste and Gonda, in preparation). Interestingly, the coding strategy of BIV *rev* is most like that of visna virus; it consists of two exons, with exon 1 occurring in the *env* ORF and in frame with the *env* gene translation and exon 2 occurring within the 3′ end of the *env* ORF but in a different reading frame. The exon assignment of *rev* in BIV has been confirmed by sequencing cDNA clones (Oberste et al., unpublished data). The identities of two other ORFs in the central region of BIV, termed W and Y, have not yet been determined, but their location suggests they may be analogous to the *vpu, vpx,* or *vpr* gene found in primate lentiviruses. A striking feature of the BIV genome is the absence of a *nef* gene; *nef* is purported to be a transcriptional silencer, although this has not been firmly established.

The organization of the BIV LTR (U3-R-U5) is similar to that of other retroviruses, although the sequences are divergent overall (Garvey et al., 1990). The LTR contains all of the regulatory signals for initiation, enhancement, and termination of transcription identified by analogy to previously described retrovirus regulatory sequences. Several *cis*-acting control sequences, whose functions have not yet been confirmed, were also identified. The proviral LTRs of BIV 127 and 106 are 589 and 587 nt, respectively. The $U_3$, R, and $U_5$ regions for BIV 127 are 384, 111, and 94 nt, respectively. These regions are 384, 109, and 94 nt, respectively, for BIV 106. The site of transcription initiation at the 5′ ends of the viral RNA has been mapped by primer extension to nucleotides 384–386 in the left LTR; this region defines the U3-R boundary. The 2 nt deletion in the R region of BIV 106 was also confirmed by the primer extension experiments.

**Transcriptional analysis and transactivation of the LTR**

Like HIV, BIV exhibits a complex transcriptional pattern with at least five recognizable size classes of viral mRNA (Oberste et al., submitted), the smaller two transcripts in HIV-infected cells have been identified as those of *rev* and *tat* (Haseltine, 1989). Viral RNA from BIV-infected cells has been cloned as cDNA; the identity of several of these cDNA clones has been determined by DNA sequencing to be putative *rev* transcripts (Oberste et al., unpublished data). Functional analysis of these BIV *rev* cDNAs has yet to be performed.

The *tat* gene product of HIV is a potent transactivator that can increase viral gene expression in cultured cells by both transcriptional and post-transcriptional mechanisms. In HIV, the target sequence for *tat* transactivation has been localized within the LTR to a region immediately downstream of the mRNA start-site (Haseltine, 1989). The *tat* gene in the BIV genome was identified by its location in the central region and by a strong conservation of amino acid residues surrounding a cysteine-rich region also present in *tat* exon 1 of HIV and SIV. To determine whether a protein is encoded by BIV *tat* that can potentiate transactivation and if a *tat*-responsive element (TAR) exists in BIV, several BIV LTR constructs were prepared in which the 5′ proviral LTR was cloned in front of a bacterial chloramphenicol acetyl transferase (CAT) reporter gene (Pallansch et al., submitted). When these LTR-CAT constructs were transfected into BIV-infected cells, a transient sixfold activation of CAT gene expression was observed, demonstrating the existence of an element within the viral LTR that is responsive to products of the viral infection; the demonstration of a direct effect of a *tat* gene product in transactivation is under investigation using *tat* mutants.

Several Cf2Th cell lines were also derived in which the BIV LTR-CAT constructs were stably integrated. Using such indicator cell lines, it was demonstrated that both the functional clones (BIV 127 and BIV 106) and parental stock from which they were derived are capable of strongly activating the LTR-CAT in Cf2Th cells (15-fold and 85-fold, respectively). This gene activation appears to be relatively virus-specific, since other bovine retroviruses (BSV and BLV) do not appear to induce significant activation of the BIV LTR-CAT gene. The BIV LTR-CAT Cf2Th cell lines may be useful in creating biologic assays to demonstrate the presence of BIV in bovine serum or cells co-cultured with them from animals suspected of harboring a BIV infection.

Computer analysis of the DNA sequence of the BIV LTR revealed the existence of a nucleotide sequence matching the glucocorticoid receptor binding site, as well as other *cis*-acting elements observed in other systems (Garvey et al., 1990). To determine whether BIV gene expression was affected by such steroids, the BIV LTR-CAT Cf2Th indicator cell lines were exposed to dexamethasone, a potent glucocorticoid analogue. Interestingly, in preliminary experiments, the addition of dexamethasone (10–50 $\mu$M) to the tissue culture medium caused a concomitant increase in CAT activity in these cells. These findings clearly indicate that, as observed in other lentiviruses, the BIV LTR contains a variety of regulatory/responsive elements. Current efforts are designed to address these features and to delineate more clearly the LTR regions responsive to various regulatory genes that characterize lentiviruses in general.

## Identification of putative structural proteins

The availability of the complete sequence of BIV has enabled us to estimate the size of the structural protein products deduced from the translation of the *gag, pol,* and *env* ORFs and compare these values to those obtained experimentally (Table 2 and Fig. 7). Various sera have been used in the serologic identification of BIV proteins by Western blotting and radioimmunoprecipitation of metabolically labeled cells and virions; these include polyvalent reagents made to purified whole virus, synthetic peptides, recombinant proteins, and sera from animals naturally or experimentally infected with BIV. For the sake of uniformity in describing the proteins of BIV, we have adopted the standardized nomenclature for retrovirus proteins proposed by Leis et al. (1988).

The BIV *gag* precursor is predicted to be approximately 53 kDa; this is consonant with the detection of the p53 antigen in BIV-infected cells by Western blot (Gonda et al., 1987) and radioimmunoprecipitation (Battles et al., sub-

TABLE 2
Structural protein products of BIV

| ORF | Standard Nomenclature [a] | Position [b] | Predicted [c] | Exp. Obs. [d] |
|---|---|---|---|---|
| *gag* | *gag* precursor | nt 316–1743 | 53440 | p53 |
| | *MA* (matrix) | aa 1–133 | 15369 | p17 |
| | *CA* (capsid) | 134–360 | 25420 | p26 |
| | *NC* (nucleocapsid) | 361–476 | 12687 | p14 |
| *pol* | *pol* precursor | nt 1581–4739 | 120658 | ? |
| | *PR* (protease) | aa 51–143 | 10564 | ? |
| | *RT* (reverse transcriptase) | 144–774 | 72157 | ? |
| | *IN* (integrase) | 775–1053 | 32054 | ? |
| *env* | *env* precursor | nt 5415–8126 | 102269[e] | gp145[f] |
| | *SU* (surface protein) | aa 1–555 | 62098[e] | gp100[f] |
| | *TM* (transmembrane protein) | 556–904 | 40189[e] | gp45[f] |

[a] Standard nomenclature and acronyms for *gag, pol,* and *env* retrovirus proteins proposed by Leis et al. (1988) have been used for BIV.
[b] Nucleotide (nt) and amino acid (aa) positions are those for BIV 127 as reported in Garvey et al. (1990).
[c] Predicted precursors and processed protein products of BIV deduced from translation of BIV 127 nucleotide sequence. Molecular weights are given in Daltons.
[d] Experimentally observed proteins. Molecular weights are in Daltons $\times$ $10^3$. Proposed nomenclature for the various BIV products is used where known.
[e] Molecular weights are of the unglycosylated form of the predicted protein product.
[f] Molecular weights are of the glycosylated form of the experimentally observed protein product.

mitted). Moreover, the entire BIV *gag* gene has been isolated and incorporated into a recombinant baculovirus for expression in insect cells; a recombinant p53 protein that is immunologically recognized by BIV-specific sera is abundantly expressed in this vector system (Rasmussen et al., 1990). The *gag* precursor is predicted to be processed into at least three functional subunits, the matrix (MA), CA, and nucleocapsid (NC) proteins, based on alignments with other known lentivirus proteins (Garvey et al., 1990; Table 2). The exact cleavage sites used for the processing of the BIV *gag* precursor remain unknown pending amino acid sequencing of mature proteins. The following putative BIV *gag* proteins have been serologically identified: p17 (MA), p26 (CA), and p14 (NC); several intermediate *gag* products in the 45–47 kDa range have also been observed (Battles et al., 1990) (Fig. 7). Immunologic cross-reactivity of the BIV, HIV, SIV, and EIAV CA proteins (Gonda et al., 1987) may be explained by the presence of a conserved sequence (N-I-H-Q-G-P-K-E-P-Y) at amino acids 289–298 (Garvey et al., 1990). It will be interesting to see if peptides made to this CA region of *gag* are reactive with sera produced against the various lentiviruses. These peptides, if immunoreactive with a variety of lentiviruses, may be useful in developing a serologic screen to detect distantly related, but as yet undiscovered, lentiviruses (Gonda et al., unpublished data).

The *pol* ORF of HIV encodes the protease (PR), RT, and endonuclease/integrase (IN) proteins (Haseltine, 1989). These proteins have been identified in the

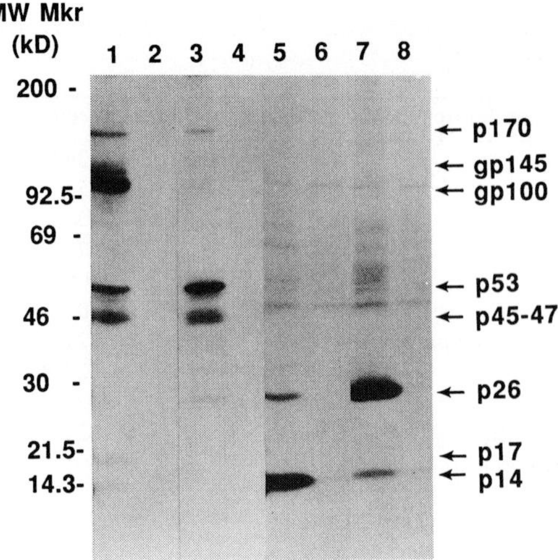


Fig. 7. Radioimmunoprecipitation of metabolically labeled BIV proteins. Lanes 1–4: infected cell lysates; lanes 5–8: virions; lanes 1 and 5: proteins precipitated by bovine serum from animals experimentally infected with BIV; lanes 2 and 6: proteins precipitated by negative control bovine serum; lanes 3 and 7: proteins precipitated by rabbit serum from an animal hyperimmunized with BIV; lanes 4 and 8: proteins precipitated by preimmune serum from a hyperimmunized rabbit. Protein designations: p170, *gag/pol* precursor; gp145 and gp100, *env* precursor and SU proteins, respectively; p53, *gag* precursor; p45–47, *gag* intermediates and TM protein; p26, *gag* CA protein; p17, *gag* MA protein; and p14, *gag* NC protein.

*pol* ORF of BIV based on amino acid alignments with the corresponding *pol* products in HIV (Garvey et al., 1990). BIV's *pol* ORF, like HIV's and other lentiviruses', overlaps the 3′ end of the *gag* ORF. The *gag* and *pol* gene products are believed to be synthesized as a polyprotein by a frameshifting event in the translation of the full-length mRNA; this polyprotein is later auto-digested into *gag* and *pol* precursors. A large protein of 170 kDa has been observed in BIV-infected cells by radioimmunoprecipitation using BIV *gag*-specific sera (Battles et al., submitted; Rasmussen et al., 1990) and in insect cells infected by a recombinant baculovirus containing the *gag/pol* genes (Rasmussen et al., unpublished data); we believe that this protein represents the *gag/pol* polyprotein. The BIV *pol* precursor is predicted to be 121 kDa and to be cleaved into mature protein products of 11 kDa (PR), 72 kDa (RT), and 32 kDa (IN) (Table 2). The BIV protease has 31% of its amino acid residues in common with HIV-1 and includes the aspartyl protease active site, D-T-G (Garvey et al., 1990; Oberste and Gonda, unpublished data). Assays developed to detect BIV-specific proteolytic cleavage of recombinant BIV p53 *gag* have demonstrated that pepstatin A, an effective aspartyl protease inhibitor that inhibits HIV's viral protease, is effective in inhibiting proteolytic activity in BIV virions (Rasmussen et al., 1990).

The *env* gene products of all retroviruses are highly glycosylated. In the case of the lentiviruses, the sugar moiety content of the surface membrane (SU) product of the *env* gene may be as much as 50%. The *env* glycoproteins are made as a precursor that is posttranslationally cleaved into the mature SU and transmembrane (TM) proteins. The non-glycosylated form of the BIV *env* precursor is estimated to be 102 kDa, and there are 21 potential glycosylation sites. We have serologically identified the putative *env* precursor, SU, and TM of BIV (gp145, gp100, and gp45, respectively) and determined by a variety of methods that they are highly glycosylated (Battles et al., 1990).

## Variability of the virus genome

Independent HIV-1 isolates may differ by as much as 25% in their *env* gene sequences (Starcich et al., 1986). In addition, with the divergent human lentiviruses, HIV-1 and HIV-2, there is only 39% homology in the SU protein (Guyader et al., 1987). Thus, it was not unexpected to find that the SUs of BIV and HIV-1 share only 13% amino acid identity (Garvey et al., 1990). Genomic variability is a striking feature of lentivirus biology; this genomic plasticity creates a heterogeneous population of genetically related but molecularly distinct genomes within the host. Individual functional proviral genomes within this quasi-species may differ not only in their sequences but also in biologic properties. Thus, genomic variability may play an important part in the persistence, pathogenesis, host range, and cellular tropisms of these constantly evolving viruses. A better understanding of, and coping with, the remarkable variability within lentiviruses is essential to developing effective vaccine strategies.

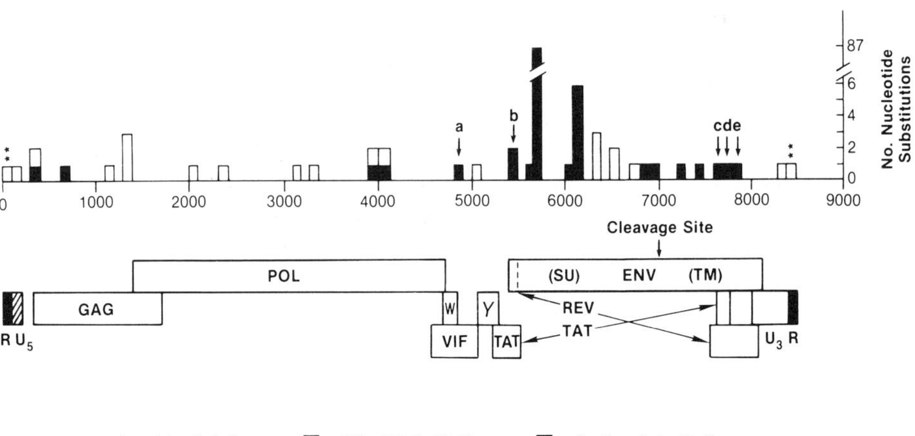


Fig. 8. Distribution of nucleotide substitutions between BIV 106 and 127. The positions of the major ORFs are shown. The arrow over the *env* segment represents the SU-TM cleavage site. Each box represents one substitution, and substitutions are cumulatively displayed every 100 nt. a: Coding substitutions in both W and *vif.* b: Two nucleotide substitutions that cause coding changes in *tat* exon 1 (only one of the two causes a coding change in *env*). c: Coding changes in *env* and *rev* exon 2 but not *tat* exon 2. d: Nucleotide substitution that causes coding changes in *rev* exon 2 and *tat* exon 2 but not in *env.* e: Nucleotide substitution that causes a coding change in *rev* exon 2 but not in *env.* (Reprinted from Garvey et al., 1990, with permission of the editors and Academic Press, Inc.).

The availability of two functional clones of BIV has allowed us to assess the amount and location of any genomic variability within its genome (Garvey et al., 1990). Since the infectious BIV proviral clones (BIV 106 and BIV 127) were derived from cellular DNA carrying proviruses from a single virus isolate (Braun et al., 1988), it was initially anticipated that differences between the two clones might be minimal. However, in the sequence comparisons, numerous point mutations were found throughout the genomes of the two infectious clones; the major difference between them is an 87 bp deletion in the 5′ end of the SU coding region of BIV 106 with respect to BIV 127 (Fig. 8). This loss of 29 amino acids does not appear to interfere with the infectivity of BIV 106 but may be a consequence of the natural polymorphism of lentivirus envelope proteins which is thought to occur by point mutations, inversions, deletions, and duplications that are further selected upon by host factors in vivo. The genomes differ by 1.7% overall, and most of the deletions and coding substitutions (75%) occur in the SU portion of the *env* gene. Recent sequence analyses of other BIV *env* clones show that most retain the 87 bp region deleted from BIV 106 (i.e., they are BIV 127-like), but contain many of the same substitutions as BIV 106 (Garvey et al., unpublished data). It is not presently known if the sequence divergence between BIV 106 and 127 is responsible for any differences in their in vivo biological activity or in antigenic properties of the infectious clones, although differences in their in vitro activity have been noted (Braun et al., 1988).

## Development of animal models

Although BIV was isolated over 15 years ago, until very recently, little attention was given to studies of its pathogenesis in naturally and experimentally infected animals. Natural BIV infections appear to cause a persistent lymphocytosis, lymphadenopathy, and limited central nervous system lesions; the animals may also appear to be weak and emaciated (Van Der Maaten et al., 1972). The clinical picture in these animals is complicated by the fact that a number of other infectious agents are concomitantly encountered, the most frequent of which are BLV and BSV (Gonda et al., unpublished data). When calves were experimentally infected with an infectious proviral clone of BIV (BIV 106; Braun et al., 1988), preliminary data indicate the induction of a mild lymphocytosis and serologic response to the virus, but no other overt signs of disease have been seen (Van Der Maaten et al., 1990).

BLV readily infects sheep and is pathogenic in this species. Therefore, we were interested in whether BIV could also infect sheep. The experimental infection of lambs with BIV (a single dose, $10^7$ infected cells), via the intraperitoneal, intratracheal, or intravenous routes, has not resulted in clinical signs of disease. Moreover, there is no evidence of seroconversion in lambs, probably indicating that they are not infected (Cockerell and Gonda, unpublished data). Realizing the limitations of extensive investigations in cattle, we have tried to infect a variety of other species, including mice, rats, guinea pigs, and rabbits, in order to

TABLE 3
Criteria for an animal model system of HIV-like infection

(1) Animal is small, readily available, inexpensive, and amenable to experimental manipulation.
(2) Pathogen is a lentivirus related to HIV with a similar genomic complexity, but does not infect humans or human cells.
(3) Functional molecular clones are available to study the molecular mechanisms of pathogenesis and level of drug or vaccine interaction.
(4) Infections are persistent with measurable pathologic lesions and recoverable virus.
(5) Measurable immunosuppression is an endpoint in the infection and may be accompanied by opportunistic infections.
(6) Diagnostic assays are available for measuring the presence of virus and accumulation of viral antigen.

develop a small animal model. Table 3 lists the criteria that we consider to be essential in an animal model of HIV-like infection for testing therapeutic drugs and vaccine strategies.

The fact that BIV readily infects EREp and rabbit peripheral blood leukocytes (Gonda et al., 1990; unpublished data) suggested to us that rabbits might be susceptible to infection. We have been able to establish persistent infections in rabbits using several infectious clones of BIV via the intraperitoneal route (Pifat et al., in preparation). BIV infection of young rabbits initially results in an enlargement of the spleen and lymphadenopathy accompanied by hyperplasia of the germinal follicles. BIV can be rescued from the spleen and lymph nodes of infected rabbits as early as 1 month and as late as 1 year post inoculation. Virus can also be isolated from peripheral blood leukocytes early in infection. The reisolated virus retains its cytopathic properties in vitro. Electron microscopy of infected cell cultures indicates that the isolate is a lentivirus and it has been more specifically identified as BIV by polymerase chain reaction (PCR) diagnostics using BIV-specific primers. We have been able to rescue virus from infected rabbits in virtually all cases. There is immunohistochemical evidence of BIV antigen accumulation in the red pulp of the spleen. A humoral immune response to BIV can be detected as early as 2 weeks post inoculation by ELISA, radioimmunoprecipitation, and Western blot techniques, and high antibody titers can be measured for at least 1 year thereafter.

## Concluding remarks

BIV is a novel lentivirus that shares many traits with HIV. We have obtained a better understanding of the molecular biology of BIV through the analysis of biologically active proviral molecular clones of BIV. The translation of their DNA sequence has enabled us to predict the major protein products of the structural genes of BIV. Putative proteins encoded by *gag* and *env* ORFs have been experimentally determined; there is a good correlation between predicted and experimentally observed results. However, the absolute serologic identification of structural and non-structural/regulatory proteins of BIV awaits the determination of their amino acid sequence and/or the application of monovalent and monoclonal antibodies to their study.

The BIV genome has a complex central region wherein five additional ORFs were identified. Several observations suggest that the central region of BIV plays an active role during the virus life cycle. First, multiple viral transcripts have been identified in BIV-infected cells. Second, a viral product(s) appears to strongly and specifically transactivate the BIV LTR. Third, we have obtained cDNA clones representative of BIV's *rev* gene. The functional proviral and cDNA clones of BIV will be of further use in dissecting the replicative cycle and molecular mechanisms of pathogenesis of BIV in vitro. Additional discoveries about the functioning of the central region ORFs of BIV will enhance our overall understanding of this region in other lentivirus systems, where parallels exist.

There is still much to be learned about the pathogenesis of BIV in cattle and surrogate hosts. At present, there is only one isolate of BIV. The uncloned stocks of this prototypic BIV isolate recently tested in in vivo studies have shown only limited pathology (Van Der Maaten et al., 1990) in comparison to that previously reported (Van Der Maaten et al., 1972). The reasons for this have not been identified. One plausible explanation, however, is that the original stocks of BIV were isolated on bovine spleen cells and passaged numerous times in vitro prior to inoculation into animals. Spleen cells may not be the normal target cell in vivo and growth on spleen or other types of fibroblast cells may select for an attenuated virus incapable of reproducing the original disease (Gonda et al., 1990). An alternative explanation may be offered. Recent experiments with cloned proviruses of FIV, obtained from in vitro passaged stocks, have failed to demonstrate any pathology or clinical disease in specific pathogen-free animals (Olmsted et al., 1989). Perhaps the pathogenic effects of BIV are initially subtle and other cofactors are needed to potentiate severe disease. It will be interesting to determine the disease-inducing capacity of virus derived from the functional BIV proviral clones inoculated singly or in combination into cattle. Moreover, it will be important to identify additional BIV-infected herds and recover new isolates for study.

Normally, the host range of lentiviruses is restricted in that only one species is naturally infected with a specific virus and only few species can be experimentally infected. The only animals susceptible to HIV-1 infection other than humans are the chimpanzee, gibbon ape, and rabbit, but an AIDS-like disease has not been reported for these species (Gardner and Luciw, 1989). The chimpanzee has been very useful for conducting vaccine studies (Arthur et al., 1989); however, the measures being taken to conserve this endangered species make expansion of its use in AIDS studies prohibitive. Thus, there is no really suitable animal model of HIV infection for vaccine and drug studies. However, based on recent information, several of the animal lentiviruses, including SIV and FIV in their natural hosts and BIV in the rabbit, offer great promise as models of

HIV-like infection (Gardner and Luciw, 1989; Gonda et al., 1990; Pifat et al., unpublished data).

The infection of rabbits with BIV appears to be a very practical alternative model of HIV-like infection in which to study the biology of lentivirus-induced disease. By successfully infecting rabbits with BIV, we have fulfilled most of the criteria outlined in Table 3. No AIDS-like disease has been observed in the BIV-infected rabbits; however, there are indications that BIV may be immunosuppressive in this species. Detailed controlled experiments are necessary to confirm this observation. The particular rabbits used in the BIV studies are from specific-pathogen-free colonies and they are kept in a clean environment; therefore, it probably is not surprising that the animals have not shown clinical signs of severe illness if cofactors are involved. It will be of interest to see whether smaller laboratory animals such as rats, mice, and guinea pigs can be infected by BIV as well. The results of these experiments are pending. Nevertheless, small animal models of BIV infection will be useful for the large-scale screening of antiviral compounds and immunomodulators, particularly when only small quantities of a drug are available. The BIV rabbit model may provide insight into effective vaccinology strategies.

## Acknowledgements

The authors would like to give special thanks to several colleagues, including M.J. Braun, A.L. Boyd, J.M. Ward, J.W. Bess, T.A. Kost, and L.O. Arthur, for scientific contributions referenced in this work that enabled us to further the development of the biology of BIV; J.E. Elser, L. Rasmussen, W. Ennis, D. Krell, M.Y. Hu, D. Hutchison, K. Noer, J. Greenwood, R. Matthai, K. Green, and C. Lackman-Smith for skilled technical assistance; and J. Hopkins for help in the preparation of the manuscript. This project has been funded at least in part with federal funds from the Department of Health and Human Services under Contract NO1-CO-74102 with Program Resources, Inc. The content of this publication does not necessarily reflect the views of policies of the Department of Health and Human Services, nor does mention of trade names, commercial products, or organizations imply endorsement by the U.S. Government.

## References

Arthur, L.O., Bess, J.W. Jr., Waters, D.J., Pyle, S.W., Kelliher, J.C., Nara, P.L., Krohn, K., Robey, W.G., Langlois, A.J., Gallo, R.C. and Fischinger, P.J. (1989) Challenge of chimpanzees (*Pan troglodytes*) immunized with human immunodeficiency virus envelope glycoprotein gp120. *J. Virol.* 63, 5046–5053.

Battles, J.K., Hu, M. and Gonda, M.A. (1990) Serologic identification of *gag* and *env* structural gene products of the bovine immunodeficiency-like virus. Submitted for publication.

Benton, C.V., Hodge, H.M. and Fine, D.L. (1978) Comparative large-scale propagation of retroviruses from Old World (Mason-Pfizer monkey virus) and New World (squirrel monkey virus) primates. *In Vitro* 14, 192–199.

Braun, M.J., Lahn, S., Boyd, A.L., Kost, T.A., Nagashima, K. and Gonda, M.A. (1988) Molecular cloning of biologically active proviruses of bovine immunodeficiency-like virus. *Virology* 167, 515–523.

Burny, A., Bruck, C., Chantrene, H., Cleuter, T., Dekegal, D., Ghysdael, J., Kettmann, R., Leclerq, M., Lennen, J., Mammerickx, M. and Portetelle, D. (1980) Bovine leukemia virus: molecular biology and epidemiology. In: G. Klein (Ed.), *Viral Oncology*. Raven Press, New York, NY, pp. 231–289.

Burny, A., Cleuter, Y., Kettmann, R., Mammerickx, M., Marbaix, G., Portetelle, D., Van Den Broeke, A., Willems, L. and Thomas, R. (1987) Bovine leukemia: facts and hypothesis from the study of an infectious cancer. *Cancer Surv.* 6, 139–159.

Desrosiers, R.C., Daniel, M.D. and Li, Y. (1989) Minireview: HIV-related lentiviruses of nonhuman primates. *AIDS Res. Human Retroviruses* 5, 465–473.

Gallo, R.C. and Wong-Staal, F. (1985) A human T-lymphotropic retrovirus (HTLV-III) as the cause of the acquired immunodeficiency syndrome. *Ann. Intern. Med.* 103, 679–689.

Gardner, M.B. and Luciw, P.A. (1989) Animal models of AIDS. *FASEB J.* 3, 2593–2606.

Garvey, K.J., Oberste, M.S., Elser, J.E., Braun, M.J. and Gonda, M.A. (1990) Nucleotide sequence and genome organization of biologically active proviruses of the bovine immunodeficiency-like virus. *Virology* 175, 391–409.

Gelderblom, H.R., Özel, M. and Pauli, G. (1989) Morphogenesis and morphology of HIV: structure-function relations. *Arch. Virol.* 106, 1–13.

Gonda, M.A. (1988) Molecular genetics and structure of the human immunodeficiency virus. *J. Electron Microsc. Tech.* 8, 17–40.

Gonda, M.A., Wong-Staal, F., Gallo, R.C., Clements, J.E., Narayan, O. and Gilden, R.V. (1985) Sequence homology and morphologic similarity of HTLV-III and visna virus, a pathogenic lentivirus. *Science* 227, 173–177.

Gonda, M.A., Braun, M.J., Clements, J.E., Pyper, J.M., Wong-Staal, F., Gallo, R.C. and Gilden, R.V. (1986) Human T-cell lymphotropic virus type III shares sequence homology with a family of pathogenic lentiviruses. *Proc. Natl. Acad. Sci. U.S.A.* 83, 4007–4011.

Gonda, M.A., Braun, M.J., Carter, S.G., Kost, T.A., Bess, J.W. Jr., Arthur, L.O. and Van Der Maaten, M.J. (1987) Characterization and molecular cloning of a bovine lentivirus related to human immunodeficiency virus. *Nature* 330, 388–391.

Gonda, M.A., Boyd, A.L., Nagashima, K. and Gilden, R.V. (1989) Pathobiology, molecular organization, and ultrastructure of HIV. *Arch. AIDS Res.* 3, 1–42.

Gonda, M.A., Oberste, M.S., Garvey, K.G., Pallansch, L.A., Battles, J.K., Pifat, D.Y., Bess, J.W. Jr. and Nagashima, K. (1990) Development of the bovine immunodeficiency-like virus as a model of lentivirus disease. In: *Progress on Animal Retroviruses, 21st Congress of the International Association of Biological Standardization* (in press).

Guyader, M., Emerman, M., Sonigo, P., Clavel, F., Montagnier, L. and Alizon, M. (1987) Genome organization and transactivation of the human immunodeficiency virus type 2. *Nature* 326, 662–669.

Haase, A. (1986) Pathogenesis of lentivirus infections. *Nature* 322, 130–136.

Haseltine, W.A. (1989) Replication and pathogenesis of the AIDS virus. *J. AIDS* 1, 217–240.

Heidecker, G., Lerche, N.W., Lowenstine, L.J., Lackner, A., Osborn, K.G., Gardner, M.B. and Marx, P. (1987) Induction of simian acquired immune deficiency syndrome (SAIDS) with a molecular clone of a type D SAIDS retrovirus. *J. Virol.* 61, 3066–3071.

Hoffman, A.D., Bonapour, B. and Levy, J.A. (1985) Characterization of the AIDS-associated retrovirus reverse transcriptase and optimal conditions for its detection in virions. *Virology* 147, 326–335.

Leis, J., Baltimore, D., Bishop, J.M., Coffin, J., Fleissner, E., Goff, S.P., Oroszlan, S., Robinson, H., Skalka, A.M., Temin, H.M. and Vogt, V. (1988) Standardized and simplified nomenclature for proteins common to all retroviruses. *J. Virol.* 62, 1808–1809.

Malmquist, W.A., Van Der Maaten, M.J. and Booth, A.D. (1969) Isolation, immunodiffusion, immunofluorescence, and electron microscopy of a syncytial virus of lymphosarcomatous and apparently normal cattle. *Cancer Res.* 29, 188–200.

McGowan, J. and Hoth, D. (1989) AIDS drug discovery and development. *J. AIDS* 2, 335–343.

Miller, J.M., Miller, L.D., Olson, C. and Gillette, K.G. (1969) Virus-like particles in phytohemagglutinin-stimulated lymphocyte cultures with reference to bovine lymphosarcoma. *J. Natl. Cancer Inst.* 43, 1297–1305.

Oberste, M.S., Greenwood, J.D. and Gonda, M.A. (1990) Analysis of the transcriptional pattern and mapping of the *rev* and *env* splice junctions of the bovine immunodeficiency virus. Submitted for publication.

Olmsted, R.A., Hirsch, V.M., Purcell, R.H. and Johnson, P.R. (1989) Nucleotide sequence analysis of feline immunodeficiency virus: genome organization and relationship to other lentiviruses. *Proc. Natl. Acad. Sci. U.S.A.* 86, 8088–8092.

Pallansch, L., Lackman-Smith, C. and Gonda, M.A. (1990) Characterization of bovine immunodeficiency-like virus gene expression: transactivation of the LTR by viral sequences in vitro. Submitted for publication.

Pedersen, N.C., Ho, E.N., Brown, M.L. and Yamamoto, J.K. (1987) Isolation of T-lymphotropic virus from domestic cats with an immunodeficiency-like syndrome. *Science* 235, 790–793.

Rasmussen, L., Battles, J.K., Ennis, W.H., Nagashima, K. and Gonda, M.A. (1990) Characterization of virus-like particles produced by a baculovirus expression vector containing the GAG gene of bovine immunodeficiency-like virus. *Virology* 178 (in press).

Starcich, B.R., Hahn, B.H., Shaw, G.M., McNeely, P.D., Modrow, S., Wolf, H., Parks, E.S. and Parks, W.P. (1986) Identification and characterization of conserved and variable regions in the envelope gene of HTLV-III/LAV, the retrovirus of AIDS. *Cell* 45, 637–648.

Van Der Maaten, M.J., Boothe, A.D. and Seger, C.L. (1972) Isolation of a virus from cattle with persistent lymphocytosis. *J. Natl. Cancer Inst.* 49, 1649–1657.

Van Der Maaten, M.J., Whetstone, C. and Miller, J. (1990) In: *Progress in Animal Retroviruses, 21st Congress of the International Association of Biological Standardization.* (in press).

Wong-Staal, F. and Gallo, R.C. (1985a) The family of human T-lymphotropic leukemia viruses: HTLV-I as the cause of adult T-cell leukemia and HTLV-III as the cause of the acquired immunodeficiency syndrome. *Blood* 65, 253–263.

Wong-Staal, F. and Gallo, R.C. (1985b) Human T-lymphotropic retroviruses. *Nature* 317, 395–403.

York, D.F., Williamson, A., Barnard, B.J.H. and Verwoerd, D.W. (1989) Some characteristics of a retrovirus isolated from transformed bovine cells. *Virology* 171, 394–400.

*Eds. H. Schellekens and M.C. Horzinek*
*Animal Models in AIDS*



# 25

# The ORF S3 protein encoded by the equine infectious anemia virus elicits a serological response in infected animals

ERIC SAMAN [1], KARIN BREUGELMANS [1], JOHAN SWINNEN [2], JOZEF MERREGAERT [2] and HUGO VAN HEUVERSWIJN [1]

[1] N.V. INNOGENETICS Research Laboratories, B-2000 Antwerp, Belgium and [2] Laboratory of Biotechnology, University of Antwerp, B-2610 Wilrijk, Belgium

## Introduction

Equine infectious anemia virus (EIAV), a member of the lentivirus subfamily of retroviridae, contains in addition to the structural retroviral genes *gag, pol* and *env* several small open reading frames (ORFs) the importance of which is being studied (Rushlow et al., 1986; Kawakami et al., 1987). For the human immunodeficiency virus (HIV), it has been demonstrated that several small regulatory proteins, involved in the control of the viral life cycle, are encoded in small ORFs and are expressed from multiple spliced messenger RNAs (Goh et al., 1986; Sodroski et al., 1986).

Recently, it has been demonstrated that a small open reading frame (ORF S1), localized between the *pol* and *env* genes of EIAV is necessary for transactivation of the viral long terminal repeat (LTR) (Sherman, 1988). Furthermore, inspection of the published sequence data on the EIAV proviral genome allows the identification of an open reading frame (ORF S3) capable of encoding 135 amino acids (Rushlow et al., 1986; Kawakami et al., 1987). This coding sequence is completely contained within the gene encoding the transmembrane protein of EIAV. This localization is similar to the one described for the second coding exons of both *tat* and *rev* genes of HIV-1 and HIV-2.

In this study, we expressed the ORF S3 information of EIAV in *E. coli* and antibodies were raised to the purified protein. These reagents allowed us to demonstrate that the ORF S3 encoded information is expressed in EIAV-infected horses and that some animals raise antibodies to this protein.

## Expression of ORF S3 in *E. coli*

The genetic information encoding the ORF S3 antigen was isolated from the proviral molecular clone 1369 of EIAV which was kindly provided by Dr. S. Aaronson (Kawakami et al., 1987). An *Apa*I-*Xba*I fragment, containing almost the entire ORF S3 information (Fig. 1B), was subcloned into the bacterial expression vector pEx (Stanley and Luzio, 1984). The pEx vectors are designed in such a way that the cloned information is fused carboxy-terminal to $\beta$-galactosidase to yield a recombinant fusion protein that can easily be detected in Coomassie blue-stained gels after electrophoretic separation of the total cellular extract. Expression of the cloned information is controlled by the lambda

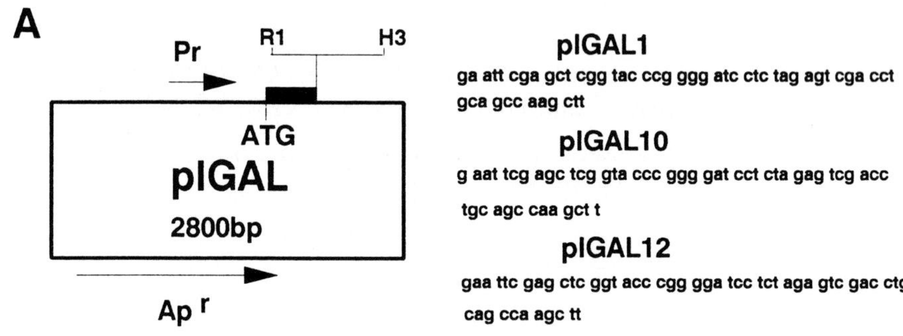


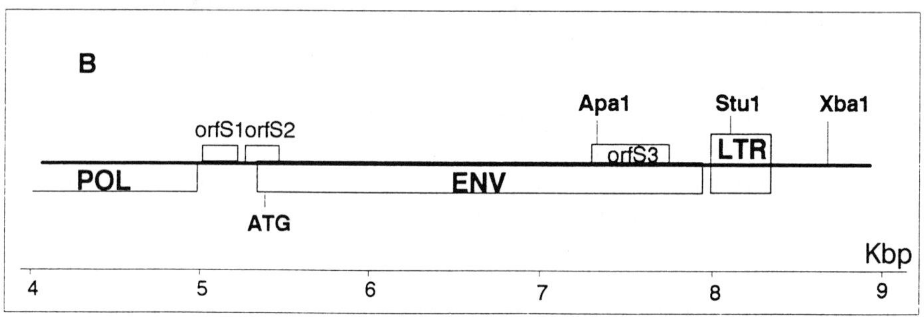


Fig. 1. (A) pIGAL vectors used for expression of EIAV proteins. The rightward lambda promotor (Pr), the *cro-lac*I peptide (box) and the polylinker are indicated. The pIGAL 1, 10 and 12 differ in reading frame relative to the *cro-lac*I peptide. R1 is *Eco*RI and H3 is *Hin*dIII. Sequences of the three different pIGAL linkers and the respective reading frames are shown. (B) Schematic representation of a part of the EIAV proviral genome. The various relevant ORFs as well as the restriction sites used for the construction of expression plasmids are shown. The *Apa*I site is located 10 bp downstream from the start of ORF S3 (position 7245). (C) Immunoblotting of ORF S35 and EIAV TM 1. *E. coli* cell lysates were analyzed for the presence of EIAV TM1 (lanes 1) or ORF S35 (lanes 2) fusion protein. The blots were incubated with an anti-EIAV horse serum (a) or a control horse serum (b). (D) Reaction of ORF S35 expression product with rabbit antiserum, raised to an ORF S3 derived synthetic peptide (a) or to an ORF S3 protein A fusion protein (b). Western blot strips were incubated with the preimmune sera (1 and 3) or with the antisera (2 and 4) and developed with an anti-rabbit alkaline phosphatase conjugate.

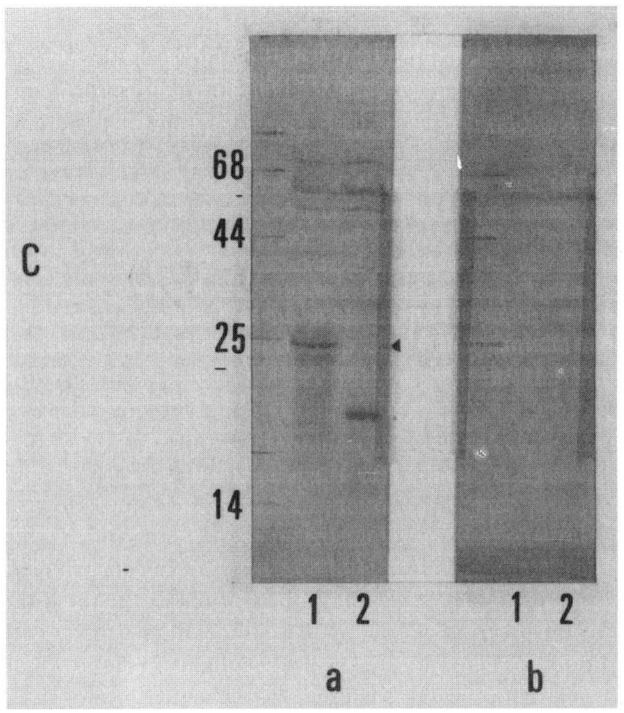


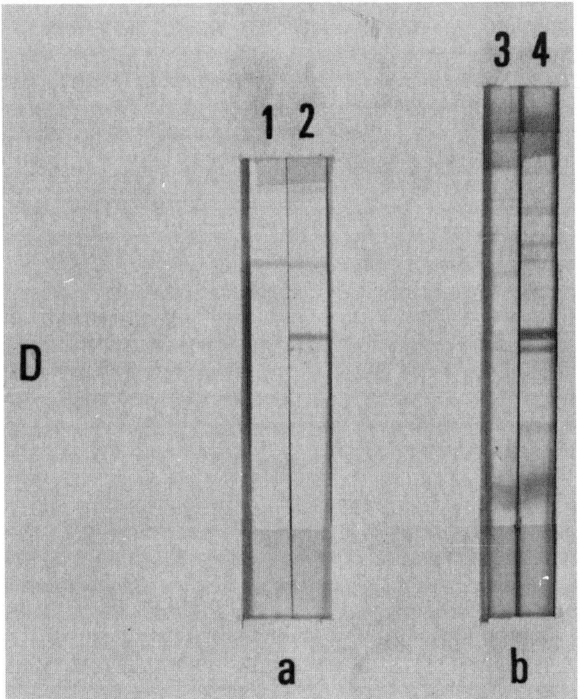


Fig. 1 (continued).

rightward promoter. Transcription can be regulated by the CI 857 repressor, provided from a compatible plasmid (Remaut et al., 1981). This repressor ts mutant is active at 28°C but can be inactivated by shifting the culture to 42°C (induction). All inductions were done over a period of 3 h and culture aliquots (1 ml) were removed every hour.

Cells were pelleted, lysed by boiling in sodium dodecyl sulfate (SDS) containing sample buffer (50 mM Tris-HCl, pH 7.5, 2% SDS, 5% β-mercaptoethanol, 10% glycerol and 0.01% bromophenolblue) and the supernatant was fractionated via SDS-PAGE (Laemmli, 1970). The gels were either stained for protein or used for Western blot transfer using the conditions described by Dunn (1986). From these preliminary experiments, it was already clear that some sera from EIAV-infected horses react with the β-galactosidase fusion protein, whereas no reaction was obtained with β-galactosidase (not shown).

To investigate this in more detail and to eliminate all cross-reaction with the β-galactosidase moiety, we expressed the ORF S3 protein in a vector of the pIGAL series (Fig. 1A). These vectors have transcription and translation control signals analogous to the pEX vectors. However, the fusion proteins synthesized contain only about 50 amino acids *cro-lac*I information at the amino terminus. Moreover, all fusion proteins produced in these vectors can be detected with a monoclonal antibody directed to the *cro-lac*I sequences (monoclonal CL).

The ORF S3 information was transferred from the pEX vector to the pIGAL-10 vector as an *Eco*RI-*Stu*I fragment. This construction should produce a fusion protein of 21 kDa, referred to as ORF S35. Since the ORF S3 is completely contained within the gene fragment, coding for the carboxy-terminal part of the transmembrane protein, expression of the overlapping part of the envelope information was achieved by introducing the same gene fragment into the appropriate reading frame of the pIGAL vector (pIGAL-1). The resulting plasmid was termed pEIAV-TM1.

Both plasmids were induced for expression in *E. coli* SG4044 [pCI857] (Gottesman et al., 1981) and cell extracts were analyzed via Western blotting with an anti-EIAV horse serum, coupled to alkaline phosphatase, as described below. This experiment shows the expression of a 25 kDa protein from pEIAV-TM1 (Fig. 1C, lane 1) and a 20 kDa protein from pORF S35 (Fig. 1C, lane 2). These experimental values are in good agreement with the calculated molecular mass of the respective fusion proteins. These results confirm that the ORF S35 construct does produce the protein encoded by the small ORF S3.

## Analysis of sera from EIAV-infected animals

To evaluate whether the ORF S3 protein is antigenic in vivo, several sera from EIAV-infected animals and normal control sera were tested for reactivity with the *E. coli*-produced protein. All sera were preincubated with extract made from induced *E. coli* SG4044 cells, without any EIAV information. The cells were concentrated from the induced culture by centrifugation, resuspended in 1/10th

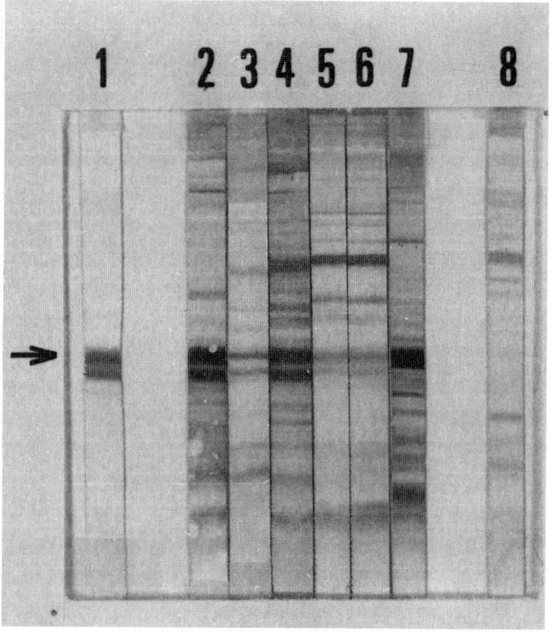


Fig. 2. Sera from experimentally infected ponies (lanes 2 and 7) or from naturally infected horses (lanes 3, 4, 5, 6) were analyzed for their reactivity with the ORF S35 protein expressed in *E. coli*. Total *E. coli* lysate was used to prepare the Western blot strips. Reaction of the ORF S35 protein with the CL monoclonal is also shown (strip 1) as well as a control with a serum from a non-infected animal (strip 8). The ORF S35 protein is indicated ( → ). This protein is often revealed as a doublet, the lower band probably representing a degradation product.

of the original volume and lysed by sonication. The soluble fraction was used for incubation with an equal volume of each serum at room temperature for 1 h. The mixture was then further diluted 50-fold in TBS (10 mM Tris-HCl, pH 7.5, containing 150 mM NaCl and 0.1% bovine serum albumin) and Western blot strips containing extract from the ORF S35-producing bacteria were incubated with this reagent for 2 h at room temperature with constant agitation. The strips were washed with TBS (3 × 10 min) and incubated with an anti-horse IgG conjugated to alkaline phosphatase (Jackson Immunoresearch, U.S.A.). After three more washes, the strips were developed with 5-bromo-4-chloro-3-indolylphosphate (BCIP) combined with nitroblue tetrazolium (NBT). The reaction was terminated by washing with water.

Fig. 2 shows some representative strips developed with EIAV-positive horse sera. Out of 40 sera from EIAV-infected horses tested, six were found to react with the ORF S3 protein (15%) whereas 29 (72%) were positive for the EIAV *gag* precursor (p55), expressed in the same configuration (not shown). The typical ORF S35 reaction was not seen when extracts from non-induced *E. coli* cultures or extracts from induced cultures not containing EIAV information were used.

Sera from non-infected animals did not react with the ORF S35 fusion protein either (11 sera).

All sera that scored positive for reaction with ORF S35 were also positive for the reaction with the EIAV *gag* precursor. These results show that in some animals an immune response towards ORF S3 protein is mounted upon infection with EIAV. The results also indicate that this protein is produced in infected animals but not all animals have detectable levels of antibodies to it. This is comparable to the results obtained for some HIV antigens, where antibodies to non-structural HIV antigens can be detected only in some AIDS patients (Arya and Gallo, 1986; Aldovin et al., 1986).

The data presented in this paper demonstrate that the ORF S3 represents a novel retroviral gene of EIAV which is expressed in infected animals. Since ORF S3 does not contain a regular initiation codon, it is most probable that expression is achieved from a spliced mRNA, although initiation at other codons has also been described (Dasso and Jackson, 1989). Recently it was shown that in maedi-visna virus an early viral protein (VEP-1) is produced from a spliced messenger composed of two coding exons, one of which is situated in front of the *env* gene while the other is located in the transmembrane protein coding sequence but read in a different frame (Mazarin et al., 1988; Davis and Clements, 1989; Sargan and Bennet, 1989).

The analogy with this other lentivirus tempts us to speculate that the ORF S3 of EIAV is spliced to the small open reading frame (ORF S2) that has been described before (Rushlow et al., 1986), which is located in front of the envelope gene (Fig. 1A). Since this ORF S2 contains an initiation codon (second codon) and a consensus splice donor site (CCCAG/GGGAAT, bp 5341–5351), it can be spliced to a splice acceptor site situated in the ORF S3 sequence (TCCTCAG/G, bp 7235–7242) (Mount, 1982). This would result in a protein of 152 amino acids (17657 Da).

In conclusion, we have shown that EIAV encodes a novel retroviral protein which is expressed during the viral life cycle in the infected animal and some animals raise antibodies to it. The predicted amino acid sequence does not show significant homology with any protein present in the NBRF and SWISS-PROT data banks. In some features, the protein resembles the VEP-1 protein described for visna virus, and in that case it was shown that the protein could be involved in trans-regulation of splicing (equivalent to HIV *rev*). If the splicing pattern described here for ORF S3 is correct, this might imply that the ORF S3 protein could encode the second exon of the EIAV *rev* protein. Although other possibilities for the expression and function of ORF S3 remain, the present model warrants further investigation.

## Acknowledgements

We thank Dr. S.A. Aaronson for the EIAV isolate 1369, Dr. J. Dahlberg for the persistently infected Cf2Th cells and Dr. S. Tronick for the anti-peptide antiserum and some of the EIAV-positive horse sera. We also thank Dr. Toma (Paris), who provided serum from an experimentally infected pony. Christiane Messiaen is acknowledged for excellent secretarial assistance. This work was partially supported by a grant to J.M. from the "Nationaal Fonds van Wetenschappelijk Onderzoek (Krediet aan navorsers)" from Belgium.

## References

Aldovin, A., Debouck, C., Feinberg, M.B., Rosenberg, M. Arya, S.K. and Wong-Staal, F. (1986) Synthesis of the complete trans-activating gene product of human T-lymphotropic virus type III in *Escherichia coli:* Demonstration of immunogenicity in vivo and expression in vitro. *Proc. Natl. Acad. Sci. U.S.A.* 83, 6672–6676.

Arya, S.K. and Gallo, R.C. (1986) Three novel genes of human T-lymphotropic virus type III: Immune reactivity of their products with sera from acquired immune deficiency syndrome patients. *Proc. Natl. Acad. Sci. U.S.A.* 83, 2209–2213.

Dasso, M.C. and Jackson, R.J. (1989) Efficient initiation of mammalian mRNA translation at a CUG codon. *Nucleic Acids Res.* 17, 6485–6497.

Davis, J.L. and Clements, J.E. (1989) Characterization of a cDNA clone encoding the visna virus transactivating protein. *Proc. Natl. Acad. Sci. U.S.A.* 86, 414–418.

Dunn, S.D. (1986) Effects of the modification of transfer buffer composition and the renaturation of proteins in gels on the recognition of proteins on Western blots by monoclonal antibodies. *Anal. Biochem.* 157, 144–153.

Goh, W.C., Rosen, C., Sodroski, J., Ho, D.D. and Haseltine, W.A. (1986) Identification of a protein encoded by the trans activator gene tat III of human T-cell lymphotropic retrovirus type III. *J. Virol.* 59, 181–184.

Gottesman, S., Gottesman, M., Shaw, E. and Pearson, M.L. (1981) Protein degradation in *E. coli:* the low mutation and bacteriophage lambda M and CII protein stability. *Cell* 24, 225–233.

Kawakami, T., Sherman, L., Dahlberg, J., Gazit, A., Yaniv, A., Tronick, S.R. and Aaronson, S.A. (1987) Nucleotide sequence analysis of equine infectious anemia virus proviral DNA. *Virology* 158, 300–312.

Laemmli, U.K. (1970) Cleavage of structural proteins during the assembly of the head of bacteriophage T4. *Nature* 227, 680–685.

Mazarin, V., Goudrou, J., Querat, G., Sauze, N. and Vigne, R. (1988) Genetic structure and function of an early transcript of Visna virus. *J. Virol.* 62, 4813–4818.

Mount, S.M. (1982) A catalogue of splice junction sequences. *Nucleic Acids Res.* 10, 459–472.

Remaut, E., Stanssens, P. and Fiers, W. (1981) Plasmid vectors for high-efficiency expression, controlled by the PL promoter of coliphage lambda. *Gene* 15, 81–93.

Rushlow, K., Olsen, K., Stiegler, G., Payne, S.L., Montelaro, R.C. and Issel, C.J. (1986) Lentivirus genomic organization: the complete nucleotide sequence of the *env* gene region of equine infectious anemia virus. *Virology* 155, 309–321.

Sargan, D.R. and Bennet, I.D. (1989) A transcriptional map of visna virus: definition of the second intron structure suggests a rev-like gene product. *J. Gen. Virol.* 70, 1995–2006.

Sherman, L., Gazit, A., Yaniv, A., Kawakami, T., Dahlberg, J.E. and Tronick, S.R. (1988) Localization of sequences responsible for trans-activation of the equine infectious anemia virus long terminal repeat. *J. Virol.* 62, 120–126.

Sodroski, J., Goh, W.C., Rosen, C., Dayton, A., Terwilliger, E. and Haseltine, W. (1986) A second post-transcriptional trans-activator gene required for HTLV-III replication. *Nature* 321, 412–417.

Stanley, K.K. and Luzio, J.P. (1984) Construction of a new family of high efficiency bacterial expression vectors: identification of cDNA clones coding for human liver proteins. *EMBO J.* 3, 1429–1434.

*Eds. H. Schellekens and M.C. Horzinek*
*Animal Models in AIDS*



# 26

# Bovine leukemia virus-infected sheep can serve as a model for the evaluation of antiretroviral compounds—the effect of treatment with suramin

S. ROSENTHAL[1], H. BURKHARDT[2], H.A. ROSENTHAL[3], E. KARGE[4] and E. DE CLERCQ[5]

[1] Zentralinstitut für Molekularbiologie, Akademie der Wissenschaften der DDR, DDR-1115 Berlin-Buch, G.D.R., [2] Sektion Tierproduktion und Veterinärmedizin, [3] Institut für Medizinische Virologie, Bereich Medizin (Charité), Humboldt-Universität, DDR-1040 Berlin, G.D.R., [4] Staatliches Institut für Epizootiologie und Tierseuchenbekämpfung, DDR-1903 Wusterhausen (Dosse), G.D.R. and [5] Rega Instituut, Katholieke Universiteit Leuven, B-3000 Leuven, Belgium

**Summary**

Bovine leukemia virus (BLV) and the human T-cell leukemia/lymphoma viruses I and II (HTLV-I, HTLV-II) represent a specific group of type C RNA tumor viruses characterized by the presence between the *env* gene and the 3′ long terminal repeat (LTR) of an "x" region or large open reading (LOR) frame, which codes for a protein that trans-activates the transcription of the viral genome. As BLV can also infect sheep and induces pre-B-cell specific tumors in these animals, we were interested in investigating whether suramin, a potent inhibitor of retrovirus-associated reverse transcriptase (RT), may inhibit the in vivo multiplication of BLV in sheep. The sheep were infected with $4 \times 10^7$ leukocytes from a BLV-infected cow. The animals were maedi-visna virus (MVV)-negative. Viral p24 antigen and RT appeared at 2 weeks and seroconversion occurred at 4 weeks after infection. Suramin was administered at 20 mg/kg/week from the 10th until the 16th week after infection. During the treatment period the expression of p24 antigen as well as the titer of anti-p24 and anti-gp51 antibodies were followed. Suramin treatment led to a significant, but transient, disappearance of p24 antigen and did not affect the titer of anti-p24 and anti-gp51 antibodies. The BLV-infected sheep may serve as a useful animal model for the investigation of retrovirus inhibitors and the evaluation of different therapeutic regimens.

## Introduction

The discovery of the human immunodeficiency virus (HIV) as the causative agent of acquired immunodeficiency syndrome (AIDS) has led to a re-evaluation of reverse transcriptase (RT) inhibitors, because (i) the virus belongs to the family of Retroviridae, genus Lentivirinae, and (ii) the RT plays a key role in establishing infection and viral expression. Some of the RT inhibitors like suramin, HPA-23, phosphonoformate and azidothymidine (AZT) have already been used for the clinical treatment of AIDS. Suramin and structurally related non-ionic polysulfonic dyes are effective competitive inhibitors of RT (De Clercq, 1979, 1986). The $ID_{50}$s of suramin, HPA-23 and AZT 5′-triphosphate for the RT of bovine leukemia virus (BLV) are 2.8, 8.0 and 0.17 $\mu$M, respectively (Reimer et al., 1989).

Usually, leukemic mice serve as animal models to assess the anti-retroviral effect of chemical substances. We now introduce BLV-infected sheep as a useful model. Together with human T-cell leukemia/lymphoma viruses I and II (HTLV-I and HTLV-II) (Wong-Staal and Gallo, 1985) BLV makes up a group of type C retroviruses which

— can be transmitted horizontally
— induce chronic leukemia/leukosis in natural populations
— do not possess endogenously inherited proviral sequences
— do not have *onc* genes but code for one or more gene products which trans-activate viral RNA synthesis and replication
— are viremic and thereby induce humoral and cell-mediated immune reactions
— cause the formation of syncytia.

On the other hand, BLV, HTLV-I, HTLV-II and lentivirus infections have certain features in common (Haase, 1986), in that they show a long lasting latency period, the chronic course of the disease and trans-activation or trans-regulation of transcription. Sheep can be experimentally infected with BLV (Wittmann et al., 1971). The virus induces pre-B-cell-specific tumors (Levy et al., 1987). Kenyon et al. (1981) reported BLV infection of sheep by using different virus sources, i.e., short-term cultivated lymphocytes from the peripheral blood of an infected cow, permanently BLV-infected lymphocyte cultures (NBC-13) and cell-free supernatant of BLV-infected bat lung cells. Forty percent of animals which were infected as newborn lambs developed lymphosarcomas between 15 and 24 months post infection (p.i.).

## Materials and methods

### Animals

The nine sheep were from one herd, they were 6 months old and female and did not have BLV p24 antigen or anti-p24 antibody. They were also negative for maedi-visna virus (MVV) infection as determined by an agar gel immunodiffusion test (AGIDT). Two sheep, serving as control animals, were neither infected nor treated. Seven sheep each received 1 ml heparinized blood from one cow with BLV-induced persistent lymphocytosis (PL) (43,000 leukocytes/$\mu$l blood). The route of infection was intraperitoneal. The donor cow was positive in all BLV tests: p24, anti-p24, anti-gp51 (all determined by means of radioimmunoassay (RIA)) and RT. Three infected animals were subjected to therapy, and four infected animals served as control.

### Therapy

Three sheep which were consistently found positive for p24 antigen were subjected to therapy at week 10 p.i. They were given suramin (Germanin, Bayer 205) intravenously at a dose of 20 mg/kg/week for a period of 6 weeks. Four days after each injection blood samples were collected from all animals. The animals received 4.2 g (no. 604), 3.9 g (no. 672) and 3.6 g (no. 728) suramin.

### Short-term cultivation of leukocytes

Leukocytes from 100 ml precooled heparinized blood were isolated according to Weinhold (1965) and cultivated according to Larsen (1979) with slight modifications using RPMI 1640 medium supplemented with 10% neonatal calf serum and 20 μg phytohemagglutinin (PHA)/ml. Cultivation was for 24 h at 37°C. A longer cultivation period did not increase the p24 synthesis in the BLV-infected sheep lymphocytes.

### Reverse transcriptase estimation

RT was determined according to Rössler et al. (1980), using the supernatant of short-term cultivated leukocytes.

### Detection of BLV p24 antigen

The p24 antigen content was estimated in lysates of short-term cultivated leukocytes by means of a competitive RIA test according to Schmerr et al. (1980).

### Detection of anti-p24 and anti-gp51 of BLV and antibodies to MVV

For the detection of the BLV antibodies we used the method described by Mammerickx et al. (1980). Detection of antibodies against MVV was accomplished by using the AGIDT described by Dawson et al. (1979).

### Infection assay

Two or three healthy recipient sheep received 5–10 ml blood s.c. of the donor sheep. Four weeks later the ovine sera of the recipients were checked for BLV-specific antibodies (AGIDT).

## Results

Seven sheep, which were MVV-free, were infected with BLV-containing lymphocytes from cattle. The infection was followed for a period of 36 weeks. The serum of all animals was examined weekly for anti-p24 by RIA. For detection of virus we used short-term (24 h) cultivated PHA-stimulated lymphocytes. RT activity was measured in the cell culture supernatant and p24 antigen in the cell lysate. The sensitivity of the p24 RIA test was such that it allowed us to detect 0.2 ng per $10^7$ cells. After it was unequivocally established that the BLV infection had taken, three animals were treated with suramin. The treatment regimen for suramin was the same as that applied for patients suffering from trypanosomiasis, that is 20 mg/kg/week, administered intravenously for 6 weeks.

The experiment comprised four periods: (i) the stage prior to virus infection, (ii) the incubation period, (ii) the treatment period, and (iv) the post-treatment period.

### Non-infectious stage of the animals

At 6 months of age, before infection with BLV, the sheep were analyzed for the absence of BLV antigen and antibodies. When using the RIA for detecting anti-BLV-p24, or, when using, after short-term cultivation of lymphocytes, the RT test or the RIA for BLV p24, neither test gave a positive result. The absence of MVV antibodies was confirmed by means of AGIDT.

### Experimental BLV infection

The seven sheep were inoculated intraperitoneally with 1 ml blood from a cow with enzootic bovine leukosis (EBL) in the stage of PL having $4.3 \times 10^4$ leukocytes per $\mu$l blood. Thus, each animal received $4.3 \times 10^7$ leukocytes. Two animals, which were neither infected nor treated, served as controls. Within the first week p.i. there were no signs of infection, but as early as 2 weeks p.i. we found p24 antigen in the lysates of the short-term cultivated cells in the seven infected animals. The RT also became detectable in the supernatant of these cells, albeit less consistently (Table 1). After week 2, six out of seven animals were RT-positive, after week 3 four out of seven, and after week 4 three out of seven animals. Only three of the seven animals were consistently positive in the RT test between week 2 and 7 p.i. One animal, though always positive for p24 antigen, never became RT-positive. The RT activity ranged from 1000 to 24,000 dpm per supernatant of $5 \times 10^7$ cells in 13 out of the 20 positive measurements (altogether 32 measurements were performed). The number of BLV-infected and BLV-expressing cells fell below the RT-detectable threshold following suramin treatment. Therefore, determination of RT activity was discontinued. However, we continued to determine the p24 antigen by the more reliable RIA.

From week 4 p.i. all sheep were anti-p24-positive, the antibody titer being 1:400. From week 8 p.i. the titer rose to 1:1200, and at week 15 p.i. the titer

TABLE 1
p24 antigen and reverse transcriptase activity of BLV-infected sheep

| Sheep no. | BLV infection | p24 1–9 weeks p.i. pos./total | Reverse transcriptase activity (dpm per supernatant of $5 \times 10^7$ cells) | | | | | | |
|---|---|---|---|---|---|---|---|---|---|
| | | | 1 (weeks p.i.) | 2 | 3 | 4 | 5 | 6 | 7 |
| 512 | – | 0/6 | 0 | 0 | 0 | 0 | 0 | n.d. | n.d. |
| 599 | – | 0/6 | 0 | 0 | 0 | 0 | 0 | n.d. | n.d. |
| 671 | + | 8/9 | 0 | 1470 | 24145 | 0 | 730 | 7045 | 8610 |
| 691 | + | 2/9 | 0 | 1070 | 8190 | 2720 | 2425 | 0 | 8540 |
| 622 | + | 6/6 | 0 | 1250 | 3345 | 0 | 0 | n.d. | n.d. |
| 735 | + | 4/6 | 0 | 3895 | 0 | 1940 | 0 | n.d. | n.d. |
| 604 | + | 6/6 | 0 | 4580 | 5625 | 1130 | 1410 | n.d. | n.d. |
| 728 | + | 6/6 | 0 | 2970 | 0 | 0 | 1725 | n.d. | n.d. |
| 672 | + | 6/6 | 0 | 0 | 0 | 0 | 0 | n.d. | n.d. |

n.d.: not determined.

reached 1:2400 to 1:3200. In the non-treated animals the titer steadily increased to 1:6000 and 1:10,000 during week 21–25 p.i. (Fig. 1).

At that time we also determined the anti-gp51 titer. In the non-treated animals the anti-gp51 titer was 1:50,000, while in the treated animals the titer was only half that (1:25,000). A similar difference between treated and non-treated animals was found with regard to the anti-p24 titer.

## Suramin therapy

After BLV infection had become apparent in the seven sheep, three animals were used for suramin treatment, and four served as controls to follow the infectious process. Suramin was administered intravenously once a week at a

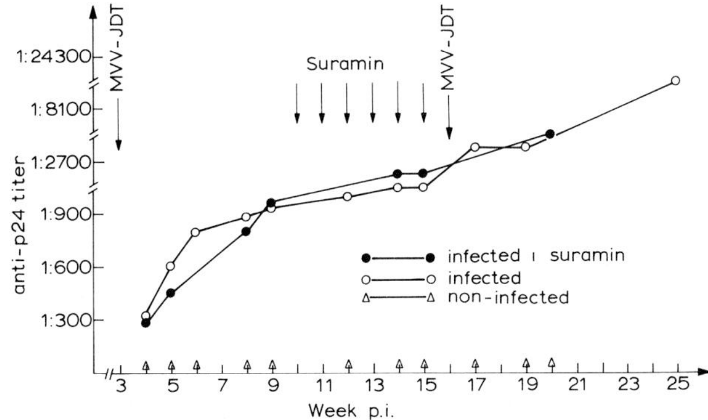


Fig. 1. Anti-p24 antibody titer in sera of BLV-infected sheep with and without suramin treatment.

TABLE 2
p24 antigen detection in lymphocytes of BLV-infected and suramin-treated sheep

| Animal no. | Pre infection | | Post infection 1–9 weeks p.i. | | Treatment p24 | | | | | | Post treatment p24 | | |
|---|---|---|---|---|---|---|---|---|---|---|---|---|---|
| | RT | p24 | RT | p24 | 10 (weeks p.i.) | 11 | 12 | 13 | 14 | 15 | 16 (weeks p.i.) | 32 | 36 |
| *Control* | | | | | | | | | | | | | |
| 512 | 0 | 0 | 0/4 | 0/6 | 0 | 0 | 0 | 0 | 0 | 0 | 0 | 0 | 0 |
| 599 | 0 | 0 | 0/4 | 0/6 | 0 | 0 | 0 | 0 | 0 | 0 | 0 | 0 | 0 |
| *Infected* | | | | | | | | | | | | | |
| 691 | 0 | 0 | 5/9 | 2/9 | 0 | n.d. | n.d. | 0 | n.d. | 0 | 0 | 0 | 0 |
| 671 | 0 | 0 | 5/9 | 8/9 | (+) | n.d. | n.d. | + | + | + | + | + | + |
| 622 | 0 | 0 | 2/4 | 6/6 | + | n.d. | + | + | + | n.d. | (+) | + | + |
| 735 | 0 | 0 | 1/4 | 4/6 | + | n.d. | n.d. | + | + | 0 | 0 | 0 | 0 |
| *Infected and treated* | | | | | | | | | | | | | |
| 604 | 0 | 0 | 4/4 | 6/6 | + | 0 | (+) | (+) | 0 | 0 | + | 0 | 0 |
| 672 | 0 | 0 | 0/4 | 6/6 | + | 0 | 0 | 0 | 0 | 0 | + | 0 | 0 |
| 728 | 0 | 0 | 2/4 | 6/6 | + | 0 | + | + | 0 | 0 | (+) | 0 | 0 |

0: negative; +: positive; (+): doubtful; n.d.: not determined.

dose of 20 mg/kg for a period of 6 weeks. Four days after each injection blood samples were collected for p24 and anti-p24 estimation. Suramin treatment led to a decrease in p24 levels. Table 2 gives a qualitative overview of the detection of p24 before, during and after suramin treatment. The course of the p24 levels during suramin treatment is presented in Fig. 2. The $t_{1/2}$ values were 2.8, 3.6, and 5.3 days respectively. The p24 levels became undetectable within 5 weeks of treatment. This points to a beneficial effect of suramin therapy. Three out of four infected non-treated control animals remained p24-positive throughout the whole period of treatment.

## Post-therapy period

During the post-treatment period again all animals were analyzed for MVV infection and found to be negative. We also followed the anti-p24 titer and found that in the seven infected animals the antibody titer was constantly high, irrespective of whether they had been subjected to suramin treatment. The treated animals again became p24 antigen-positive 1 week after treatment was stopped (week 16). At weeks 32 and 36 these animals were again p24-negative. Yet they turned out to be infectious: transmission of 5–10 ml blood to recipient sheep resulted in an infection of the recipients. The non-treated control animals also proved to be infectious as monitored by this transmission experiment,

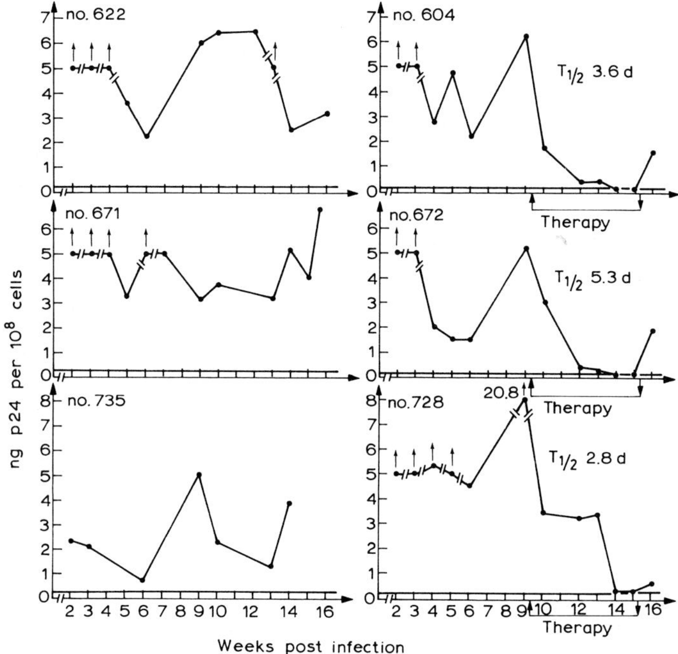


Fig. 2. p24 antigen expression in lymphocytes of BLV-infected sheep with and without suramin treatment. Nos. 622, 671, 735: non-treated control sheep; Nos. 604, 672, 728: sheep subjected to suramin treatment from week 10 to week 15 p.i. The small arrows starting from some black dots indicate p24 values which were significantly higher than 5 ng/$10^8$ cells. The background level of p24 was 0.2 ng (horizontal line just above the abscissa). The treatment period is indicated by large arrows. No. 728: 20.8 ng p24/$10^8$ cells at week 9 p.i.

irrespective of whether they were p24 antigen-positive. Only the non-infected control animals remained non-infectious throughout.

### Hematology

We did not see changes in leukocyte numbers during the experiment, the cell numbers ranging from 4.5 to $10 \times 10^3/\mu l$ blood. The seven BLV-infected individuals showed a small increase in leukocyte counts up to $7–10 \times 10^3/\mu l$ blood during the first 3 weeks p.i. Cell counts returned to the original values thereafter regardless of treatment or non-treatment. The lymphocyte percentage was about 70% in the non-infected control animals and 74% in the infected animals.

## Discussion

Mammerickx et al. (1987) estimated that for sheep the minimal infectious dose of lymphocytes from cattle with EBL was about 1000 cells (corresponding to about 300 infected cells). We decided to inoculate a high dose ($4 \times 10^7$ leukocytes (about $10^7$ infected cells)) in order to achieve infection within a short period of time.

Lymphocytes must be cultivated for a short period of time to allow detection of antigen and RT. Assuming that one BLV virion contains 3000 p24 molecules (A. Burny, personal communication), 0.2 ng p24, the amount which could still be reliably detected by RIA, refers to $6.23 \times 10^8$ p24 molecules or $2 \times 10^5$ BLV particles per $10^7$ cells. Thus, detection of BLV p24 antigen is one order of magnitude more sensitive than detection of RT (Rössler et al., 1980). The detection method of p24 is so sensitive that one can still find one BLV-infected cell among 50 non-infected lymphocytes (2%).

As early as 1979 De Clercq showed that suramin, a polyanionic compound used for the treatment of sleeping sickness, is efficacious in inhibiting the RT of a number of retroviruses. The $ID_{50}$ of suramin for avian myeloblastosis virus (AMV) RT is about 0.1 $\mu$M (De Clercq, 1979). The RT of BLV is blocked at an $ID_{50}$ of about 2.8 $\mu$M suramin (Reimer et al., 1989), 2.2 $\mu$M 3′-FTTP (Matthes, personal communication), 0.17 $\mu$M AZT and 8.0 $\mu$M HPA-23 (Reimer et al., 1989). BLV RT is less sensitive to the above-mentioned RT inhibitors than is HIV RT (Matthes et al., 1987).

In our experiment suramin was administered following the same regimen as used in the treatment of humans suffering from protozoal infections, that is at 20 mg/kg/week intravenously for 6 weeks. Under these conditions we observed a suppression of p24-positive cells in the peripheral blood.

Our tests do not permit the detection of those cells that are infected but do not express the viral proteins. Suramin only inhibits infection of new cells by the actively virus-producing cells. So, only after a certain period of time do infected cells begin to produce virus, making them on the one hand detectable by our tests and on the other hand susceptible to suramin, which then blocks the spread of the infection to new cells. However, infected cells that do not express antigen survive and can express antigen after termination of therapy. The animals, therefore, remain infectious, as was shown by the transmission experiments.

Our data could be interpreted as an indication for a positive effect of suramin, which together with the immunological response led to a drastic decrease of BLV-infected cells. The BLV-infected sheep may indeed serve as an animal model for the exploration of other retrovirus inhibitors or other therapeutic regimens. They may also serve as a model for the study of the pathogenesis of retroviral diseases in vivo.

## Acknowledgements

We thank Mrs. E. Kinder for skillful technical assistance and Mrs. G. Klöss, Dr. H. Schlüter and Dipl. Vet. Med. T. Sellmann for their help with the animal experiments. Dr. J.G. Reich followed the course of the p24 levels calculating the

$t_{1/2}$ values. Suramin was a gift of Bayer (Leverkusen, F.R.G.). We thank Dr. Roberts for the gift of MVV antigen and control sera.

## References

Dawson, H., Chasey, D., King, A.A., Flowers, H.J., Day, R.H., Lucas, M.H. and Roberts, D.H. (1979) The demonstration of maedi/visna virus in sheep in Great Britain. *Vet. Rec.* 105, 220.

De Clercq, E. (1979) Suramin: a potent inhibitor of the reverse transcriptase of RNA tumor viruses. *Cancer Lett.* 8, 9.

De Clercq, E. (1986) Chemotherapeutic approaches to the treatment of the acquired immune deficiency syndrome (AIDS). *J. Med. Chem.* 29, 1561.

Haase, A.T. (1986) Pathogenesis of lentivirus infections. *Nature* 322, 130.

Kenyon, S.J., Ferrer, J.F., McFeely, R.A. and Graves, D.C. (1981) Induction of lymphosarcoma in sheep by bovine leukemia virus. *J. Natl. Cancer Inst.* 67, 1157.

Larsen, H.J. (1979) A whole blood method for measuring mitogen-induced transformation of sheep lymphocytes. *Res. Vet. Sci.* 27, 334.

Levy, D., Kettmann, R., Marchand, P., Djilali, S. and Parodi, E.L. (1987) Selective tropism of BLV for surface immunoglobulin bearing ovine B lymphocytes. *Leukemia* 1, 463.

Mammerickx, M., Portetelle, D., Burny, A. and Leunen, J. (1980) Detection by immunodiffusion- and radioimmunoassay of antibodies to bovine leukemia virus antigens in sera of experimentally infected sheep and cattle. *Zbl. Vet. Med.* B27, 291.

Mammerickx, M., Portetelle, D., De Clercq, K. and Burny, A. (1987) Experimental transmission of enzootic bovine leukosis to cattle, sheep and goats: infectious doses of blood and incubation period of the disease. *Leukemia Res.* 11, 353.

Matthes, E., Lehmann, Ch., Scholz, D., von Janta-Lipinski, M., Gaertner, K., Rosenthal, H.A. and Langen, P. (1987) Inhibition of HIV-associated reverse transcriptase by sugar-modified derivatives of thymidine 5′-triphosphate in comparison to cellular DNA polymerases alpha and beta. *Biochem. Biophys. Res. Commun.* 148, 78.

Reimer, K., Matthes, E., Scholz, D. and Rosenthal, H.A. (1989) Effects of suramin, HPA-23 and 3′-azidothymidine triphosphate on the reverse transcriptase of bovine leukemia virus. *Acta Virol.* 33, 43.

Rössler, H., Werner, O., Drescher, B., Wittmann, W., Venker, P. and Rosenthal, S. (1980) Improved assay for detection of reverse transcriptase of bovine leukosis virus. *Arch. Exp. Vet. Med.* 34, 595.

Schmerr, M.J.F., Van Der Maaten, M.J. and Miller, J.M. (1980) Application of a radioimmunoassay for detection of the major internal antigen (p24) of bovine leukemia virus from cultured lymphocytes of cattle. *Comp. Immun. Microbiol. Infect. Dis.* 3, 327.

Weinhold, E. (1965) Gewinnung weisser Blutkörperchen des Rindes für die Zellkultur. *Tierärztl. Wschr.* 78, 406.

Wittmann, W., Urbaneck, D., Seils, H. and Beyer, J. (1971) Untersuchungen zur Ätiologie der Rinderleukose. 10. Gesamtauswertung erster Übertragungsversuche mit Blut leukosekranker Rinder auf Schaflämmer unter besonderer Berücksichtigung klinischer und hämatologischer Befunde. *Arch. Exp. Vet. Med.* 25, 587.

Wong-Staal, F. and Gallo, R.C. (1985) Human T-lymphotropic retroviruses. *Nature* 317, 395.

*Eds. H. Schellekens and M.C. Horzinek*
*Animal Models in AIDS*



# 27

# Pathogenesis of lentiviral infections

OPENDRA NARAYAN and MICHAEL F. McENTEE

Johns Hopkins University School of Medicine, Division of Comparative Medicine, Baltimore, MD 21205, U.S.A.

**Summary**

Persistent infection in cells of the macrophage lineage combined with loss of helper T (T-4) lymphocytes and proliferation of cytotoxic T and B lymphocytes are key events in the pathogenesis of lentiviral infections in small ruminants (sheep and goats) and primates (macaques and humans). The disease endpoint in these infections is usually cachexia but the pathological effects of the infection vary greatly between ruminants and primates. Lesions in the former are characterized by active-chronic inflammation in specific organ systems and in the latter by initial lymphoproliferation followed by depletion of lymphoid elements and loss of cells from parenchymal organs such as the brain. These cell losses in primates may or may not be complicated with other diseases. This presentation will review both types of infection and identify points of congruence and departure in pathogenesis that lead to different syndromes.

Current data indicate that the lentiviruses are maintained in vivo in cells of the macrophages lineage and disease develops when viral gene expression becomes enhanced in these cells. In ruminant animals, such enhancement occurs in specific groups of macrophages which are located in specific tissues. The enhancement is caused by a combination of a number of factors that include maturation–differentiation–activation of the macrophages, breed and tissue specific factors of the host, age and hormonal elements and tissue tropism of the virus. Enhancement of the virus life cycle, whatever the cause, leads to local inflammation such as encephalitis, arthritis, pneumonia and mastitis. Cellular and humoral immune responses mediate the lesions. On the cellular side, infected macrophages present synthesized viral antigens to T-4 cells in a class 2 restricted manner and responses of the T-4 cells lead to proliferation of T-8 and B lymphocytes. The T-8 cells produce interferon and kill virus-producing macrophages. The cells do not kill latently infected monocytes that are recruited continuously from the bone marrow. B lymphocytes–plasma cells produce large amounts of immunoglobulin, some of which are antiviral antibodies. On the humoral side, virus proteins, especially viral glycoproteins, produced by the infected macrophages induce antibody production locally (by the plasma cells mentioned above) and immune complexes are formed. Most of the antibodies produced do not neutralize virus infectivity but rather combine with virus particles and potentiate or enhance infection in mature macrophages by Fc receptor-mediated endocytosis. These cause inflammation. The net results of these two types of immune responses are proliferation of macrophages, B and T-8 lymphocytes and, for inexplicable reasons, disappearance of most of the T-4 cells. The active-chronic local inflammation parallels the development of cachexia in the animal.

Two types of diseases occur in primates. One type seems to revolve around the virus life cycle in macrophages similar to that seen in ruminant animals. Examples of this in humans are the encephalopathy in adults and lymphoid interstitial pneumonia in infants, both of which are thought to be mediated immunopathologically by the virus or the virus-infected macrophages. Such cells have been identified in tissue sections. Presumably because of the susceptibility of T-4 cells to lysis by infected macrophages (see below) lesions on the brain and lungs are not nearly as inflammatory as those seen in ruminant animals. The second type of disease relates to the loss of T-4 cells which leads to the well-known profound immunosuppression that in turn allows development of other types of infectious and non-infectious diseases. The cellular pathogenesis of this type of disease lies in the phenomenally high susceptibility of T-4 cells of primates to fusion and lysis by the primate lentiviruses. However, this phenomenon presents a paradox. In vivo, virus expression has been recognized mainly in macrophages rather than T-4 cells. Yet, T-4 cells disappear in vivo. In vitro, inoculation of virus into cultures of macrophages and T-4 cells separately leads to persistent, minimally productive infection in the macrophages and fulminant, productive and cytopathic replication of the virus in the lymphocytes. This latter event is not paralleled by similar observations in vivo. Recent studies on co-cultures of macrophages and T-4 lymphocytes have shown that the infected macrophages can kill the T-4 cells. Such cells coming into contact with the infected macrophages underwent rapid fusion and lysis and the debris was phagocytized by the macrophages. This occurred before the lymphocytes could produce virus. This provides an accurate reflection of events occurring in vivo. Thus, in lentivirus-infected macaques and humans both types of diseases are probably initiated by the persistent infection in macrophages. Loss of the T-4 cells in these infections may occur as a result of innocent bystander effects because of the high affinity of the fusogenic virus glycoprotein for the CD4 receptor of the T-4 cells. Since cachexia results in all of the lentiviral diseases irrespective of susceptibility of T-4 lymphocytes to infection, this clinical entity may be a direct or indirect result of infection in macrophages. Also, since T-4 cells disappear in vivo, irrespective of their susceptibility to infection with the virus, the loss of the cells in primates may be the result of a two-hit phenomenon. First, virus-induced down-regulation of maturity of the cells, similar to that postulated to occur in sheep and goats, may occur also in primates. However, this may not be obvious because of the second effect: the selective kill-off of the activated T-4 cells when they contact the infected macrophages in lymphoid tissues. This combined mechanism for elimination of the T-4 cells results in the profound immunosuppression seen in primate hosts.

# *Mouse models*

*Eds. H. Schellekens and M.C. Horzinek*
*Animal Models in AIDS*



# 28

# Murine models of AIDS

MURRAY B. GARDNER

Department of Medical Pathology, University of California at Davis, Davis, CA 95616, U.S.A.

**Summary**

The murine models of acquired immunodeficiency syndrome (AIDS) consist of several different oncovirus infections of laboratory mice, allogeneic disease, human immunodeficiency virus (HIV) infection of human lymphoid cells in SCID:hu mice and HIV transgenic mice. Although none of these models offers an exact replica of the human disease each of them does provide useful knowledge about mechanisms of pathogenesis that may have relevance to AIDS. Several of the oncovirus models are now in use for testing of antiretroviral therapy. The beginning search for a murine lentivirus model of AIDS is also summarized.

## Introduction

A mouse model of acquired immunodeficiency syndrome (AIDS) would be very useful because of its practicality and the ready availability of knowledge, reagents and expertise bearing upon mouse retroviruses and immunogenetics. With cancer as the main driving force during this century an immense amount of scientific information was gained by studying the oncovirus subfamily of retroviruses in inbred and wild mice and other animals (for summary see Gardner, 1980). This knowledge facilitated the discovery in 1980 of the first human oncovirus, the human T-lymphotropic retrovirus, type I (HTLV-I), and the subsequent characterization of the associated adult T cell leukemia and spastic paraparesis. Ironically, the lentivirus subfamily of retroviruses was relatively ignored during these earlier years because these agents did not cause cancer and were then known to exist in only certain large farm animals. With the onset of the AIDS pandemic in the early 1980s and the discovery that the causative human immunodeficiency virus type 1 (HIV-1) was a lentivirus, attention became focused on the biology of this specific retrovirus subfamily. Again, the huge base of knowledge and material resources gained by study of animal oncoviruses paid off by making possible the rapid scientific progress experienced in characterizing the biology and pathogenesis of HIV and in discovering new animal retrovirus models of AIDS. In particular, during the past few years, naturally occurring T cell tropic lentiviruses and associated fatal AIDS-like syndromes were discovered in monkeys and cats (for summaries, see Gardner et al., 1988; Pedersen et al., 1989). The complex biology of the lentivirus infections in animals and man, in particular the lifelong persistence of infectious virus despite an initial vigorous host immune response and the T cell tropism and cytopathology, poses a tremendous challenge for efforts at treatment and immunoprevention (for summary see Pearson et al., 1989). Animal models of retroviral (onco- and lentiviral) induced chronic disease resembling AIDS are therefore essential if we are to better understand mechanisms of pathogenesis and develop more effective therapies and vaccines. In this paper, I briefly review the current mouse models being used in AIDS-related research and describe an ongoing search in wild mice for an, as yet undiscovered, murine lentivirus and associated disease.

The current murine models of AIDS will be discussed in the order outlined in Table 1. They can be divided into three groups: (I) laboratory mice infected by murine leukemia virus (MuLV) with associated immunodeficiency and/or neuropathology, (II) genetically immune deficient laboratory mice reconstituted with human immune cells and infected with HIV-1, and (III) transgenic laboratory mice carrying the HIV-1 transactivating gene (*tat*), the entire HIV-1 provirus or only the HIV-1 long terminal repeat (LTR) linked to a "reporter" gene.

## Mouse oncovirus models

### Immunosuppressive strains of MuLV

#### *Friend, Rauscher and Moloney MuLVs*

The immunosuppressive effects of murine retroviruses was first documented in the 1960s when the Friend MuLV (F-MuLV) was shown to decrease antibody production to various antigens (for summary see Salaman and Wedderburn, 1966). This depressed response occurs before onset of virus induced erythroleukemia and is due, at least in part, to failure of the MuLV-infected precursor B cells to develop into plasma cells. T cell numbers are also decreased and their function impaired as evidenced by suppression of various cell mediated host responses and increased susceptibility to pathogens. Certain macrophage functions such as phagocytosis are impaired while suppressor function may be enhanced. Natural killer (NK) function and antibody dependent cellular cytotoxicity (ADCC) are also severely depressed. The mechanisms underlying these deficiencies in humoral and cellular immunity brought on by F-MuLV and certain other murine oncoviruses are not entirely clear because these viruses are not cytolytic to infected target cells. Their immunosuppressive effects probably involve defects in cytokine production as well as failure of normal T and B cell maturation from direct infection of precursor cells (for summary see Bendinelli et al., 1985).

TABLE 1
Murine models of AIDS

| Model | References |
|---|---|
| *Mouse oncovirus models: murine leukemia virus (MuLV):* | |
| Immunosuppressive strains of MuLV | |
| Friend, Rauscher and Moloney strains | Salaman and Wedderburn, 1966 |
| | Lilly and Pincus, 1973 |
| | Chesebro and Wehrly, 1976 |
| | Bendinelli et al., 1985 |
| | Sharpe et al., 1985 |
| | Ruprecht, 1989 |
| LP-BM5 strain | Mosier et al., 1985, 1986 |
| | Yetter et al., 1985 |
| | Aziz et al., 1989 |
| | Chattopadhyay et al., 1989 |
| Neuropathic strains of MuLV | |
| Cas-Br-E strain | Gardner et al., 1973, 1979, 1980 |
| | Jolicoeur et al., 1983 |
| | Gardner, 1985, 1987, 1989 |
| | Dandekar et al., 1987 |
| | Portis et al., 1987 |
| Moloney TS-1 strain | Prasad et al., 1989 |
| | Wong et al., 1989 |
| Allogeneic diseases | |
| Graft vs. host and host vs. graft syndromes | Hirsch et al., 1970 |
| | Hard and Cross, 1983 |
| | Via and Shearer, 1988 |
| MRL autoimmune mice | Shearer et al., 1986 |
| | Via and Shearer, 1986 |
| *New mouse models of HIV infection* | |
| SCID:hu/hematolymphoid mice | McCune et al., 1988 |
| | Namikawa et al., 1988 |
| SCID:hu/PBL mice | Mosier et al., 1988 |
| Bg/Nu/xid:hu/myeloid mice | Kamel-Reid and Dick, 1988 |
| *HIV transgenic mice* | |
| *tat* gene | Vogel et al., 1988 |
| | Ensoli et al., 1989 |
| Whole proviral DNA | Leonard et al., 1988 |
| LTR/CAT | Leonard et al., 1989 |
| *Search for a murine lentivirus* | |
| PCR screen of wild mouse DNA | Shih et al., 1989 |

The Friend and closely related Rauscher strains of MuLV are a mixture of replication defective and replication competent helper viruses. The virus complex infects immature erythrocytes and causes an acute erythroleukemia in adult mice. Susceptibility is governed by various host genes which interfere with virus replication (e.g., FV-1) (for summary see Lilly and Pincus, 1973) or direct a strong antiviral humoral immune response (e.g., RFV-3) (Chesebro and Wehrly, 1976).

As a model for AIDS treatment these immunosuppressive MuLV strains can be conveniently and cost effectively used to test candidate antiretroviral agents directed at universal retroviral functions such as reverse transcription because the viruses are pathogenic in adult mice, have a very short incubation period and induce splenomegaly proportional to virus titer. For potential inhibitors targeted at specialized lentivirus genes, such as *tat, rev* and *vif,* other models must be used because these regulatory genes are not present in MuLV. Early therapeutic intervention (4 h after virus exposure) with effective antiviral regimes, e.g., azidothymidine (AZT) combined with recombinant human interferon $\alpha$, dramatically prevented F-MuLV infection and disease in Balb/c mice without toxicity (Ruprecht, 1989). These mice were also very effectively immunized by the pharmacologically attenuated live MuLV used in this study.

The Moloney strain of MuLV (M-MuLV), although not markedly immunosuppressive, is activated prenatally in M-MuLV transgenic mice and is transmitted from viremic mothers to offspring, primarily by milk. These murine models have therefore also been used for evaluating transplacental and perinatal antiretroviral therapy (Sharpe et al., 1985).

*LP-BM5 MuLV*

The LP-BM5 strain of MuLV was derived from the bone marrow of C57Bl/6 mice infected with the radiation induced Dupan-Laterjet strain of MuLV isolated many years ago. This virus causes non T cell lymphomas and immunodeficiency in adult mice (Mosier et al., 1986). The virus was recently shown to be a mixture of ecotropic, recombinant and defective MuLVs, the latter apparently responsible for the immunosuppressive effect. The virus is not directly immunosuppressive when added to normal cells in vitro (Aziz et al., 1989; Chattopadhyay et al., 1989). Inoculation of adult C57Bl/6 mice with this virus complex leads rapidly to an acquired immunodeficiency syndrome called "MAIDS" (Mosier et al., 1985) showing similar physiological abnormalities to those seen in early stages of AIDS. The disease exhibits profound T lymphocyte and polyclonal B cell proliferation, progressive lymphadenopathy and splenomegaly, hypergammaglobulinemia and marked depression of essentially all facets of humoral and cellular immunity with death occurring 16–26 weeks after infection. Advanced stages of the disease are associated with enhanced susceptibility to infection and development of B cell lymphomas. The disease is dependent upon the presence of functional CD4 + T lymphocytes which are not infected or decreased in numbers. Indeed, there is a significant increase in the total number of both T and B blast cells in the spleen. Athymic nude mice are thus resistant to the disease (Yetter et al., 1988). MAIDS appears to result from a retroviral induced polyclonal activation of both T and B cells preempting their normal functions and leading to secondary immune dysregulation. The initial step in this pathogenic pathway is still unknown. Whether or not the 60 kDa protein expressed by the defective MuLV component has a pathogenic effect on immune cell function is not known. The relevance of such complex defective pseudotype and recombinant MuLV strains present as high titered viremia, and the rapidly induced immunoproliferation, to the long latency period immunodeficiency induced by the mostly cell associated lentiviruses is not clear. This "MAIDS" model has been used to show the beneficial effect of diethyldithiocarbamate in controlling this retroviral disease but only as long as the drug is administered (Hersh et al., 1990).

## Neuropathic strains of MuLV

### *Cas-Br-E strain*

The prototype neuropathic strain of infectious (ecotropic) MuLV (Cas-Br-E) was discovered about 20 years ago in wild mice living at a squab farm near Lake Casitas (LC) in southern California (Gardner et al., 1973). This virus was acquired at birth, primarily in mother's milk, and the infected mice were immunologically tolerant to the virus. The virus was present throughout life as a systemic infection with high titers of cell free virus in the bloodstream and central nervous system. However, general immunity is intact and the mice do not suffer from an AIDS-like disease. Instead, they are prone after 1 year of age to develop pre-B cell lymphomas and, independently, a fatal neurologic disease with hind leg paralysis (Gardner, 1985). The paralysis is caused by loss of anterior horn neurons in the lower spinal cord secondary to intraneuronal abortive virus replication as well as other more indirect mechanisms of virus injury. This is a non-inflammatory process with prominent intra- and extracellular vacuolar changes in the spinal cord and brain stem, prompting the label "spongiform polioencephalomyelopathy". Molecular studies indicated that the neurotropic property of this virus was attributed to its envelope polypeptide composition. This is the only example to date of a molecularly cloned retrovirus causing both lymphoma and a non neoplastic neurologic disease (Jolicoeur et al., 1983). Genetic resistance to this virus disease in nature is attributed to a dominant gene called FV-4 (formerly Akvr-1) which segregated in LC wild mice (Gardner et al., 1980). FV-4 represents a defective endogenous MuLV provirus expressing an ecotropic viral envelope glycoprotein which interferes at the cell surface with entry of exogenous pathogenic strains of related ecotropic virus (Dandekar et al., 1987). The pathology of this murine disease differs from that of other retroviral neurologic diseases of animal and man, in that in none of the other examples has virus been shown to directly infect neurons or cause a non inflammatory spongiosis as seen in the wild mouse model (Gardner, 1989). The experimental high reproducibility ($\sim 100\%$) and shortened latent period (2–4 months) of the neurologic disease induced by these neuropathic strains of MuLV in newborn laboratory mice of susceptible FV-$1^n$ genotype make this model ideally suited for testing antiretroviral drugs against transplacental spread of virus and for testing effectiveness of such agents across the blood-brain barrier. For example, AZT treatment during pregnancy and in the perinatal period markedly retarded the onset and course of Cas-Br-E-MuLV induced neurologic disease in SWR/J mice (Ruprecht, 1989).

Interestingly, venereal transmission of MuLV was also shown to occur from LC wild mice to susceptible laboratory mice (Gardner et al., 1979; Portis et al., 1987) and, to this day, this represents the only established model for testing antiviral agents against the sexual route of retrovirus spread. In retrospect, the natural history of infectious MuLV in wild mice observed 20 years ago proved different in many respects from infectious MuLV in inbred mice and served as a harbinger of events to come a decade later with the advent of retrovirus infections of man (Gardner, 1987).

*Moloney TS-1 strain*

A temperature sensitive mutant of the Moloney strain of MuLV (M-MuLV) induces a very similar paralytic disease to that caused by the wild mouse ecotropic viruses (Wong et al., 1989). This is not surprising insofar as the M-MuLV strain is genetically most closely related to the ecotropic MuLV of LC wild mice. However, the Ts-1 virus appears to differ from the wild mouse virus by infecting and destroying T lymphocytes and causing a dramatic immunodeficiency in addition to the neurologic disease. The thymus and functional T lymphocytes played a key role in the Ts-1 induced neurologic disorder (Prasad et al., 1989). Although not a homology of HIV induced AIDS, this murine model could also be useful for investigating the pathogenesis of retroviral induced dysfunction of the murine and nervous systems.

## Allogeneic disease

*Graft vs. host (GVH) and host vs. graft (HVG)*

GVH and HVG syndromes are immunologic diseases induced experimentally in certain strains of inbred mice by the inoculation of related $F_1$ or parental T cells (Hard and Cross, 1983; Via and Shearer, 1988). Depending on several variables including the inbred strains crossed and the major histocompatibility complex (MHC) class I or II incompatibility created by the cross the resulting immunologic disease can be rapidly immunosuppressive and fatal with decreased T cells and B cells or stimulatory of T cells and B cells leading to an autoimmune disorder resembling lupus erythematosis in humans. In both syndromes ecotropic and non infectious (xenotropic) MuLV may be activated from either donor or recipient cells (Hirsch et al., 1970). In some versions of these allogeneic diseases T cell depletion and B cell stimulation resemble certain stages of HIV infection. It is not known how the severe allogeneic reactions cause T cell depletion and lymphoid atrophy and the role of activated MuLV in the pathogenesis of these disorders also remains unknown. There is evidence that the lupus-like condition in these allografted mice may result from deficient cytotoxic T cell responses that are unable to control the proliferation of autoantibody producing B cells (Via and Shearer, 1988). The deficient T cell responses are apparently related to the activation of a suppressor T cell that is selective for MHC-self restricted T-helper cell responses (Shearer et al., 1986).

*MRL autoimmune mice*

This inbred strain develops a lupus-like disease with age. A suppressor cell induced loss of MHC restricted function of T-helper cells also occurs in aging MRL mice, perhaps as a compensatory mechanism to down regulate excessive T-helper cell activity (Via and Shearer, 1986). A similar defect in CD4+ dependent MHC restricted responses precedes the reduction of CD4+ cell number in HIV-1 seropositive healthy humans and suggests a common pathogenic mechanism with these allogeneic disease syndromes in mice. A better understanding of these allogeneic disorders of inbred mice could provide further insight into the mechanisms (e.g., role of specific lymphokines) underlying the B cell stimulation and T cell depletion occurring during HIV infection.

## New mouse models of HIV infection

Recently six new mouse models have been described that may facilitate HIV research. Three of these models use congenitally immunodeficient inbred mice reconstituted with human cells and infected with HIV, and three models are based on HIV transgenic mice.

### SCID:HU / HEMATOLYMPHOID MICE

In this model inbred mice with genetically determined combined immunodeficiency (SCID) are reconstituted with fetal human liver, thymus and lymph node (McCune et al., 1988). These mice thus support the growth and differentiation of functional human T and B lymphoid cells which, after differentiation in the human thymus and lymph node implants, respectively, are released into the general circulation. The T4/T8 ratio of the human lymphoid cells is normal and these cells persist as long as 18 months. Human B cells also differentiate to IgG and IgM secreting plasma cells. These mice show no signs of graft versus host disease and appear protected against opportunistic infections, presumably because of the functioning human immune system which is also tolerant of murine elements. Reconstitution of these mice with human bone marrow and thymus allows for the growth in vivo of all myeloid as well as lymphoid elements; only erythroid elements are not produced.

The human thymus and lymph node transplants in SCID mice support infection with cloned HIV-1 (Namikawa et al., 1988). Almost 100% of SCID:hu mice become infected after either intravenous or intraperitoneal inoculation of HIV-1. It remains to be seen whether these mice will develop an AIDS-like disease. AZT, given prophylactically or soon after infection, blocks HIV-1 replication in the SCID : hu mouse. This is therefore an excellent model for testing of antiviral drugs.

## SCID:hu / PBL mice

These mice receive a reconstituted functional human immune system by injection of adult human peripheral blood leukocytes (PBLs) (Mosier et al., 1988). Low dose irradiation of the mice facilitates this engraftment of human cells. The human PBLs, mostly T4 + cells, survive for at least 6 months. T8 + cells and monocytes decline sooner. A secondary antibody response to tetanus toxoid lasts for at least 36 weeks. It is assumed that functioning human T and B lymphocytes in these SCID mice are derived from long-lived recirculating mature cells. The Burkitt lymphomas that develop in SCID:hu mice transplanted with $\geqslant 50 \times 10^6$ PBLs from Epstein-Bar virus (EBV) seropositive donors resemble the sporadic Burkitt lymphomas that arise in AIDS patients. The tumors are all EBV + , monoclonal or oligoclonal, with rearranged JH immunoglobulin genes on chromosome 14 and translocation of the *c-myc* oncogene.

These SCID/PBL mice are readily infected with HIV-1 given cell free or as infected human cell lines. The virus can be isolated from spleen, lymph node and PBLs and shown by in situ hybridization in the human T cells and mononuclear cells in the spleen. A depletion of the human T cells occurs 6–8 weeks post inoculation such that the animals histologically resemble unconstituted SCID mice (D. Mosier, personal communication). Although a decrease in human Ig may be noted, human B cells are still present and most of the mice are still clinically healthy. However, about 15% of the HIV infected SCID:hu mice develop a wasting syndrome with increased levels of tumor necrosis factor (TNF) in their plasma. This is also an excellent model for testing of anti-HIV drugs.

## Bg / Nu / xid:hu / myeloid mice

These genetically immune deficient mice are engrafted with adult human bone marrow containing hematopoietic stem cells (Kamel-Reid and Dick, 1988). Increasing numbers of human macrophage progenitors, dependent on human growth factors, are present during more than 5 weeks of in vivo growth, indicating that seeding, proliferation and differentiation of human stem cells has occurred. These mice have not as yet been inoculated with HIV.

Although it remains uncertain how closely HIV infection of human cells in these reconstituted mice will simulate the human disease these new mouse models will prove useful for basic studies on differentiation of human lymphoid and other hematopoietic cells, the effect of HIV on these functions, the development of assays for growth factors, chemotherapy and vaccines and for study of other human infectious agents and genetic disease that affect the hematopoietic and immune systems.

## HIV transgenic mice

### TAT GENE

Three founder lines of transgenic mice bearing the HIV-1 *tat* gene under control of the homologous viral LTR develop skin tumors that resemble Kaposi's sarcoma (KS) (Vogel et al., 1988). The skin tumors develop only in male mice after 1 year of age and the mice are not immunosuppressed. The *tat* gene is expressed only in skin and not in the tumor cells or other organs. The detection of *tat* expression only in epidermis and not in the adjacent dermal tumor parallels the same observations with KS and HIV infection and supports a common mechanism such as HIV *tat* stimulated secretion of autocrine and paracrine growth factors (Ensoli et al., 1989). This promises to be a very useful model for better understanding the pathogenesis of KS.

### WHOLE PROVIRAL DNA

A single founder line of transgenic mice containing intact copies of HIV-1 proviral DNA developed a rapidly fatal disease characterized by epidermal hyperplasia, lymphadenopathy, splenomegaly, pulmonary lymphoid infiltrates and growth retardation (Leonard et al., 1988). HIV expression was detected in the epidermis and infectious virus was recovered from the spleen, lymph nodes and skin. Immune suppression was not a prominent feature and infection or depletion of T cells was not seen. The usefulness of this model remains uncertain and the single founder line was lost by accident.

### LTR/CAT

Four lines of transgenic mice were constructed containing the HIV-1 LTR linked to the bacterial gene encoding chloramphenicol acetyltransferase (CAT) (Leonard et al., 1989). Characteristic tissue patterns of CAT expression were observed and low levels of CAT activity in circulating lymphocytes and monocytes could be augmented by mitogens or various lymphokines. Langerhans cells in the skin showed unusually high levels of CAT activity. These animals may help identify cell specific determinants of LTR directed gene activity and exogenous cofactors that promote the progression of HIV disease.

## Search for a murine lentivirus

### PCR SCREEN OF WILD MOUSE DNA

Although oncoviruses are abundant in laboratory and wild mice (*Mus musculus*) a murine lentivirus has never been described. Discovery of such a virus in mice might provide a very useful and practical model for AIDS. Therefore we have started to search for evidence of a lentivirus in DNA of newly trapped LC wild mice using the polymerase chain reaction (PCR) technique. As primers we have used synthetic oligonucleotides homologous to highly conserved regions of retro- and lentiviral and hepadnaviral reverse transcriptase. A similar PCR approach was recently used to clone and sequence primate retrovirus related *pol* genes from human tissue (Shih et al., 1989). As a probe to detect the amplified template (and primers) of 126 nucleotides we used a 44mer oligonucleotide sequence in the corresponding region of the caprine arthritis encephalitis lentivirus. We have amplified and sequenced two 126 base pair clones and found one to resemble an hepadnavirus polymerase and the other to resemble a new endogenous Type B/Type D polymerase (R. Cardiff and M. Gardner, unpublished observation). We have as yet found no evidence of an infectious virus, lentivirus or otherwise. However, this appears to be a reasonable strategy to screen wild mice for evidence of an indigenous lentivirus. Discovery of a murine lentivirus could lead to yet another murine model of AIDS, supplementary to and perhaps more relevant in some respects than the existing murine oncovirus models.

## References


Aziz, D.C., Hanna, Z. and Jolicoeur, P. (1989) Severe immunodeficiency disease induced by a defective murine leukemia virus. *Nature* 338, 505–508.

Bendinelli, M.D., Matteucci, D. and Friedman, H. (1985) Retrovirus induced acquired immunodeficiencies. *Adv. Cancer. Res.* 45, 125–181.

Chattopadhyay, S.K., Morse, H.C. III, Makino, M., Ruscetti, S.K. and Hartley, J.W. (1989) Defective virus is associated with induction of murine retroviruses-induced immunodeficiency syndrome. *Proc. Natl. Acad. Sci. U.S.A.* 86, 3862–3866.

Chesebro, B. and Wehrly, K. (1976) Studies on the role of the host immune response in recovery from Friend virus leukemia. I. Antiviral and antileukemia cell antibodies. *J. Exp. Med.* 143, 73–84.

Dandekar, S., Rossitto, P., Picket, S., Mockli, G., Bradshaw, H., Cardiff, R. and Gardner, M. (1987) Molecular characterization of the Akvr-1 restriction gene: a defective endogenous retrovirus identical to Fv-$4^R$. *J. Virol.* 61, 308–314.

Ensoli, B., Nakahmura, S., Salahuddin, S.Z., Biberfeld, P., Larsson, L., Beaver, B., Wong-Staal, F. and Gallo, R.C. (1989) AIDS-Kaposi sarcoma-derived cells express cytokines with autocrine and paracrine growth effects. *Science* 244, 223–226.

Gardner, M.B. (1980) Historical background. In: J.R. Stephenson (Ed.), *Molecular Biology of RNA Tumor Viruses,* Chapter 1. Academic Press, New York, NY, pp. 1–46.

Gardner, M.B. (1985) Retroviral spongiform polioencephalomyelopathy. *Rev. Infect. Dis.* 7, 99–110.

Gardner, M.B. (1987) Naturally occurring leukaemia viruses in wild mice: how good a model for humans. *Cancer Surv.* 6, 55–71.

Gardner, M.B. (1989) Retroviral infection of the nervous system in animals and man. In: *Neuroimmune Networks: Physiology and Diseases.* Alan R. Liss, New York, NY, pp. 179–192.

Gardner, M.B., Henderson, B.E., Officer, J.G., Rongey, P.W., Parker, J.C., Oliver, C., Estes, J.D. and Huebner, R.J. (1973) A spontaneous lower motor neuron disease apparently caused by indigenous type C RNA tumor virus in wild mice. *J. Natl. Cancer Inst.* 51, 1243–1254.

Gardner, M.B., Chiri, A., Dougherty, M.F., Casagrande, J. and Estes, J.D. (1979) Congenital transmission of murine leukemia virus from wild mice prone to the development of lymphoma and paralysis. *J. Natl. Cancer Inst.* 62, 63–70.

Gardner, M.B., Rasheed, S., Pal, B.K., Estes, J.D. and O'Brien S.J. (1980) Akvr-1, a dominant MuLV restriction gene is polymorphic in leukemia-prone wild mice. *Proc. Natl. Acad. Sci. U.S.A.* 77, 531–535.

Gardner, M.B., Luciw, P., Lerche, N. and Marx, P.E. (1988) Nonhuman primate retrovirus isolates and AIDS. In: K. Perk (Ed.), *Immunodeficiency Disorders and Retroviruses.* Academic Press, New York, NY, pp. 285–299.

Hard, R.C. Jr. and Cross, S.S. (1983) Pathology, immunology and virology of the host versus graft syndrome. *Surv. Immunol. Res.* 2, 1–11.

Hersh, E.M., Funk, C.Y., Ryschon, K.L., Petersen, E.A., and Mosier, D.E. (1990). Effective therapy of the LP-BM5 murine retrovirus induced lymphoproliferative immunodeficiency disease with diethyldithiocarbamate. *AIDS Res.* (in press).

Hirsch, M.S., Black, P.H., Tracey, G.S., Leibowitz, S. and Schwartz, R.S. (1970). Leukemia virus activation in chronic allogenic disease. *Proc. Natl. Acad. Sci. U.S.A.* 67, 1914–1917.

Jolicoeur, P., Nicolaiew, N., DesGroseillers, L. and Rassart, E. (1983) Molecular cloning of infectious viral DNA from ecotropic neurotropic wild mouse retrovirus. *J. Virol.* 56, 639–643.

Kamel-Reid, S. and Dick, J.E. (1988) Engraftment of immune-deficient mice with human hematopoietic stem cells. *Science* 242, 1706–1709.

Leonard, J.M., Abramczuk, J.W., Pozen, D.S., Rutledge, R., Belcher, I.H., Hakim, F., Shearer, G., Lamperth, L., Travis, W., Fredrickson, T., Notkins, A.L. and Martin, M.A. (1988) Development of disease and virus recovery in transgenic mice containing HIV proviral DNA. *Science* 242, 1665–1670.

Leonard, J., Khillan, J.S., Gendelman, H.E., Adachi, A., Lorenzo, S., Wesphal, H., Martin, M.A. and Meltzer, M.S. (1989) The human immunodeficiency virus long terminal repeat is preferentially expressed in Langerhans cells in transgenic mice. *AIDS Res. Human Retroviruses* 5, 421–430.

Lilly, F. and Pincus, T. (1973) Genetic control of murine viral leukemogenesis. *Adv. Cancer Res.* 17, 231–277.

McCune, J.M., Namikawa, R., Kanashima, H., Schultz, L.P., Lieberman, M. and Weissman, I.L. (1988) The SCID-hu mouse: murine model for the analysis of human hematolymphoid differentiation and function. *Science* 241, 1632–1638.

Mosier, D.E., Yetter, R.A. and Morse, H.C. III (1985) Retroviral induction of acute lymphoproliferative disease and profound immunosuppression in adult C57Bl/6 mice. *J. Exp. Med.* 161, 766–784.

Mosier, D.E., Yetter, R.A. and Morse, H.C. III (1986) Retrovirus induction of immunodeficiency and lymphoproliferative disease in mice. In: L.A. Salzman (Ed.), *Animal Models of Retrovirus Infection and Their Relationship to AIDS.* Academic Press, New York, NY, pp. 285–294.

Mosier, D.E., Gulizia, R.J., Baird, S.M. and Wilson, D.B. (1988) Transfer of a functional human immune system to mice with severe combined immunodeficiency. *Nature* 335, 256–259.

Namikawa, R., Kanashima, H., Lieberman, M., Weissman, I.L. and McCune, J.M. (1988) Infection of the SCID-hu mouse by HIV-1. *Science* 242, 1684–1686.

Pearson, L.D., Poss, M.L. and Demartini, J.C. (1989) Animal lentivirus vaccines: problems and prospects. *Vet. Immunol. Immunopathol.* 20, 183–212.

Pedersen. N.C., Yamamoto, J.K., Ishido, T. and Hauser, H. (1989) Feline immunodeficiency virus infection. *Vet. Immunol. Immunopathol.* 21, 111–129.

Portis, J.L., McAtee, F.T., and Hayes, S.F. (1987) Horizontal transmission of murine retroviruses. *J. Virol.* 61, 1037–1044.

Prasad, G., Stoica, G. and Wong, P.K.Y. (1989) The role of the thymus in the pathogenesis of hind leg paralysis induced by Ts-1, a mutant of murine leukemia virus-TB. *Virology* 169, 332–340.

Ruprecht, R.M. (1989) Murine models for antiretroviral therapy. *Intervirology* 30 (Suppl. 1), 2–11.

Salaman, M.H. and Wedderburn, N. (1966) The immunodepressive effects of Friend virus. *Immunology* 10, 445–448.

Sharpe, A.S., Jaenisch, R. and Ruprecht, R.M. (1985) Retroviruses and mouse embryos: a rapid model for neurovirulence and transplacental antiviral therapy. *Science* 236, 1671–1679.

Shearer, G.M., Bernstein, D.B., Tung, K.S.K. et al. (1986) A model for the selective loss of major histocompatibility complex self-restricted T cell immune responses during the development of acquired immune deficiency syndrome (AIDS). *J. Immunol.* 137, 2514–2521.

Shih, A., Misra, R. and Rush, M.G. (1989) Detection of multiple, novel reverse transcriptase coding sequences in human nucleic acids: relation to primate retroviruses. *J. Virol.* 63, 64–75.

Via, C.S., and Shearer, G.M. (1986) Functional heterogeneity of L3T4+ T cells in MRL-lpr/lpr mice. *J. Exp. Med.* 168, 2165–2181.

Via, C.S. and Shearer, G.M. (1988) T-cell interactions in autoimmunity: insights from a murine model of graft-versus-host disease. *Immunol. Today* 9, 207–213.

Vogel, J., Hinrichs, S.H., Reynolds, R.K., Luciw, P.A. and Jay, G. (1988) The HIV Tat gene induces dermal lesions resembling Kaposi sarcoma in transgenic mice. *Nature* 335, 606–611.

Wong, P.K.Y., Prasad, G., Hansen, J. and Yuen, P.H. (1989) Ts-1, a mutant of Moloney murine leukemia virus-TB, causes both immunodeficiency and neurologic disorders in Balb/c mice. *Virology* 170, 450–459.

Yetter, R.A., Buller, R.M.L., Lee, J.S., Elkins, K.L., Mosier, D.E., Fredrickson, T.V. and Morse, H.C. III (1988) CD4+ T cells are required for development of a murine retrovirus induced immunodeficiency syndrome (MAIDS). *J. Exp. Med.* 168, 623–635.

*Eds. H. Schellekens and M.C. Horzinek*
*Animal Models in AIDS*


# 29

# The development of HIV-1 p24 antigenemia in the athymic "nude" mouse

NEAL T. WETHERALL

Department of Pathology, Vanderbilt University School of Medicine, Nashville, TN 37232-2561, U.S.A.

## Introduction

Recent developments toward defining animal models of human immunodeficiency virus (HIV) disease or acquired immunodeficiency syndrome (AIDS) include the successful infection of mice with the etiological agent, HIV-1. Leonard et al. (1988) have produced transgenic mice incorporating full length HIV-1 proviruses which produce offspring with infectious HIV. Namikawa et al. (1988) have reported on severe combined immunodeficiency (SCID) mice transplanted with human fetal tissue which produce infectious HIV-1. Another approach involving SCID mice, reported by Mosier et al. (1988), in which human peripheral blood lymphocytes are transplanted to reconstitute the immune system of the mice, can also support HIV-1 replication (Mosier et al., 1989).

The athymic or "nude" mouse has had utility for the study of several human infectious diseases of bacterial and parasitic (Armstrong and Walzer, 1978), mycobacterial (Colson and Kohsaka, 1982) or viral origin (Iwaski, 1978). In addition, through the process of "viral xenogenization" (Kobayashi, 1989) infectious human RNA (mumps) virus has successfully been recovered from nude mice (Reid et al., 1979). Using a similar approach, we now report the establishment of a persistent HIV-1 antigenemia in irradiated athymic mice through the xenotransplantation of virus in infected human CD4 + receptor positive (CEM) lymphoma cells. Many different human cell lines of various origins have been successfully infected with HIV-1 (Weiss, 1985). In preparation for future studies, we have transplanted and determined in vivo growth patterns for six other cell lines which may also be capable of producing a similar antigenemic state.

## Materials and methods

### Cell lines and virus cultures

All cells of human T-cell (CCRF-CEM or CEM, Jurkat, Molt-4), monocytic (U937, THP-1), or promyelo(mono)cytic (HL-60) origin were acquired from the American Type Culture Collection, Rockville, MD, and maintained in RPMI 1640 medium with 15–20% fetal calf serum. HeLa T4+ epithelial cells were acquired from the NIH AIDS Research and Reference Reagent Program and maintained in DMEM medium with 10% fetal calf serum. The cells were propagated at 37°C in a humid 5% $CO_2$ atmosphere. All of these cell lines are capable of producing infectious HIV-1 in vitro (Chesebro and Wehrley, 1988). The $TCID_{50}$ values of the human T-lymphocyte leukemia virus type III (HTLV-III) strain of HIV-1 were determined by endpoint titration of viral culture supernatants on MT-2 cells (Montefiori et al., 1988), and were standardized to produce $10^6$ infectious units/ml.

### Mice and cell transplantation

Athymic 3–4 week old (nu/nu) nude mice were purchased from Harlan Sprague Dawley, Inc. and were housed, maintained and inoculated as previously described (Johnson et al., 1989). All mice were exposed to 609 (± 15) R at the body surface using a $^{137}$Cesium source 24 h prior to cell transplantation. Additional precautions as outlined for biosafety level 3 were adhered to (CDC, 1988). To avoid the use of HIV-1 infected needles, a 22 gauge teflon catheter (FLASH-CATH, Travenol Labs, Inc., Deerfield, IL, U.S.A.) was inserted at the inoculation site subcutaneously, and the syringe containing 0.2 ml of CEM/HIV-1 cell suspension in serum-free RPMI 1640 medium was luer locked onto the catheter prior to injection. The animals were monitored 5 days a week for body weight and tumor presence or progression. The tumor volume was calculated from measurements in two dimensions using the formula for a prolate ellipsoid, $\pi/6\ LW^2$ (Skarlin et al., 1988). Significance of differences between groups was evaluated by the unpaired Student *t*-test. Probability values are specified in two tails.

### DNA and RNA analysis

The nucleic acids were extracted from tumor tissue, rapidly frozen in liquid nitrogen and stored at −70°C until use for DNA and RNA isolation and fractionation by methods previously described (Johnson et al., 1989). The DNA and RNA blots are modifications of the procedure of Southern (1975) and Vrati et al. (1988) respectively. The pBH10R3 plasmid is available from the NIH AIDS Research and Reference Reagent Program.

HIV-1 P24 ANTIGEN ASSAYS

The HIV-1 antigen enzyme immunoassay (EIA) is manufactured by Abbott Laboratories (Chicago, IL, U.S.A.) and is utilized on both tissue culture supernatants and heparinized mouse plasma (200 $\mu$l), acquired by exsanguination. The procedure was followed without modification (Allain et al., 1986), except that 1000 units of antigen were translated to 200 pg/ml. Background levels of reactivity using undiluted mouse plasma are similar to those of human plasma. Tumor tissue was processed for immunohistochemistry by the method described by Casey et al. (1988). The sheep anti-p24 polyclonal antibodies were purchased from Accurate Chemical and Scientific Corp., Westbury, NY, U.S.A.

## Results and discussion

Our initial experiments were designed to determine if the HIV-1 permissive (Dalgleish et al., 1984), tumorigenic (Fodstad et al., 1984), CD4+ receptor positive cell line CCRF-CEM, or CEM (Foley et al., 1965), could be transplanted into gamma-irradiated nude mice and provide predictable tumor incidence and progression with minimal morbidity from irradiation or tumor burden. Various cell inocula ($0.5 \times 10^7$, $1.0 \times 10^7$, $2.0 \times 10^7$, and $5.0 \times 10^7$ cells) were injected subcutaneously (s.c.) into the interscapular region of irradiated and non-irradia-

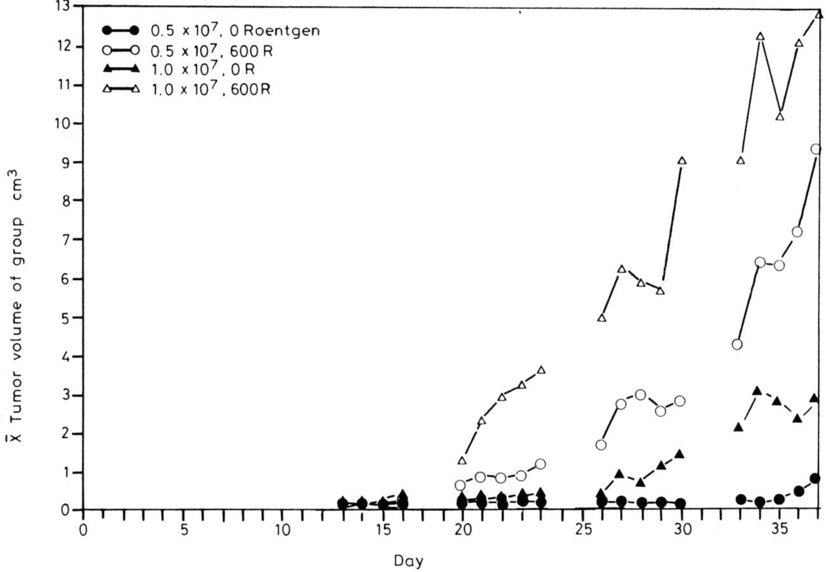


Fig. 1. Comparison of tumor volumes of CEM heterotransplants in irradiated and non-irradiated "nude" mice. Populations (n = 6) of mice were inoculated with $0.5 \times 10^7$ or $1.0 \times 10^7$ CEM cells. One group of each inoculum received 600 R $^{137}$Cesium irradiation 1 day prior to inoculation.

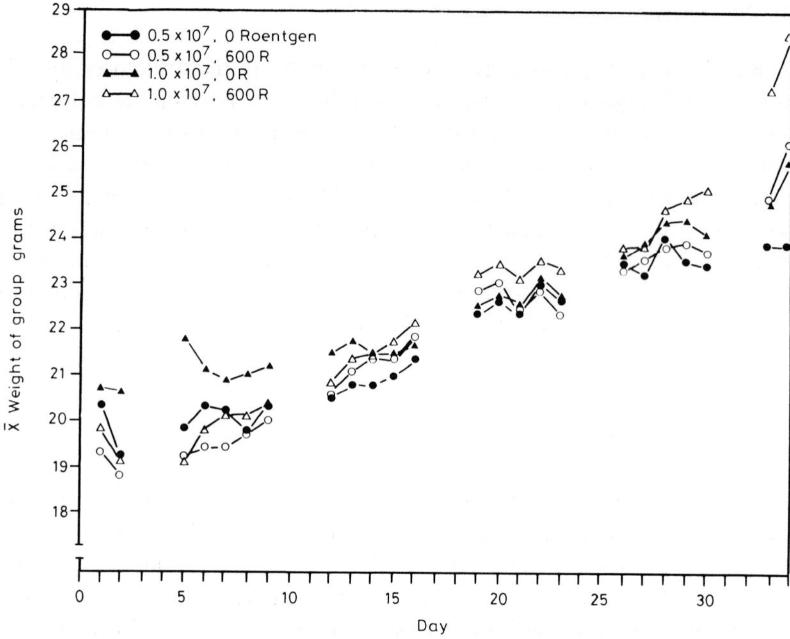


Fig. 2. Comparison of total body weight gain in irradiated and non-irradiated "nude" mice heterotransplanted with CEM cells. One group of each inoculum received 600 R $^{137}$Cesium irradiation 1 day prior to inoculation.

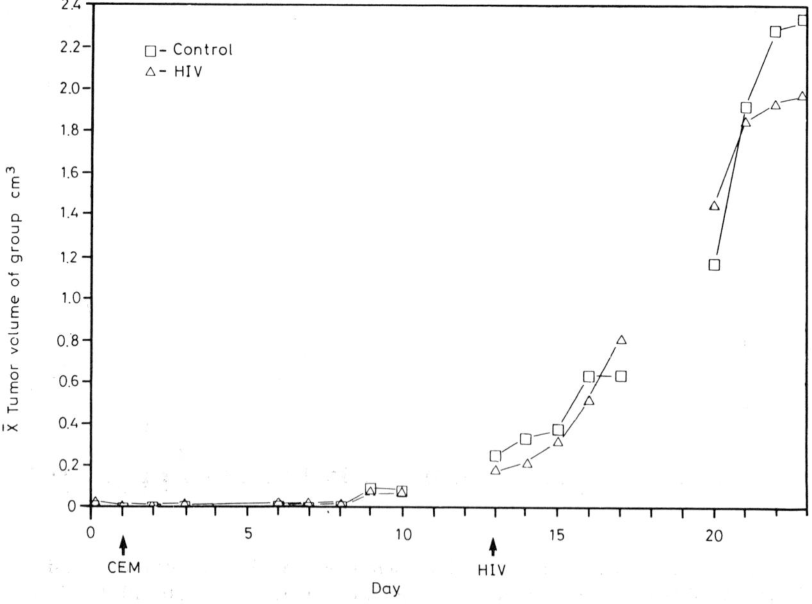


Fig. 3. Effect of HIV-1 challenge on tumor growth in "nude" mice with pre-existing CEM tumor.

ted mice. Weights and tumor volumes were monitored for 37 days. Tumors were detectable in all groups 12–14 days after inoculation. The exponential phase of tumor development was delayed by approximately 5 days in all non-irradiated groups. Regression of individual tumors occurred in 16 out of 20 non-irradiated animals. Fig. 1 shows the effects of irradiation on tumor growth in mice injected with $0.5 \times 10^7$ cells, and the optimum $1 \times 10^7$ cells. Significant differences ($P \geqslant 0.05$) were found between the 0.5 and $1.0 \times 10^7$ groups, and between the 1.0 and $5.0 \times 10^7$ groups. No significant differences were found between the 1.0 and

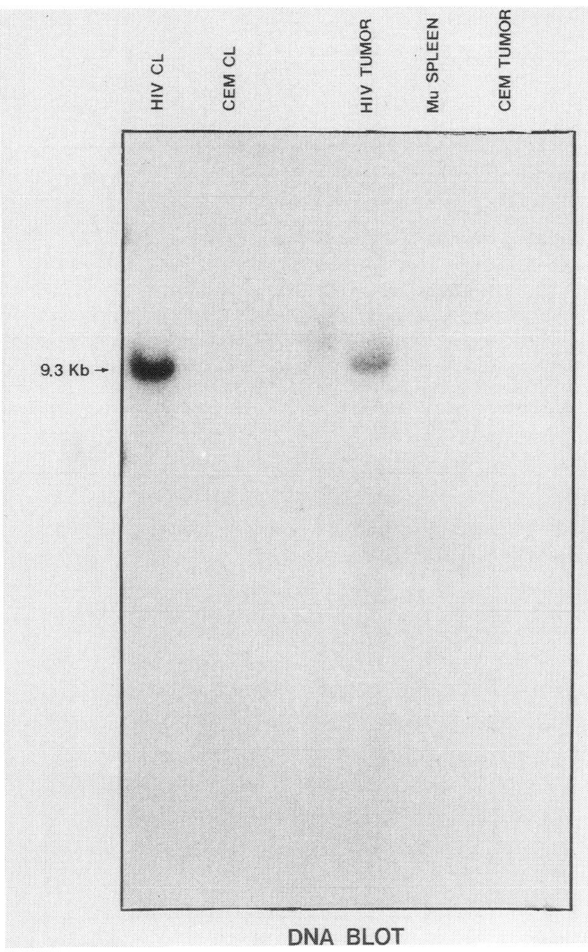


Fig. 4. Southern blot analysis of DNA extracted from HIV challenged CCRF-CEM heterotransplanted tumor. Each sample (10 μg) was digested ON at 37°C with *Sst*1 restriction endonuclease. Probe used was $^{32}$P-labeled 1.1 kb HIV *nef* sequence from pBH10R3 plasmid. lane 1, CEM cell line infected with HTLV-IIIB strain of HIV-1; lane 2, uninfected CEM cell line; lane 3, tumor from infected cells; lane 4, mouse spleen; lane 5, tumor from uninfected cells.

$2.0 \times 10^7$ groups, however the $1 \times 10^7$ inoculum produced consistent tumor growth without tumor necrosis. Fig. 2 shows the weight gain and the ability of the animals to thrive in these same groups of mice was similar, indicating that there were no harmful effects from the irradiation.

In order to determine if an established transplant could support the replication of HIV-1, six mice were challenged with HIV-1 chronically infected CEM cells. An inoculum was injected directly into the palpable mass created by inoculating $1 \times 10^7$ uninfected CEM cells s.c. 13 days earlier. The mice were followed for 10 days. Fig. 3 indicated that using this approach, the virus had no effect on tumor

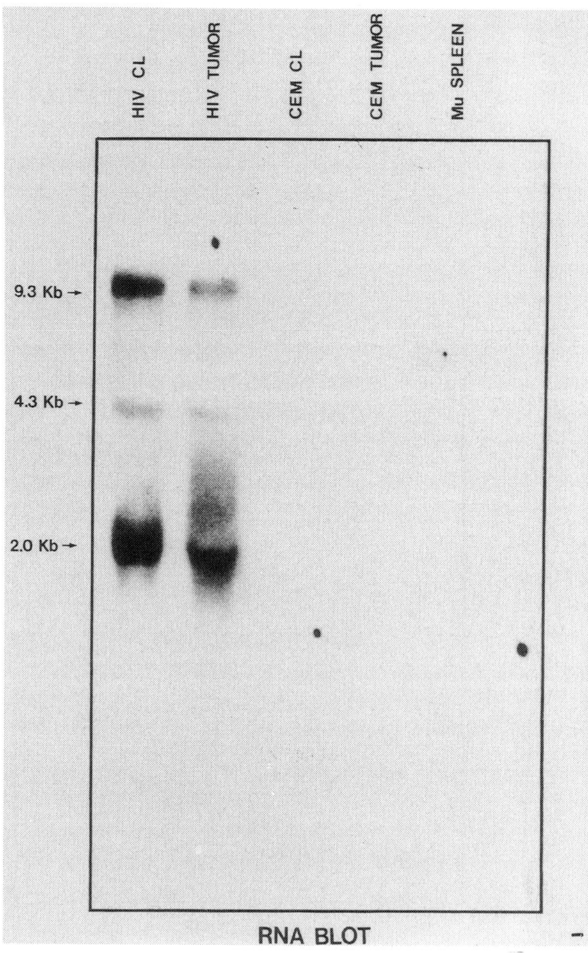


Fig. 5. Northern blot analysis of total cellular RNA from HIV challenged CCRF-CEM heterotransplanted tumor. Blot was probed with the same $^{32}$P-labeled *nef* sequence used for Southern analysis. Lane 1, CEM cell line infected with HTLV-IIIB strain of HIV-1; lane 2, tumor produced in "nude" mouse with infected cells; Lane 3, CEM uninfected cell line; lane 4, tumor from uninfected cells; Lane 5, mouse spleen. All samples were 20 $\mu$g of total cellular RNA.

progression. Previous reports (Ratner et al., 1985; Wain-Hobson et al., 1985) indicate that homology exists between the HTLV-III/LAV strains of HIV-1 and the Moloney murine leukemia virus (Mo-MuLV). To determine the integrity of the 1.1 kb *nef* gene probe, a Southern blot of infected and non-infected CEM tumor and nude mouse spleen DNA was performed. The findings displayed in Fig. 4 indicate that HIV-1 proviral DNA can be detected in the tumor mass, without cross-reacting with murine cells or potentially present murine retrovirus. Viral replication, and not solely integration, was determined by performing a Northern blot (Fig. 5) on the RNA from the same tissues. The four mRNA moieties, i.e., from the 9.3 kb genomic, 4.3 kb envelope, and the approximately 2.0 kb *tat* and *nef* genes, are expressed only in the control cell line and the infected tumor tissue. The findings offered by the nucleic acid analyses strongly suggest that non-murine antibodies raised against HIV-1 proteins should be specific, and would not cross-react with other potentially present retroviral proteins.

Presence of the major core p24 *gag* protein of the HIV-1, p24 *gag*, circulating in the bloodstream, as detected by antigen capture assays, has significant clinical implications. Variations in the plasma antigen levels in HIV-1 infected individuals is accepted as an important indicator of disease progression in both hemo-

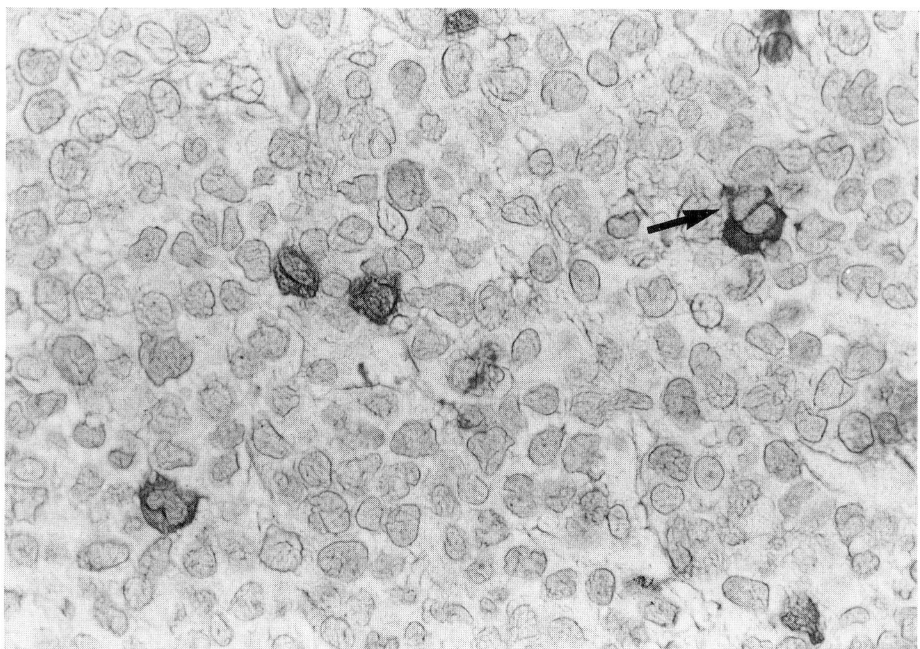

Fig. 6. Stained tissue section of HIV-1 infected CEM tumor transplanted into a "nude" mouse reacted with a sheep polyclonal antibody to p24 HIV core protein. Peroxidase conjugated secondary antibody was developed with diaminobenzidine as substrate.

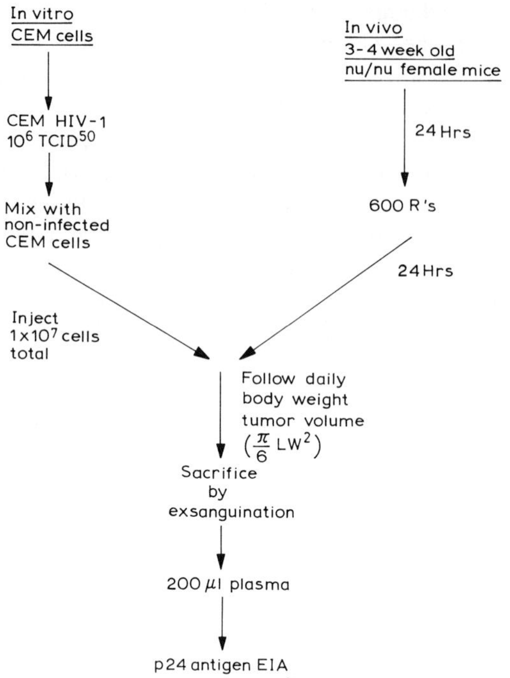


Fig. 7. Scheme for the production of HIV p24 anigenemia in "nude" mice.

philiac (Allain et al., 1986) and homosexual (Lange et al., 1986) populations. In addition, a suppression in plasma levels of p24 antigen is associated with a positive therapeutic response to candidate antiviral agents (Chaisson et al., 1986). Therefore, we determined the presence of p24 antigen in tumor tissue by immunohistochemistry and in plasma by EIA with antibodies raised in sheep and rabbits respectively. The tumors from the animals infected in the initial experiments were stained using an immunoperoxidase method and revealed numerous cells with cytoplasmic positivity for p24 antigen (Fig. 6). Control tissue was negative and without background (not shown).

An approach was developed to determine if p24 antigen could readily be detected in mouse plasma, and is depicted in Fig. 7. This scheme was followed by preparing irradiated 4 week old nude mice, and injecting the optimum $1 \times 10^7$ inoculum of CEM cells, which were first mixed in a ratio of 90% uninfected and 10% HIV-1 infected cells. We determined the course of antigenemia over a 9 week period in matched groups of six HIV-1 infected nude mice (total of 48 infected and six control animals). At each test point, one group of six mice was exsanguinated and killed by cardiac puncture and plasma p24 antigen levels were determined at various time points. Fig. 8 shows the average antigen level of the group at each time point. Antigen was detectable at 3 days after inoculation (28

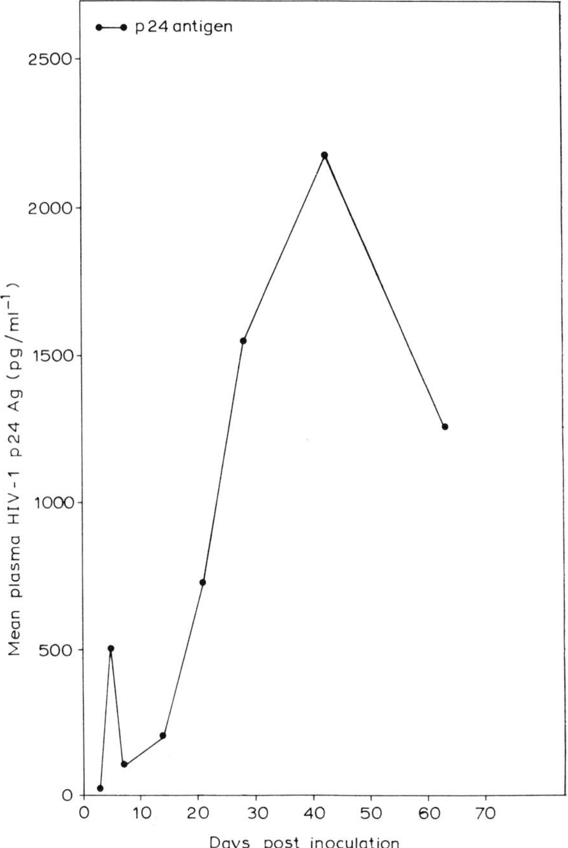


Fig. 8. Average antigen plasma levels of mice heterotransplanted wih HIV-infected CCRF-CEM cells. Each point represents the average of six animals.

pg/ml), spiked at 5 days (514 pg/ml), rose steadily from 7 to 42 days (90–2181 pg/ml), then dropped off at day 63 (1269 pg/ml). It is not clear at this time what is responsible for this dynamic antigenemic state, but it could be due to either the mouse immune system (Holub, 1989), the viral replicative cycle (Gallo et al., 1984), or CD4 + receptor regulation by the CEM cells (Salmon et al., 1988), however the antigen curve indicates a strong similarity to in vitro HIV-1 replication (Montefiori and Mitchell, 1987). No mortality or disease symptoms from HIV-1 infection were observed in any of these mice.

The pathogenesis of HIV disease is complex and the course of the disease may be influenced by the type of cells which are infected with the virus (Levy, 1989). Therefore, using $1 \times 10^7$ cells as an inoculum, we determined if other HIV permissive cell lines could produce successful heterotransplants in the irradiated nude mouse system. Seven cell lines (including CEM) of four different cell lineages were injected into populations of six mice each, and the tumor progres-

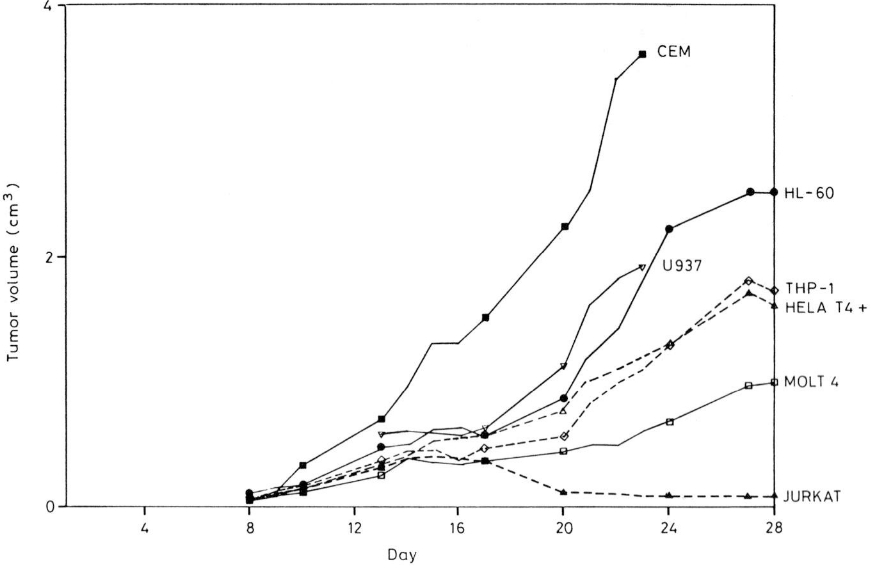


Fig. 9. Tumor progression of several HIV permissive cell lines heterotransplanted into "nude" mice. All mice received 600 R $^{137}$Cesium irradiation and $1 \times 10^7$ cells.

sion is shown in Fig. 9. All of the cell lines developed palpable masses by day 8 and progressively grew except for the CD4 + positive lymphoma derived Jurkat, which regressed starting at day 17. The T-cell derived Molt-4 did progress in tumor volume, however not in a similar manner to the CEM cells. These findings indicate that differences exist among these cells which may influence the antigenemic state when infected cells are transplanted. Although several titers of inocula need to be assayed, the other cells of hematopoietic or epithelial origin which were utilized in this study all developed progressively expanding masses in the mice with a $1 \times 10^7$ cell inoculum, and should prove to have utility to study the role of HIV infection and therapy in cells of differing phenotypes.

The results reported here demonstrate a system for the infection of nude mice with HIV-1 which produces a dynamic measurable antigenemic state. This clinically relevant parameter provides the means to investigate several aspects of HIV infection. We anticipate this model system will prove useful to assay and study candidate anti-HIV therapies as well as offer insight into other aspects of HIV disease such as host immunomodulation, passive immunotherapy, host/HIV strain isolate interaction, and in vivo virus mutation.

## Acknowledgements

We wish to thank Drs. D. Montefiori for providing HIV-1 infected cell cultures, T. Casey for the immunohistochemistry, and J. Stewart (Abbott Diagnostics) for information and suggestions on the Abbott p24 EIA. We would also like to acknowledge the receipt of the HeLa T4 + cell line through the AIDS Research and Reference Reagent Program. This work is supported by the U.S. Army Medical Research and Development Command under Contract DAMD17-88-C-8071, and the opinions, interpretations, conclusions and recommendations are those of the authors and are not necessarily endorsed by the U.S. Army.

In conducting research using animals, the investigators adhered to the "Guide for the Care and Use of Laboratory Animals," prepared by the committee on Care and Use of Laboratory Animals of the Institute of Laboratory Animal Resources, National Research Council (NIH Publication No. 86-23, Revised 1985).

## References

Allain, J.P., Lauriam, U., Paul, D. and Senn, D. (1986) Serological markers in early stages of human immunodeficiency virus infection in hemophiliacs. *Lancet* ii, 1233–1236.

Armstrong, D. and Walzer, P. (1978) Experimental infections in the nude mouse. In: J. Fogh and B.C. Giovanella (Eds.), *The Nude Mouse in Experimental and Clinical Research.* Academic Press, New York, NY, pp. 477–489.

Casey, T.T., Cousar, J.B. and Collins, R.D. (1988) A simplified plastic embedding and immunohistologic technique for the immunophenotype analysis of human hematopoetic and lymphoid tissues. *Am. J. Path.* 131, 183–189.

Centers for Disease Control (CDC) (1988) Agent summary statement for human immunodeficiency virus and report on laboratory-acquired infection with human immunodeficiency virus. *MMWR* 37 (S-4), pp. 11–15.

Chaisson, R.E., Allain, J.P. and Volberding, P.A. (1986) Significant changes in HIV antigen level in the serum of patients treated with azidothymidine. *N. Engl. J. Med.* 315, 1610–1611.

Cheseboro, B. and Wehrley, K. (1988) Development of a sensitive quantitative focal assay for human immunodeficiency virus infectivity. *J. Virol.* 62, 3779–3788.

Colson, J.J. and Kohsaka, K. (1982) The nude mouse in studies of leprosy. In: J. Fogh and B.C. Giovanella (Eds.), *The Nude Mouse in Experimental and Clinical Research,* Vol. 2. Academic Press, New York, NY, pp. 247–266.

Dalgleish, A.G., Beverley, P.C.L., Clapham, P.R., Crawford, D.H., Greaves, M.F. and Weiss, R.A. (1984) The CD4(T4) antigen is an essential component of the receptor for the AIDS retrovirus (HTLV-3). *Nature* 312, 736–767.

Fodstad, O., Hansen, C.T., Cannon, G.B., Statham, C.N., Lichtensten, G.R. and Boyd, M.R. (1984) Lack of correlation between natural killer activity and tumor growth in nude mice with different immune defects. *Cancer Res.* 44, 4403–4408.

Foley, G.E., Lazarus, H., Farber, S., Uzman, B.G., Boone, B.A. and McCarthy, R.E. (1965) Continuous culture of human lymphoblasts from peripheral blood of a child with acute leukemia. *Cancer* 8, 522–529.

Gallo, R.C., Salahuddin, S.Z., Popovic, M., Shearer, G.M., Kaplan, M., Haynes, B.F., Palker, T.J., Redfield, R., Oleske, J., Safai, B., White, G., Foster, P. and Markham, P.D. (1984) Frequent detection and isolation of cytopathic retroviruses (HTLV-III) from patients with AIDS and at risk for AIDS. *Science* 224, 500–503.

Holub, M. (1989) *Immunology of Nude Mice.* CRC Press, Boca Raton, FL, pp. 53–82.

Iwaski, Y. (1978) Experimental virus infections in nude mice. In: J. Fogh and B.C. Giovanella (Eds.), *The Nude Mouse in Experimental and Clinical Research.* Academic Press, New York, NY, pp. 453–475.

Johnson, M.D., Davis, B.W. and Wetherall, N.T. (1989) Production of proto-oncogene expressing control tissues for in situ hybridization and immunohistochemical studies. *J. Environ. Path. Toxicol. Oncol.* 9, 171–190.

Kobayashi, H. (1986) The biological modification of tumor cells as a means of inducing their regression: an overview. *J. Biol. Resp. Mod.* 5, 1–11.

Lange, J.M.A., Paul, D.A., Huisman, H.G., DeWolf, F., Van den Berg, H., Coutinho, R.A., Danner, S.A., Van der Noorda, J. and Goudsmit, J. (1986) Persistent HIV antigenaemia and decline of HIV antibodies associated with transition to AIDS. *Br. Med. J.* 293, 1459–1462.

Leonard, J.M., Abranczuk, J.W., Pezen, D.S., Rutledge, R., Belcher, J.H., Hakim, F., Shearer, G., Lamperth, L., Travis, W., Fredrickson, R., Notkins, A.L. and Martin, M.A. (1988) Development of disease and virus recovery in transgenic mice containing HIV proviral DNA. *Science* 242, 1665–1670.

Levy, J.A. (1989) The human immunodeficiency viruses: detection and pathogenesis. In: J.A. Levy (Ed.), *AIDS Pathogenesis and Treatment.* Marcel Dekker, New York, NY, pp. 159–229.

Montefiori, D.C. and Mitchell, W.M. (1987) Persistent coinfection of T-lymphocytes with HTLV-1 and HIV and the role of synctium formation in HIV-induced cytopathic effect. *Virology* 160, 372–378.

Montefiori, D.C., Robinson, E., Shuffman, S.S. and Mitchell, W.M. (1988) Evaluation of antiviral drugs and neutralizing antibodies to human immunodeficiency virus by a rapid and sensitive microtiter infection assay. *J. Clin. Microbiol.* 26, 231–235.

Mosier, D.E., Gulizia, R.J., Baird, S.M. and Wilson, D.B. (1988) Transfer of a functional human immune system to mice with severe combined immunodeficiency. *Nature* 335, 256–259.

Mosier, D.E., Gulizia, R.J., Spector, S.A., Baird, S.M., and Wilson, D.B. (1989) HIV-1 infection of PBL-reconstituted SCID mice. In: *V International Conference on AIDS,* Montreal, Quebec, p. 522 (Abstract).

Namikawa, R., Kaneshima, H., Lieberman, M., Wiessman, I.L. and McCune, J.M. (1988) Infection of the SCID-hu mouse by HIV-1. *Science* 242, 1684.

Ratner, L., Haseltine, W., Patarca, R., Livak, K.J., Starcich, B., Josephs, S.F., Doran, E.R., Rafalski, J.A., Whitehorn, E.A., Baumeister, K., Ivanoff, L., Petteway, S.R., Pearson, M.L., Latenberger, J.A., Papas, T.S., Ghrayeb, J., Chang, N.T., Gallo, R.C. and Wong-Staal, F. (1985) Complete nucleotide sequence of the AIDS virus, HTLV-III. *Nature* 313, 277–284.

Reid, L.M., Jones, C.L. and Holland, J. (1979) Virus carrier state suppresses tumorigenicity of tumor cells in athymic (nude) mice. *J. Gen Virol.* 42, 609–614.

Salmon, P., Olivier, R., Riviere, Y., Brisson, E., Gluckman, J.-C., Kieny, M.-P., Montagnier, L. and Klatzmann, D. (1988) Loss of CD4 membrane expression and CD4 mRNA during acute human immunodeficiency virus replication. *J. Exp. Med.* 168, 1953–1969.

Skarlin, N.T., Chahinian, A.P., Feuer, E.J., Lahman, L.A., Szrajer, L. and Holland, J.F. (1988) Augmentation of activity of *cis*-diamminedichloroplatinum and mitomycin C by interferon in human malignant mesothelioma xenografts in nude mice. *Cancer Res.* 48, 64–67.

Southern, E.M. (1975) Detection of specific sequences among DNA fragments separated by gel electrophoresis. *J. Mol. Biol.* 98, 503–517.

Vrati, S., Mann, D.A. and Reed, K.C. (1988) Alkaline Northern blots: Transfer of RNA from agarose gels to zeta-probe membrane in dilute NaOH. *Bio-Rad Bull.* 1393.

Wain-Hobson, S., Sonigo, P., Danos, D., Cole, S. and Allizon, M. (1985) Nucleotide sequence of the AIDS virus, LAV. *Cell* 40, 9–17.

Weiss, R. (1985) Human T-cell retroviruses. In: R. Weiss, N. Teich, H. Varmus and J. Coffin (Eds.), *RNA Tumor Viruses.* Cold Spring Harbor Laboratory Press, Cold Spring Harbor, NY, pp. 405–485.

*Eds. H. Schellekens and M.C. Horzinek*
*Animal Models in AIDS*



# 30

# Mechanisms of immunosuppression by the murine Friend leukemia complex

MAURO BENDINELLI, DONATELLA MATTEUCCI and ELISABETTA SOLDAINI

Department of Biomedicine, Section of Virology, University of Pisa, Pisa, Italy

## Introduction

The first description of a retrovirus induced immune deficiency goes back to 30 years ago when Old and coworkers (1959) made a passing reference to the fact that the murine Friend leukemia virus (FLV) suppressed the antibody responsiveness of infected mice. Since then, many other murine retroviruses, both acutely and chronically oncogenic, have been shown to produce variable degrees of immunodepression (Bendinelli et al., 1985). The system most extensively investigated remains, however, FLV which is now more properly referred to as Friend leukemia complex (FLC) because it has been shown to consist of two viral entities, known as Friend murine leukemia virus (F-MuLV) and spleen focus forming virus (SFFV). F-MuLV is replication competent and, when injected into adult mice of susceptible genotypes, induces an early mild lymphoid hyperplasia followed by leukemias of varied histotype after a latency of 10 or more months. SFFV is replication defective and is responsible for the hematological changes as well as for the rapidly evolving splenic erythroblastosis and erythroleukemia which develop within a few days after inoculation of the entire viral complex.

We have worked on the FLC model of retrovirus induced immune deficiency for over 2 decades and here highlight some of the results obtained.

## Phenomenology

Table 1 shows the many immune functions measurable at the organism level that have been found suppressed in FLC infected mice of susceptible strains. It is clear from the changes observed that FLC viruses induce a generalized immune deficiency, involving both humoral and cell mediated immune responses. It is important to note, however, that many factors can affect the extent of immunosuppression. They encompass variables concerning the immunization challenge

TABLE 1
Major immunological functions suppressed by FLC in BALB/c mice

| |
|---|
| Primary and secondary immune responses |
| Age dependent immunological maturation |
| Delayed hypersensitivity |
| Contact sensitivity |
| T cell mediated cytotoxic responses |
| Graft rejection |
| Resistance to superinfections |
| Resistance to tumor grafts |

used to monitor the immune responsiveness such as the timing and route of immunization, the nature and dose of immunogen, the use of adjuvants, etc., as well as host variables such as genetics, age, pre-existing immunological deficits, concomitant activations of the immune system, etc. (Bendinelli et al., 1985). Most interestingly, depression of immune responsiveness is observed also in mice genetically resistant to the leukemogenic activity of FLC, although the impairment is generally transient and mild (especially with regard to cell mediated immunity) compared to the effects seen in susceptible animals. Accordingly, reports indicate that susceptibility to immunosuppression is controlled not only by loci that regulate host susceptibility to FLC induced leukemogenesis but also by independent genes (Morrison et al., 1986).

In addition, extent and kinetics of the immune deficiency are considerably different depending on whether the animals are infected with the entire viral complex or with F-MuLV alone. For example, following infection with the entire FLC the antibody responsiveness declines steadily and remains at zero level until the infected animals die a few weeks later, whereas mice infected with F-MuLV alone show an early peak of immunosuppression which is followed by a partial recovery and then the responsiveness stabilizes at about half the normal level for the life span of the animals (Bendinelli and Nardini, 1973). Cell-mediated immune responses are also less affected by F-MuLV than by the entire viral complex. On the other hand, F-MuLV represents 90–99% of the viral infectivity of FLC preparations and is therefore likely to play an important role in the immunodepressive effects as well as in other aspects of FLC pathogenesis (Jones et al., 1988). In fact, despite such differences, both viral preparations lead to a marked reduction of host resistance to a variety of protozoa, fungi, bacteria, and viruses and to a faster growth of transplanted tumors. The pathology produced by these superinfecting agents can also be profoundly modified (Specter et al., 1987).

## Cellular basis of the immune deficiency

We have made considerable efforts to understand the cellular mechanisms responsible for the immune defects of mice infected with FLC viruses. Tables

TABLE 2
Alterations of T lymphocytes observed in FLC infected BALB/c mice

| |
|---|
| Decreased number |
| Altered circulation |
| Decreased expression of differentiation antigens |
| Reduced antigen and mitogen driven proliferation |
| Decreased ability to mediate allogeneic effects |
| Reduced production of IL 2 |
| Reduced production of interferon-γ |
| Reduced responsiveness to cytokines |

2–5 summarize the major alterations observed in immunocompetent cell functions in vivo or in vitro. The changes of T lymphocytes range from altered migratory activity to reduced production and responsiveness to soluble mediators (Table 2). For example, the decrease of lectin driven interleukin-2 (IL-2) production begins early after infection and shows a kinetics which is remarkably similar to that of the immunosuppressions induced by FLC and F-MuLV: after FLC infection the deficit becomes progressively more severe with time, until IL-2 production is completely ablated in a few weeks; in contrast, after F-MuLV infection the amount of IL-2 produced remains at a lowered but constant level irrespective of the time elapsed (Matteucci et al., 1989). Such divergence is not due solely to dilution of IL-2 producing cells by the neoplastic erythroid cells which invade the spleen of FLC but not of F-MuLV infected animals, as cell separation experiments have clearly evidenced an intrinsic defect of lymphocytes (Lopez-Cepero et al., 1988b). Interferon-γ production follows a similar pattern during infection, suggesting the existence of a general defect at this level (unpublished results).

TABLE 3
Responsiveness of spleen cells to con A and A23187 + TPA at different times of infection with FLC viruses

| Stimulation | Days after infection | | | | | |
|---|---|---|---|---|---|---|
| | FLC | | | F-MuLV | | |
| | 8 | 14 | 21 | 8 | 14 | 21 |
| IL-2 production | | | | | | |
| Con A | R[a] | RR | RRR | R | RR | RR |
| A23187+TPA | N | N | RRR | N | N | RR |
| Interferon-γ production | | | | | | |
| Con A | R | RR | RRR | R | RR | RR |
| A23187+TPA | N | N | RRR | N | N | RR |
| Proliferation | | | | | | |
| Con A | R | RR | RRR | R | RR | RR |
| A23187+TPA | N | R | RRR | N | R | RR |

[a] N: normal; R, RR, RRR: reduction of increasing severity.

TABLE 4
Alterations of B lymphocytes observed in FLC infected BALB/c mice

| |
|---|
| Reduced antibody responsiveness |
| Reduced mitogen driven proliferation |
| Reduced surface immunoglobulin expression and capping |
| Ability to suppress antibody responses by normal cells |
| Polyclonal activation |

Interestingly, during the early stages of infection lymphokine production is normal if the cells are stimulated by a combination of the calcium ionophore A23187 and the phorbol ester TPA, while at later stages of infection this stimulation is even less effective than concanavalin A (con A). The proliferative response to A23187 + TPA also is less readily suppressed by infection than that to con A (Table 3), suggesting that a defect of signal transduction across the cell membrane contributes to T lymphocyte hyporeactivity. The responsiveness to IL-2 is also reduced very soon after infection, as shown by a reduced ability of con A co-stimulated lymphoid cells to proliferate in response to it (Matteucci et al., 1989).

Table 4 shows that B lymphocytes also undergo alterations which are reminiscent of what is observed in human immunodeficiency virus (HIV) infected patients while Table 5 lists the numerous functional modifications found in macrophages. Among the latter, one potentially very important change is the reduced ability to cooperate with lymphocytes in the generation of immune responses.

A straightforward and very informative piece of evidence was provided by cross recombination experiments in vitro between macrophages and lymphocytes of normal and infected mice. For example, the mixture of infected macrophages and normal lymphocytes produced much fewer antibody forming cells than the reciprocal combination, thus indicating that impairment of macrophage accessory functions contributes considerably to the reduced antibody responsiveness seen in infected mice (Bendinelli et al., 1986).

TABLE 5
Alterations of macrophages observed in FLC infected BALB/c mice

| |
|---|
| Reduced ability to spread on surfaces |
| Reduced motility |
| Reduced accumulation at sites of inflammation |
| Reduced killing of ingested bacteria |
| Reduced antibody dependent cytotoxicity |
| Enhanced stimulation of erythropoiesis |
| Reduced ability to cooperate with lymphocytes |
| Suppression of NK activity |
| Suppression of IL-2 dependent proliferation of CTLL2 cells |

TABLE 6
Major mechanisms of immunocompetent cell alteration in FLC infected BALB/c mice

| |
|---|
| Virus replication within immunocompetent cells |
| Immunodepressive virion components |
| Derangements of immunoregulatory circuits |
| Tumor dependent mechanisms (late) |

Constitutive antimicrobial host defenses are also severely compromised. Natural killer (NK) cell activity, for example, remains strongly suppressed even when boosted with interferon (Moody et al., 1984).

It can be concluded from the above results that the immune deficiency induced by viruses of the FLC is a complex phenomenon resulting from multiple alterations of many immunocompetent cell classes. It is, however, essential to keep in mind that we still do not know which immunocompetent cell change(s) described is more directly due to the viral infection and, therefore, primarily responsible for the immune deficiency. As the immune system is highly integrated, some changes may not only be secondary to others but may have a compensatory role.

## Mechanisms of immunocompetent cell alteration

While trying to understand how the cellular alterations described in the previous section are generated, we have come across four major mechanisms (Table 6).

Viruses of the FLC replicate extensively in immunocompetent cells. They grow in lymphocytes, possibly with a preference for B cells (Cerny et al., 1976; Bendinelli et al., unpublished results). In addition, they readily replicate in macrophages that are among the earliest cells where FLC viruses are replicated, at least in the spleen (Toniolo et al., 1980).

The importance of immunocompetent cell infection is demonstrated by results showing that mixing infected with normal spleen cells results in a dose dependent reduction of antibody responsiveness by the latter cells. The cells responsible for the inhibition are B lymphocytes and their activity is entirely prevented by the presence of neutralizing antiviral antibody in the culture medium, indicating that the effect is mediated by viral products (Bendinelli et al., 1979).

The second mechanism is exemplified by experiments where a cell free semipurified virus inhibited the antibody response of normal spleen cells in a dose dependent manner. The effect was neutralized by antiviral antibody. Moreover, inactivation of infectivity by UV irradiation reduced but by no means abolished it, thus indicating that the virus does not need to be viable to modulate immunocompetent cell functions (Bendinelli et al., 1985). These results are in line with findings showing that the envelope protein p15(E) of many retroviruses has strong immunomodulatory activities (Schmidt et al., 1987). A powerfully immunosuppressive oligopeptide from this retroviral component has also been synthesized (Kleinerman et al., 1987).

On the other hand, the role of perturbation of immunoregulatory circuits as a mechanism of immune derangement is proved by a number of findings, such as:

(i) infected spleen cells suppress NK activity of normal lymphoid cells. This effect is due to macrophages, is not prevented by antiviral antibody, and is markedly reduced by indometacin, suggesting that it is prostaglandin mediated (Moody et al., 1984);

(ii) infected cells suppress IL-2 production by normal spleen cells. The effect is antiviral antibody resistant, suggesting that it is not mediated by viral products, but the cell type responsible has not been identified yet (Matteucci et al., 1989);

(iii) infected spleen cells suppress the proliferative response to IL-2 of the IL-2 dependent CTLL2 cell line. The cells responsible for this effect co-purify with macrophages and their action is not prevented by antiviral antibody (Matteucci et al., 1989).

Most changes described above develop prior to any significant neoplastic proliferation and are also induced by the late leukemia inducer F-MuLV. However, there are also some tumor associated effects which are only observed in the late stages of infection with the acutely oncogenic FLC or are strictly dependent on the presence of neoplastic cells (Lopez-Cepero et al., 1988a). Such tumor dependent mechanisms will not be discussed here.

Thus, available evidence indicates that pathogenetic routes leading to altered immunocompetent cell behavior in FLC infected mice are manyfold. However, we still do not know which mechanism is the first to go into action or is the most important in the generation of the immune deficiency. It is also feasible that the relative importance of the different mechanisms varies with time following infection.

## Attempts to alleviate the immune deficiency

We have tried a number of immunological manipulations in the attempt to reverse or reduce the severity of the immunodepressed state induced by FLC. So far, the few manipulations that have proved efficacious are those which ameliorate the accessory functions of macrophages. For example, we could show that the addition of small numbers of exogenous syngeneic macrophages restores the antibody responsiveness of infected spleen cell cultures. Even in vivo moderate numbers of macrophages given together with the antigen enhanced the antibody response significantly though not as markedly as in vitro.

More recently, we have studied the mechanism whereby bacterial endotoxins (lipopolysaccharides, LPS) greatly enhance the antibody response of infected mice and of infected spleen cells in vitro, bringing it back to almost normal levels. Briefly, we found that the effect is mediated by macrophages as shown by

TABLE 7
Some areas of AIDS research that can benefit most from investigation of the murine FLC model

| |
|---|
| Basic mechanisms of retroviral immune deficiencies |
| Co-factor involvement in pathogenesis |
| Screening of antiretroviral drugs |
| Possible usefulness of biological response modifiers |
| Vaccine development strategies |

a number of data (Bendinelli et al., 1986) showing that preincubating infected macrophages with LPS entirely restores their accessory functions. In addition, a recent brief report indicates that tumor necrosis factor-$\alpha$, a macrophage product that has many immunoregulatory functions, may exert beneficial effects in FLC infected mice (Johnson and Furmanski, 1987). Interestingly, abnormalities of accessory cell functions are increasingly recognized as crucial events in the immune deficiency caused by HIV (Folks et al., 1988; Rich et al., 1988). It might be worth investigating the effect of macrophage stimulatory treatments on the evolution and severity of HIV infections.

## Concluding remarks

The murine retroviruses of the FLC present marked genetic, biological, and pathogenetic differences from HIV. However, the immune deficiency state they induce presents interesting analogies with human acquired immunodeficiency syndrome (AIDS). Investigation of the FLC model can therefore provide valuable information in several areas of AIDS research where there is still much to be learned (Table 7). The major advantages of this model of retrovirus induced immune deficiency may be summarized as follows: (1) it is fairly well characterized; (2) it is rapid in onset and progression; (3) its severity can be modulated by infecting with FLC or F-MuLV as well as by varying the infecting dose; (4) it is caused by viruses well known in many respects; (5) it affects an animal host whose immune system is known in great detail.

## Acknowledgements

This work was supported in part by grants from the Italian National Research Council and Ministry of Health (Istituto Superiore di Sanitá) Project AIDS 1989.

## References

Bendinelli, M. and Nardini, L. (1973) Immunodepression by Rowson-Parr virus in mice. 2. Effect of Rowson-Parr virus infection on the antibody response to sheep red cells in vivo and in vitro. *Infect. Immunol.* 7, 160–166.

Bendinelli, M., Matteucci, D., Toniolo, A. and Friedman, H. (1979) Suppression of in vitro antibody response by spleen cells of mice infected with Friend-associated lymphatic leukemia virus. *Infect. Immunol.* 24, 1–6.

Bendinelli, M., Matteucci, D. and Friedman, H. (1985) Retrovirus-induced acquired immunodeficiencies. *Adv. Cancer Res.* 45, 125–181.

Bendinelli, M., Matteucci, D., Giangregorio, A.M. and Conaldi, P.G., (1986) Restoration of antibody responsiveness by endotoxin in retrovirus immunosuppressed mice: role of macrophages. In: A. Szentivanyi, H. Friedman and A. Nowotny (Eds.), *Biological Effects of Endotoxin.* Plenum Press, New York, NY, pp. 465–478.

Cerny, J., Hensgen, P.A., Fistel, S.H. and Demler, L.M. (1976) Interactions of murine leukemia virus with isolated lymphocytes. II. Infection of B and T cells with Friend virus complex in diffusion chambers and in vitro: effect of polyclonal mitogens. *Int. J. Cancer* 18, 189–196.

Folks, T.M., Kessler, S.W., Orenstein, J.M., Justement, J.S., Jaffe, E.S. and Fauci, A.S. (1988) Infection and replication of HIV-1 in purified progenitor cells of normal human bone marrow. *Science* 242, 919–922.

Johnson, C.S. and Furmanski, P. (1987) In vivo effects of tumor necrosis factor on normal and leukemic erythropoiesis. *Proc. Annu. Meet. Am. Ass. Cancer Res.* 28, 399.

Jones, K.S., Ruscetti, S. and Lilly, F. (1988) Loss of pathogenicity of spleen focus-forming virus after pseudotyping with Akv. *J. Virol.* 62, 511–518.

Kleinerman, E.S., Lachman, L.B., Knowles, R.D., Snyderman, R. and Cianciolo, G.J. (1987). A synthetic peptide homologous to the envelope proteins of retroviruses inhibits monocyte-mediated killing by inactivating interleukin 1. *J. Immunol.* 139, 2329–2337.

Lopez-Cepero, M., Specter, S., Friedman, H. and Bendinelli, M. (1988a) Altered IL 2 production during murine retrovirus infection. *Proc. Annu. Meet. Am. Soc. Microbiol.* 88, 109.

Lopez-Cepero, M., Specter, S., Matteucci, D., Friedman, H. and Bendinelli, M. (1988b) Altered interleukin production during Friend leukemia virus infection. *Proc. Soc. Exp. Biol. Med.* 188, 353–363.

Matteucci, D., Giangregorio, A.M., Lopez-Cepero, M., Specter, S., Bendinelli, M. and Friedman, H. (1989) Interleukins 1 and 2: production and responsiveness in the early stages of retrovirus infection of mice. *Cell. Immunol.* 120, 10–20.

Moody, D.J., Specter, S., Bendinelli, M. and Friedman, H. (1984) Suppression of natural killer cell activity by Friend murine leukemia virus. *J. Natl. Cancer Inst.* 72, 1349–1356.

Morrison, R.P., Nishio, J. and Chesebro, B. (1986) Influence of the murine MHC (H-2) on Friend leukemia virus-induced immunosuppression. *J. Exp. Med.* 163, 301–314.

Old, L.J., Clarke, D.A., Benaceraff, B. and Goldsmith, M. (1959) The reticuloendothelial system and the neoplastic process. *Ann. NY Acad. Sci.,* 88, 264–280.

Rich, E.A., Toossi, Z., Fujiwara, H., Hanigosky, R., Lederman, M.M. and Ellner, J.J. (1988) Defective accessory function of monocytes in human immunodeficiency virus-related disease syndromes. *J. Lab. Clin. Med.* 112, 174–181.

Schmidt, D.M., Sidhu, N.K., Cianciolo, G.J. and Snyderman, R., (1987) Recombinant hydrophilic region of murine retroviral protein p15E inhibits stimulated T-lymphocyte proliferation. *Proc. Natl. Acad. Sci. U.S.A.* 84, 7290–7294.

Specter, S., Basolo, F. and Bendinelli, M., (1987) Retroviruses as immunosuppressive agents. In: R.A. Good and E. Lindenlaub (Eds.) *The Nature, Cellular and Biochemical Basis of Management of Immunodeficiencies.* Schattauer Verlag, Stuttgart, pp. 127–145.

Toniolo, A., Matteucci, D., Pistillo, M.P., Gori, Z. and Bendinelli, M. (1980) Early replication of Friend leukemia viruses in spleen macrophages. *J. Gen. Virol.* 49, 203–208.

*Eds. H. Schellekens and M.C. Horzinek*
*Animal Models in AIDS*



# 31

# Mouse model of retroviral infection: early combination therapy of azidothymidine with synthetic double-stranded RNA (poly I).(poly C)

O. LAUNAY [1], M. SINET [1], P. VARLET [2] and J.J. POCIDALO [1]

[1] INSERM U13, Hôpital Claude Bernard, Paris, France and [2] INSERM U 152, Hôpital Cochin, Paris, France

**Summary**

Friend murine leukemia virus (F-MuLV) infection of DBA2 mice causes erythroleukemia with polycythemia and splenomegaly, leading to death in 4–8 weeks. Viral infection was performed by retro-orbital inoculation of $10^2$ ffu F-MuLV. Mice were treated for 14 days with different therapeutic schedules, starting at either 4 or 48 h post infection. Azidothymidine (AZT) was given twice daily at 40, 60 or 80 mg/kg/day; synthetic double-stranded RNA (poly I).(poly C) at 5 mg/kg every 48 h; the combination therapy associated AZT at 40 mg/kg/day with (poly I).(poly C). Treatment efficacy was evaluated by determination of splenic weight and infectious virus titer on day 14 (half of the mice were killed) and by following survival times of the remaining animals.

We showed that each treatment prevented development of splenomegaly and polycythemia at day 14. All regimens led to at least 70% reduction of splenomegaly whether the treatment was started at 4 or 48 h post infection. In spite of over 90% inhibition of splenomegaly after AZT monotherapy, no significant prolongation of survival time was observed compared to infected control animals. Only combination therapy of AZT with (poly I).(poly C) started at 4 h post inoculation substantially prolonged survival time of the infected mice.

These results suggest that early administration of AZT in combination with an interferon inducer could protect against retroviral infection. This information may be considered for the prophylaxis of human immunodeficiency virus infection following accidental exposure.

## Introduction

For the treatment of human immunodeficiency virus (HIV) infection we need to develop a safe and effective drug to treat infected subjects, and also to stop HIV transmission after accidental exposure, and finally, if possible, to cure HIV infected individuals. Numerous new therapies have been developed (De Clercq,

1989) and some encouraging results of azidothymidine (AZT) treatment in HIV infection (Fischl et al., 1987; Dournon et al., 1988) suggest that it should be possible to stop progression of the disease and even to prevent HIV infection.

Significant numbers of health care workers and researchers are at risk of accidental exposure to HIV (CDC, 1988). Therefore, it is essential to examine if candidate compounds can be used effectively to block viral infection after exposure. Considering the difficulties related to the management of clinical trials in this field, therapeutic intervention in man may be based on preclinical research. In the present work, an animal model program has been developed to examine the possibility of finding a therapeutic schedule providing prophylactic efficacy.

Combination of AZT with other compounds has been shown to be synergistic against HIV replication in cell cultures in vitro (Hartshorn et al., 1987; Mitchell et al., 1987; Wong et al., 1988). This was especially the case for Ampligen (a mismatched polymer of double-stranded RNA) which was shown to reduce the concentration of AZT required for inhibitory activity against HIV in vitro (Mitchell et al., 1987).

The aim of this work was to examine if an early and short course of therapy could stop virus replication and prevent the development of disease. A mouse model of retroviral infection was used to evaluate in vivo the synergy of drugs in combination for their potential use in chemoprophylaxis. The efficiency of a combination therapy of AZT and synthetic double-stranded RNA (poly I).(poly C), was tested in mice experimentally infected with polycythemia-inducing Friend leukemia virus (FLV-P).

## Materials and methods

### Animals

Male DBA2 mice aged of 6 weeks were obtained from Iffa Credo Laboratories, Grenoble, France. Animals were acclimatized for 1 week prior to experimental use. The animals were housed in a protected unit at 21–25°C and supplied with food and water ad libitum.

### Viruses and virus titration

The polycythemia-inducing Friend virus (FLV-P) was obtained through the courtesy of Dr. P. Tambourin, Paris. High titer virus stocks of FLV-P were prepared from the spleens of mice taken 4 weeks after infection. A 10% w/v spleen homogenate in cold Dulbecco's modified Eagle's Medium (DMEM, Flow Laboratories) was centrifuged at 8000 × g for 15 min. The supernatant fluid was filtered through a 0.45 $\mu$m Millipore filter and aliquots of virus suspension were stored at −80°C until use.

To measure total virus in vivo, the spleen focus assay was used (Axelrad and Steeves, 1964). Briefly, 0.2 ml of virus suspension, serially diluted ($10^{-1}$–$10^{-6}$), was inoculated by retro-orbital injection. Mice were killed 9 days later, and, after being weighed, the spleens were fixed in Bouin's solution. Yellow focal lesions on the planar surface of the spleen were counted macroscopically, and SFFV virus titer (mean number of foci per spleen × dilution factor) were expressed in focus-forming units/ml (ffu/ml).

### Drugs

Zidovudine (AZT, 3′-azido-3′-deoxythymidine, Retrovir) was kindly provided by Laboratoires Wellcome, France. Synthetic double-stranded RNA polyinosinic-polycytidylic acid ((poly I).(poly C)) was purchased from Boehringer Mannheim, France.

### Experimental schedule

On day 0, mice were inoculated intravenously with 0.2 ml of virus suspension at different viral titers (about $10^2$ ffu). Treatment was initiated either 4 or 48 h after viral challenge. Drugs were given subcutaneously, either alone or in combination: AZT twice daily at 40 mg/kg/day and (poly I).(poly C) every 48 h at 5 mg/kg, until day 14 after inoculation.

At day 14 after infection, half the mice were killed, the spleens were weighed and stored at −80°C for further titration. The inhibitory effect of treatment on the development of splenomegaly was calculated as follows:

$$(\%)\ \text{Inhibition} = \left(1 - \frac{\text{Net spleen weight increase in the presence of drug}}{\text{Net spleen weight increase in the absence of drug}}\right) \times 100$$

The remaining mice were observed for mortality. Determination of weight and hematocrit were carried out once a week.

## Results

### Evaluation of efficacy of AZT and (poly I).(poly C) alone or in combination against FLV-P infection: effect of starting time of antiviral therapy

Preliminary experiments were carried out to study the dose effect of AZT therapy on the inhibition of splenomegaly of infected mice at day 14. No significant differences between spleen weights of treated mice were seen when AZT was given twice daily in doses of 40, 60 or 80 mg/kg/day and inhibition of splenomegaly was always above 85% (data not shown). Therefore, the 40 mg/kg/day dosage schedule was selected.

TABLE 1
Effects of AZT and (poly I).(poly C) (pIpC) alone or in combination on splenomegaly induced by FLV-P in mice

| Drug | 4 h | | | 48 h | | |
|---|---|---|---|---|---|---|
| | Spleen weight mean (mg) | | Inhibition % | Spleen weight mean (mg) | | Inhibition % |
| | infected | control | | infected | control | |
| AZT | 136 ± 31 | 88 ± 8 | 95.8 | 187 ± 41 | 83 ± 7 | 90.9 |
| pIpC | 484 ± 91 | 150 ± 4 | 70.9 | 450 ± 86 | 150 ± 4 | 73.8 |
| AZT-pIpC | 144 ± 10 | 134 ± 9 | 99.1 | 227 ± 52 | 130 ± 7 | 91.5 |
| Placebo | 1234 ± 160 | 87 ± 8 | | | | |

Average spleen weights for four mice from each group are expressed in mg ± SEM.

The drugs, alone or in combination, appeared to be non-toxic at the doses used, as assessed by weight gain and clinical examination of treated uninfected mice. No hematological toxicity of AZT was seen since mean hematocrit was 44.5 ± 0.7 in the AZT treated group versus 47.0 ± 0.9 in the untreated group after 14 days of treatment. Spleen weights were measured at day 14 after viral inoculation. In each treated group, splenomegaly was highly reduced as shown in Table 1. Treatment with (poly I).(poly C) alone, started either 4 or 48 h after infection, led to only about 70% inhibition whereas AZT alone or in combination induced over 90% inhibition.

In spite of the almost complete inhibition of splenomegaly at the end of treatment by AZT with or without (poly I).(poly C), disease progression in the remaining mice depended on the therapeutic schedule: polycythemia (mean hematocrit > 65%) appeared 3 weeks post infection in the untreated group, this delay was unchanged in the groups treated with (poly I).(poly C) alone or with AZT starting 48 h after infection; it was increased by only 1 or 2 weeks in the group treated with AZT alone started 4 h post infection and with the combination therapy started at 48 h post infection, respectively. Only mice treated with the combination therapy started early exhibited a substantial delay in the onset of polycythemia (10 weeks after virus inoculation). This delay in disease progression was confirmed by the prolongation of survival rate in this group, as shown in Fig. 1.

### Evaluation of efficacy of AZT and (poly I).(poly C) alone or in combination against FLV-P infection: effect of virus inoculum

In the first experiment, combination therapy of AZT and (poly I).(poly C) improved the survival rate after a short course of therapy (14 days), provided it was started early after inoculation (4 h). We therefore investigated to what extent differences in virus inoculum could influence therapeutic efficiency. Two experiments were selected, in which the mean spleen weight of untreated infected mice

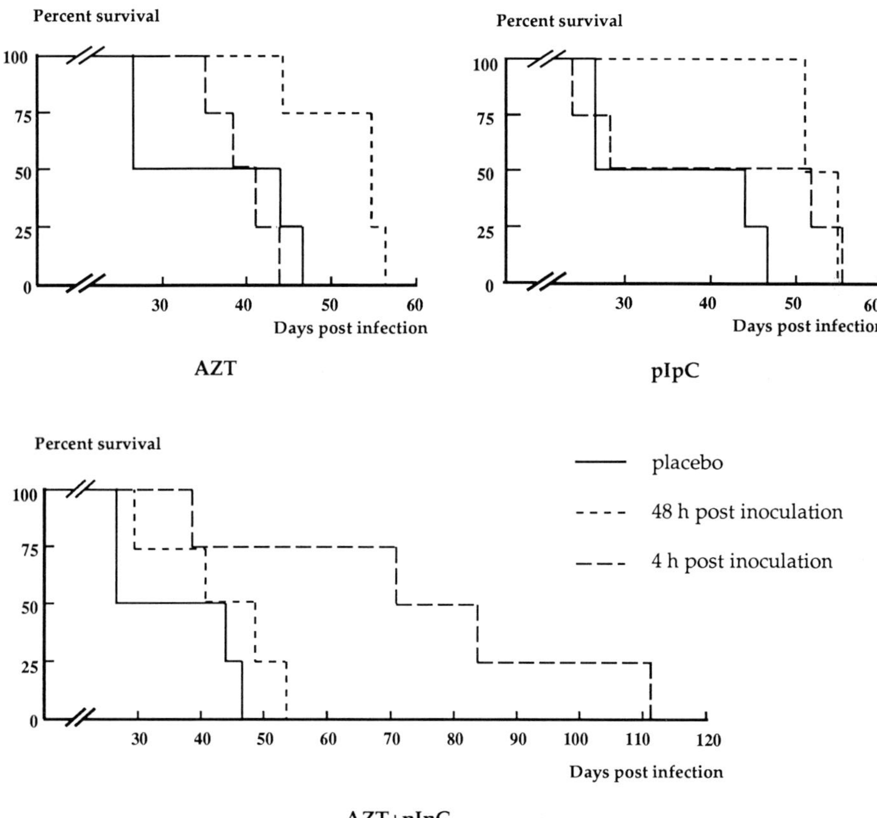


Fig. 1. Survival of FLV-P infected mice. Kaplan-Meier plots of virus infected untreated mice (placebo) or infected mice treated with AZT, (poly I).(poly C) or the two drugs in combination, starting 4 or 48 h post inoculation. Each group contained four mice; all animals were treated until day 14 post inoculation.

at day 14 post inoculation was either 1669 ± 125 mg or 718 ± 263 mg, for high and low inoculum respectively. Treatment was started 4 h post infection, with either AZT alone or combined with (poly I).(poly C) using the same dosages as in the first experiment. The inhibitory effect of treatment on splenomegaly was evaluated both at the end of therapy (day 14) and 1 week later (day 21). Fig. 2 shows average spleen weights at day 14 and day 21 in the different groups of infected mice and the results of subsequent titrations of supernatants of these spleen extracts. In the high inoculum experiment, indicator mice that received spleen homogenates from virus infected animals developed significant splenomegaly in the three groups. In this case, inhibition of splenomegaly in treated mice was achieved, and it was better in mice receiving combination therapy; nevertheless, low dilutions of spleen extracts still produced spleen foci in indicator mice. In the low inoculum experiment, indicator mice that received spleen homogenates at day 14 from virus infected animals developed significant

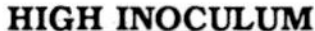


LOW INOCULUM

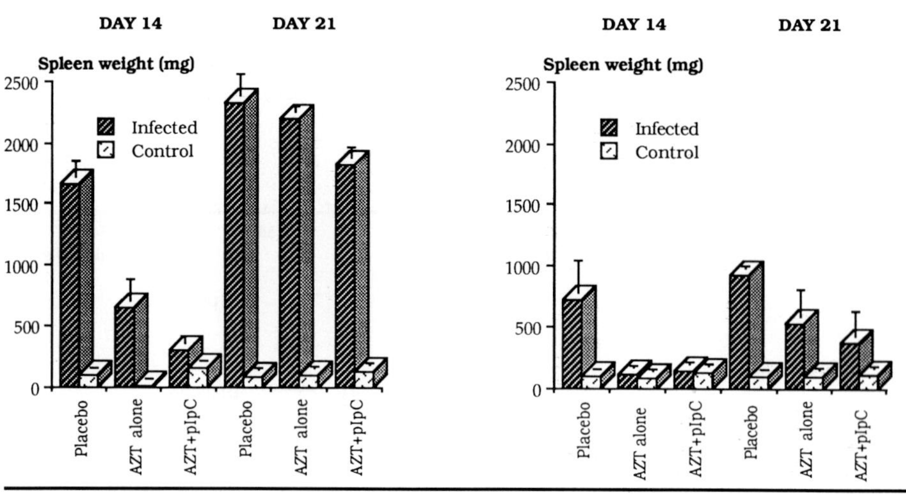


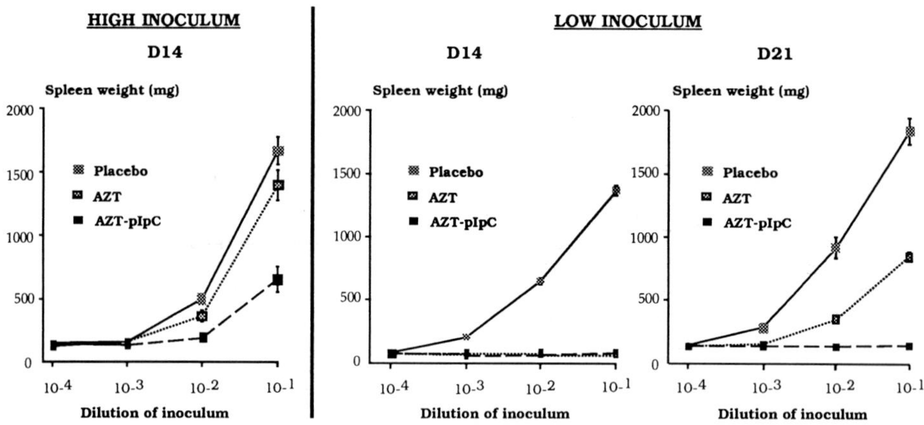


Fig. 2. Effects of AZT alone or in combination with (poly I).(poly C) on splenomegaly induced by FLV-P in mice: comparison between high and low inoculum. Top: mean spleen weights of infected and control mice. Bottom: splenomegaly bioassay in indicator mice inoculated with 10-fold dilutions of spleen homogenates from mice killed at day 14 or day 21.

splenomegaly only in the group receiving placebo. No infectious virus was detected in the spleen of treated mice. Spleen homogenates of treated mice at day 21 induced splenomegaly only in the AZT treated group; the virus titers were $2 \times 10^5$, $2 \times 10^4$ and 40 ffu/ml for placebo, AZT and AZT + (poly I).(poly C) treated mice respectively.

Survival of infected mice with low and high inoculum is shown in Fig. 3. In the high inoculum experiment, mean survival times (days) were 38.8, 37.4 and 46.7 for the placebo, AZT and AZT + (poly I).(poly C) groups respectively; only

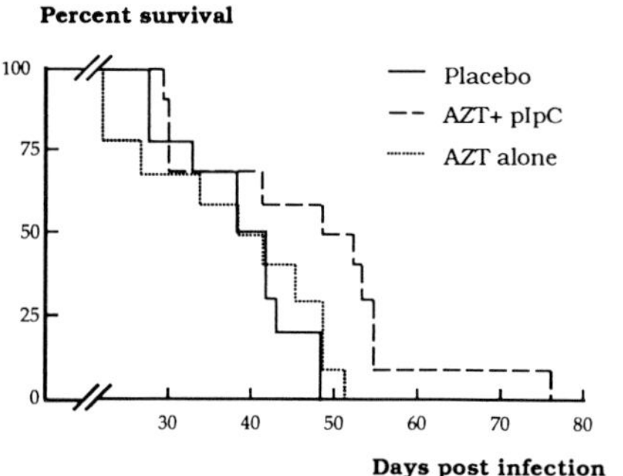




Fig. 3. Survival of FLV-P infected mice. Kaplan-Meier plots of virus infected untreated mice (placebo) or infected mice treated with AZT alone or in combination with (poly I).(poly C) in high and low inoculum experiments. Each group contained 10 mice.

combination therapy led to a significant increase in survival time. In the low inoculum experiment, the mean survival time in the placebo group was 47.8; it was significantly increased with AZT alone (66.9). Combination therapy led to a further increase of survival time (86.4).

## Discussion

Accidental exposure to blood and body fluids in the work place is common. Some health care workers have been infected with HIV through occupational exposure, and at least one of them developed acquired immunodeficiency syndrome (AIDS) (CDC, 1988). In view of the extreme gravity of this disease, it is becoming increasingly common for health care workers, following accidental exposure to HIV, to take AZT for a short time as prophylaxis (Meylan et al., 1988). However, the efficacy of AZT is very difficult to evaluate in humans. Since the risk of becoming infected after work related accidental exposure is less than

0.5% (Marcus et al., 1988), a huge number of patients would be required to do a control study to test the prophylactic efficacy of AZT. Therefore, the usefulness of developing experimental protocols on animal models becomes evident. Even if conclusions of these experiments have to be interpreted with caution, they may provide guidelines for subsequent clinical trials.

There is no animal model that completely fulfills the requirements for the study of potential drugs and strategies to use in the treatment of HIV infection (Schlumberger and Schrinner, 1989). However, mouse models of retroviral infection provide a screening procedure that allows the rapid detection in vivo of useful antiretroviral therapies. Murine leukemia virus (MuLV) infection shares numerous features with HIV infection and, especially, it leads to various degrees of immunodeficiency (Dent, 1972; Bendinelli et al., 1985). This model is suitable when using drugs known for their ability to prevent both HIV and MuLV replication in vitro and provides an in vivo test for different therapeutic strategies. Therefore, the murine model might improve the evaluation of early therapy using drugs targeted to viral reverse transcriptase in combination with agents modulating the host defense against infection. Experimental infection of mice with FLV-P was chosen because of the short latency period for disease induction, the possibility to evaluate antiretroviral activity by quantification of spleen foci and splenomegaly which are proportional to the virus titer, and the possibility to evaluate progression of the disease through the appearance of polycythemia. Death usually occurs between 30 and 50 days after inoculation.

In the present work, we used a combination of two drugs, simultaneously breaking the viral life cycle by means of AZT and stimulating the host defense against infection using the interferon inducer (poly I).(poly C). In vitro, it was shown that AZT inhibits the cytopathic effect of HIV and other retroviruses including Friend-MuLV (Mitsuya et al., 1985; Furman and Berry, 1988). AZT is the only drug that has been licensed as an antiretroviral agent for the treatment of AIDS and it is the first to demonstrate clinical efficacy in the treatment of AIDS-related complex (ARC) and AIDS (Fischl et al., 1987). However, AZT was shown to be toxic for hematopoietic progenitor cells in vitro (Sommadossi and Carlisle, 1987) and the most common adverse effect met during AZT therapy is the occurrence of anemia and neutropenia (Richman et al., 1987); especially in the case of prophylactic intervention, the need for non-toxic therapy is evident. Due to their minimal level of side effects, immunomodulating compounds are good candidates to potentiate the activity of an antiretroviral agent such as zidovudine. The combination of AZT and Ampligen (a mismatched double-stranded RNA) has been shown to be highly synergistic against HIV infection in vitro (Furman and Berry, 1988), therefore the synthetic double-stranded RNA (poly I).(poly C) was used in combination with a short low dose regimen of AZT.

In the FLV-P infected mouse model, we showed that (poly I).(poly C) had a potent inhibitory activity on splenomegaly and improved the survival rate of infected mice when it was used in combination with a short course of AZT therapy. This effect was observed provided the treatment was started early (4 h) after virus inoculation. This study showed differences in treatment efficacy depending on the importance of the disease in the untreated mice: AZT alone led to a substantial inhibition of splenomegaly on day 14 post infection, however, a short course of monotherapy with AZT at moderate dose achieved a prolongation of survival time only after the low virus inoculum infection.

Ruprecht et al. (1986) have shown in a mouse model of infection with Rauscher leukemia virus (RLV) that AZT is capable of suppressing infection and disease in mice treated 4 h after infection, but efficient doses led to severe hematological depression after prolonged therapy. With lower doses of AZT, a prolongation of survival time was observed in mice chronically treated. We have shown that a short and non-toxic course of AZT therapy led to a recurrence of retroviral illness after cessation of treatment, undetectable in the presence of AZT. Therefore, the capacity of antiretroviral and immunomodulating combination treatment to achieve prevention of retrovirus spreading after *de novo* infection had to be examined. It has been reported that combination therapy of AZT with interferon $\alpha$ (IFN-$\alpha$) was effective, synergistic and non-toxic in RLV infected mice (Ruprecht et al., 1988). The authors concluded that a 20 day course of 15 mg/kg/day of AZT in drinking water +10,000 U IFN-$\alpha$ twice daily prevented infection (absence of infectious virus in either plasma or spleen at the end of treatment). However, the survival of treated mice was not determined. Another biological response modifier, FK-565, was used in combination with AZT against FLV infection in mice (Yokota et al., 1988). A longer prolongation of survival time than with monotherapy was observed with a 25 day course of combination therapy starting 4 h post inoculation.

The results of the present work show a beneficial effect of combination therapy of AZT with double-stranded RNA (poly I).(poly C), providing in vivo arguments for the synergistic action observed in vitro with the combination AZT + Ampligen against HIV replication in human cell lines. The possible mechanisms of this beneficial effect of (poly I).(poly C) may involve both antiviral activity, probably mediated through the 2′-5′A-synthetase pathway (Hearl and Johnston, 1986), and immunomodulatory properties, including induction of interferon and other cytokines (De Clercq and De Somer, 1971; Carter and De Clercq, 1974). It may also be possible that some adverse effects of AZT are cancelled by combination with (poly I).(poly C). The present work also showed that the importance of the disease affected the efficacy of treatment. First, therapy had to be started early after virus inoculation and became less efficient if started later; second, improvement in survival time after infection was better in the low inoculum experiment, suggesting that after accidental exposure it should be possible to find a therapeutic schedule able to prevent retrovirus spreading. It should be underlined that, although the presence of infectious virus was not evidenced at the end of therapy (Ruprecht et al., 1988; the present work), a prolongation of survival time was observed but the animals were not cured.

In conclusion, the present work describes an animal model to test the efficacy of chemotherapeutic prevention of retroviral disease through combination drug treatment. The results suggest that AZT, with high in vivo toxicity, could be given at rather low doses if combined with double-stranded RNA (poly I).(poly

C). Combination therapy may both reduce the effective dose of AZT, thereby reducing its toxicity, and improve the absolute antiviral effect as a result of attacking the virus through multiple mechanisms. The experiments described in this report address whether therapeutic efficacy will be affected by virus inoculum and it was shown that the therapeutic schedule necessary for optimal effect may be dependent on the importance of the disease. Finally, since the beneficial effect of adding double-stranded RNA to AZT therapy has been confirmed in vivo, the combination of AZT with Ampligen appears to offer potential clinical effectiveness in the prevention of HIV infection after accidental exposure.

## References

Axelrad, A.A. and Steeves, R.A. (1964) Assay for Friend leukemia virus: rapid quantitative method based on enumeration of macroscopic spleen foci in mice. *Virology* 24, 513–518.

Bendinelli, M., Matteuci, D. and Friedman, H. (1985) Retrovirus-induced acquired immunodeficiencies. *Adv. Cancer Res.* 45, 125–181.

Carter, W.A. and De Clercq, E. (1974) Viral infection and host defense. *Science* 186, 1172–1178.

Centers for Disease Control (1988) Update: Acquired immunodeficiency syndrome and human immunodeficiency virus infection among health care workers. *MMWR* 37, 229–239.

De Clercq, E. (1989) Perspectives for chemotherapy of HIV infection. *AIDS/HIV Exp. Treat. Directory* 3, 21–28.

De Clercq, E. and De Somer, P. (1971) Role of interferon in the protective effect of the double stranded RNApoly ribonucleotide against murine tumors induced by Moloney sarcoma virus. *J. Natl. Cancer Inst.* 47, 1345–1355.

Dent, P.B. (1972) Immunodepression by oncogenic viruses. *Progr. Med. Virol.* 14, 1–35.

Dournon, E., Matheron S., Rozenbaum, W., Gharakhanian, S. et al. (1988) Effects of Zidovudine in 365 consecutive patients with AIDS or AIDS-related complex. *Lancet* 3, 1297–1302.

Fischl, M.A., Richman, D.D., Griego, M.H. et al. (1987) The efficacy of azidothymidine (AZT) in the treatment of patients with AIDS and AIDS-related complex. A double blind, placebo-controlled trial. *N. Engl. J. Med.* 317, 185–191.

Furman, P.A. and Barry, D.W. (1988) Spectrum of antiviral activity and mechanism of action of Zidovudine. *Am. J. Med.* 85 (Suppl. 2A), 176–181.

Hartshorn, K.L., Vogt, M.W., Chou, T.-C., Blumberg, R.S., Byington, R., Schooley, R.T. and Hirsch, M.S. (1987) Synergistic inhibition of human immunodeficiency virus in vitro by azidothymidine and recombinant alpha A interferon. *Antimicrob. Agents Chemother.* 31, 168–172.

Hearl, W.G. and Johnston, M.I. (1986) A misaligned double-stranded RNA, Poly (I).Poly (C12,U), induces accumulation of 2′,5′-oligoadenylates in mouse tissues. *Biochem. Biophys. Res. Commun.* 138, 40–46.

Marcus, R. and Cooperative Needlestick Surveillance Group (1988) Surveillance of health care workers exposed to blood from patients infected with the human immunodeficiency virus. *N. Engl. J. Med.* 319, 1118–1123.

Meylan, P.R., Francioli, P., Decrey, H., Chave, J.P. and Glauser, M.P. (1988) Post exposure prophylaxis against HIV infection in health care workers. *Lancet* i, 481.

Mitchell, W.M., Montefiori, D.C. and Robinson, W.E. (1987) Mismatched double stranded RNA (Ampligen) reduces concentration of zidovudine (azidothymidine) required for in vitro inhibition of human immunodeficiency virus. *Lancet* i, 890–892.

Mitsuya, H., Weinhold, K.J., Furman P.A. et al. (1985) 3′-Azido-3′-deoxythymidine (BW A509U): an antiviral agent that inhibits the infectivity and cytopathic effect of human T-lymphotropic virus type III/lymphadenopathy-associated virus in vitro. *Proc. Natl. Acad. Sci. U.S.A.* 82, 7096–7100.

Richman, D.D., Fischl, M.A., Grieco, M.H. et al. (1987) The toxicity of azidothymidine (AZT) in the treatment of patients with AIDS and AIDS-related complex. A double blind, placebo-controlled trial. *N. Engl. J. Med.* 317, 192–197.

Ruprecht, R.M., Gama-Sosa, M.A. and Rosas, H.D. (1988) Combination therapy after viral inoculation. *Lancet* i, 239–240.

Ruprecht, R.M., O'Brien, L.G., Rossoni, L.D. and Nusinoff-Lehrman, S. (1986) Suppression of mouse viremia and retroviral disease by 3′-azido-3′-deoxythymidine. *Nature* 323, 467–469.

Schlumberger, H.D. and Schrinner, E. (1989) *Intervirology* 30 (Suppl.), 1–72.

Sommadossi, J.-P. and Carlisle, R. (1987) Toxicity of 3′-azido-3′-deoxythymidine and 9-(1,3-dihydroxy-2-propoxymethyl)guanine for normal human hematopoietic progenitor cells in vitro. *Antimicrob. Agents Chemother.* 31, 452–454.

Wong, G.H., Krowka, J.F., Stites, D.P. and Goeddel, D.V. (1988) In vitro anti-human immunodeficiency virus activities of tumor necrosis factor-$\alpha$ and interferon-$\beta$. *J. Immunol.* 140, 120–124.

Yokota, Y., Wakai, Y., Watanabe, Y. and Mine, Y. (1988) Inhibitory effect of FK-565 alone or in combination with zidovudine on retroviral infection by Friend leukemia virus in mice. *J. Antibiot.* 41, 1479–1487.

*Eds. H. Schellekens and M.C. Horzinek*
*Animal Models in AIDS*



# 32

# Murine AIDS: effect of the muramyl-tripeptide derivative, MTP-PE, and interferon α against herpes simplex virus superinfection

R.M. COZENS and H.-K. HOCHKEPPEL

Research Department, Pharmaceutical Division, Ciba-Geigy Ltd., CH-4002 Basel, Switzerland

## Introduction

The advent of the acquired immunodeficiency syndrome (AIDS) pandemic has led to a requirement for new animal models not only relevant to the therapy of the human immunodeficiency virus (HIV) itself but also models of immunosuppression which may be useful to assess the efficacy of treatment regimens against the opportunistic infections characteristic of AIDS. Immunosuppression in laboratory animals may be achieved by a variety of methods. Agents such as cyclosporin, cyclophosphamide and dextran sulfate (e.g., Hahn, 1974; Blyth et al., 1980; Mattson et al., 1980; Fraser-Smith et al., 1982; Lawson et al., 1989) may be administered to deplete various cells of the immune system. Thymectomy or splenectomy, often combined with whole body irradiation or injection of antilymphocyte antibodies, has been similarly employed (e.g., Müller et al., 1987). Animals, particularly mice, are available which have a variety of congenital defects in the immune system, e.g., SCID, nude and beige mice.

While experimental infections in such models can provide much useful information they may be considered unnatural to varying degrees, in that the many interactions between the components of the immune system may be artificially distorted. In addition the models may produce technical problems in terms of treatment schedules and, for example, potential drug-drug interactions.

The LP-BM5 virus complex (Haas and Meshorer, 1979; Haas and Reschef, 1980) causes a profound immunosuppression in susceptible mice (Mosier, 1986; Mosier et al., 1985). As the manifestations of the disease are similar in many respects to those of AIDS (Klinken et al., 1988; Mosier, 1986; Mosier et al., 1985; Pattengale et al., 1982) the disease is conveniently known as murine AIDS (MAIDS). We describe here the use of this model to assess the efficacy of the immunomodulator muramyl tripeptide phosphatidyl ethanolamine (MTP-PE), a recombinant human interferon-$\alpha$ BDBB hybrid (rhuIFN$\alpha$B/D) and the chemotherapeutic agents acyclovir and 9-(2-phosphonyl-methoxyethyl) adenine (PMEA; De Clercq et al., 1986, 1987) against experimental herpes simplex virus (HSV) type 1 superinfections.

## Materials and methods

### Viruses and animals

LP-BM5 virus was kindly provided by Dr. Robert Yetter, VA Hospital, Baltimore, MD, and was maintained in a persistently infected SC-1 cell line (TC 2110). Working stocks of virus were prepared by overlaying TC 2110 cells with rapidly growing uninfected SC-1 cells maintained in Eagle's minimal essential medium (MEM) supplemented with 5% fetal calf serum, penicillin and streptomycin. These cultures were incubated for 24 h and supernatant fluids harvested, centrifuged at $1000 \times g$ for 30 min and filtered through a 0.22 $\mu$m membrane filter. Virus stocks were stored at $-80°C$ for up to 6 months prior to use. Female C57Bl/6 mice (28–33 days old; Ciba-Geigy, Sisseln, Switzerland) were infected intraperitoneally with 0.5 ml of undilute virus. A complete description of the

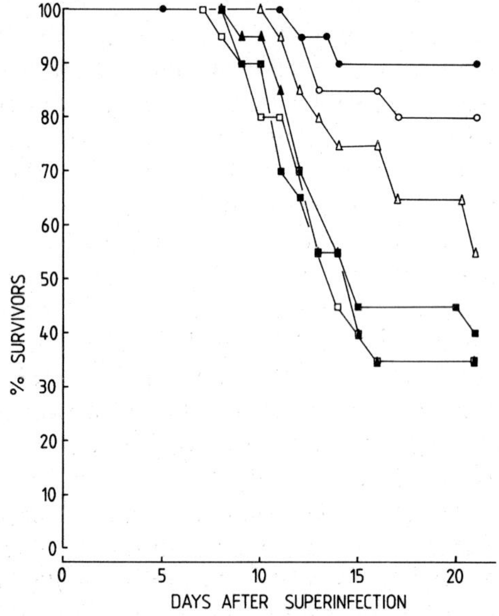


Fig. 1. Survival of LP-BM5 virus infected mice following challenge (62 days post LP-BM5 virus infection) with HSV-1/MacIntyre and treatment with MTP-PE/MLV. Mice were infected intraperitoneally ($5 \times 10^5$ pfu) and treated with one dose of MTP-PE/MLV (i.p.) 3 h after the superinfection with HSV. Immunocompetent controls (●); immunosuppressed controls (no drug) (▲); MLVs alone (■), $P \geqslant 0.1$; 1.0 mg/kg (○) $P \leqslant 0.01$; 0.1 mg/kg (△) $P \geqslant 0.1$; 0.01 mg/kg (□) $P \geqslant 0.1$.

LP-BM5 virus complex and the immunosuppression which occurs following infection has been reported elsewhere (Hartley et al., 1977; Haas and Meshorer, 1979; Haas and Reschef, 1980; Klinken et al., 1988; Mosier, 1988; Mosier et al., 1985).

A neurovirulent strain of HSV-1 (MacIntyre) was obtained from the American Type Culture Collection (ATCC VR-539) and propagated in human embryonic foreskin cells (7000, Flow Laboratories Inc., McLean, VA). Culture supernatants were harvested at 72 h after infection, clarified by centrifugation ($1000 \times g$ for 20 min) and stored at $-80°C$. The virus titer, as assessed on Vero cells, was $1.0 \times 10^8$ pfu/ml.

### Drugs

MTP-PE incorporated in multilamellar vesicles (MLV) composed of phosphatidylcholine and phosphatidylserine (MTP-PE/MLV; ratio of drug to phospholipid was 1:250) was produced at Ciba-Geigy, Basel, Switzerland. The drug containing liposomes were reconstituted in phosphate-buffered saline (PBS) prior to intraperitoneal injection.

rhuIFNαB/D (CGP 35269) was produced in yeast and purified as previously described (Meister et al., 1986). This interferon was biologically active in at least

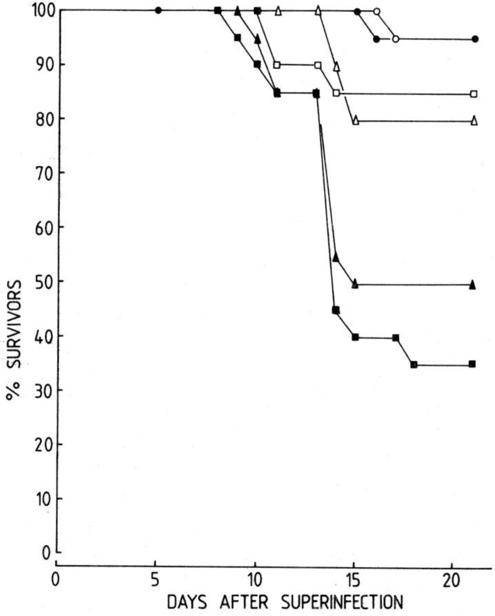


Fig. 2. Survival of LP-BM5 virus infected mice following challenge (62 days post LP-BM5 virus infection) with HSV-1/MacIntyre and treatment with MTP-PE/MLV. Mice were infected intraperitoneally ($5 \times 10^5$ pfu) and treated with three doses of MTP-PE/MLV (i.p.) 3, 24 and 48 h after the superinfection with HSV. Immunocompetent controls (●); immunosuppressed controls (no drug) (▲) MLVs alone (■), $P \geqslant 0.1$; 1.0 mg/kg (○) $P \leqslant 0.005$; 0.1 mg/kg (△) $P \leqslant 0.05$; 0.01 mg/kg (□) $P \leqslant 0.05$.

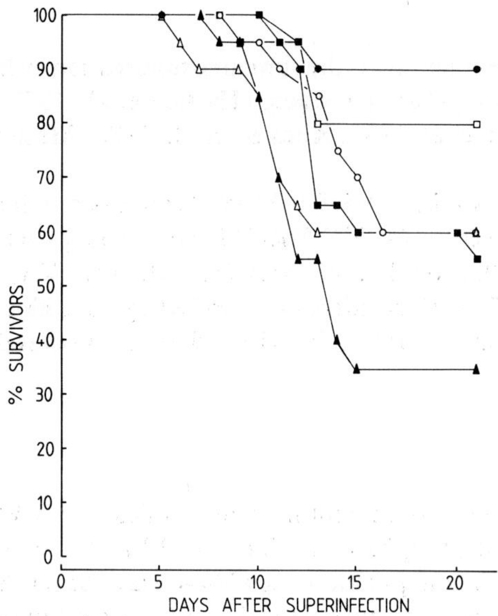


Fig. 3. Survival of LP-BM5 virus infected mice following challenge (62 days post LP-BM5 virus infection) with HSV-1/MacIntyre and treatment with MTP-PE/MLV. Mice were infected intraperitoneally ($5 \times 10^5$ pfu) and treated every second day for 21 days with MTP-PE/MLV (i.p.) starting 3 h after the superinfection with HSV. Immunocompetent controls (●); immunosuppressed controls (no drug) (▲); MLVs alone (■), $0.05 \leqslant P \leqslant 0.1$; 1.0 mg/kg (○) $P \leqslant 0.05$; 0.1 mg/kg (△) $P \geqslant 0.1$; 0.01 mg/kg (□) $P \leqslant 0.01$.

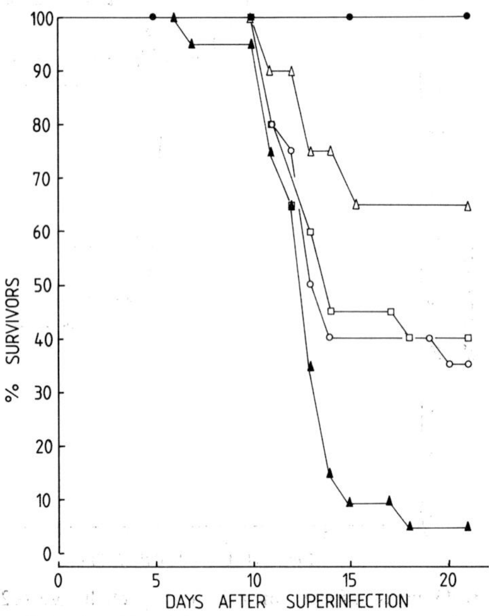


Fig. 4. Survival of LP-BM5 virus infected mice following challenge (60 days post LP-BM5 virus infection) with HSV-1/MacIntyre and treatment with rhuIFNαB/D. Mice were infected intraperitoneally ($5 \times 10^5$ pfu) and treated after 3 h with $5 \times 10^7$ U/kg of rhuIFNαB/D. Mice received no further treatment (○), $P \geqslant 0.1$; two further doses 24 and 48 h later (△), $P \leqslant 0.001$; or received drug every second day for 21 days (□), $P \leqslant 0.02$. Immunocompetent controls (●); immunosuppressed controls (no drug) (▲).

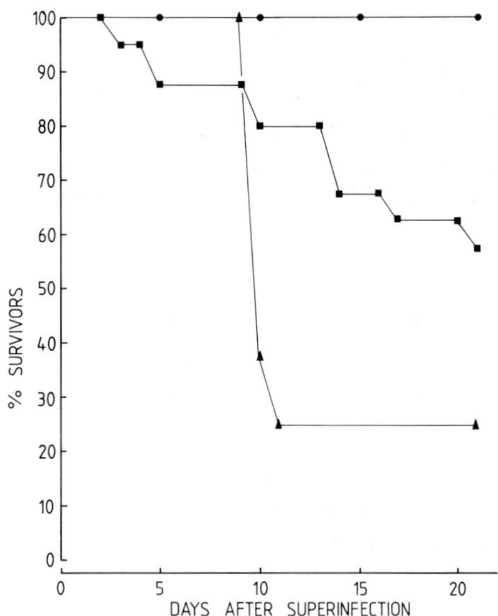


Fig. 5. Survival of LP-BM5 virus infected mice following challenge (65 days post LP-BM5 virus infection) with HSV-1/MacIntyre and treatment with acyclovir. Mice were infected intraperitoneally ($5 \times 10^5$ pfu) and treated with 200 mg/kg i.p. of acyclovir beginning on the day of virus infection and again on days 2, 4 and 6 following infection. Immunocompetent controls (●); immunosuppressed controls (no drug) (▲); acyclovir treated (■), $P \leqslant 0.05$.

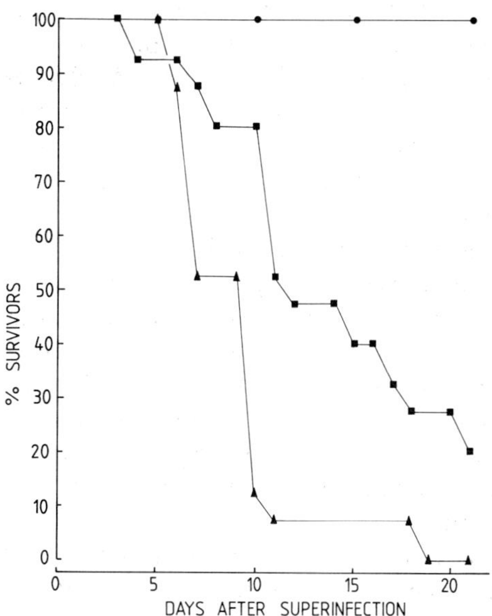


Fig. 6. Survival of LP-BM5 virus infected mice following challenge (65 days post LP-BM5 virus infection) with HSV-1/MacIntyre and treatment with PMEA. Mice were infected intraperitoneally ($5 \times 10^5$ pfu) and treated with 100 mg/kg i.p. of PMEA beginning on the day of virus infection and again on days 2, 4, and 6 following infection. Immunocompetent controls (●); immunosuppressed controls (no drug) (▲); PMEA treated (▲), $P \leqslant 0.05$.

12 species including mice. The final formulation was stored carrier-free in PBS at 4°C at a concentration of 0.2 mg/ml ($3 \times 10^7$ international units). The drug was diluted in pyrogen-free saline shortly before subcutaneous administration.

PMEA was kindly provided by Dr. A. Holy (Institute of Organic Chemistry and Biochemistry, Czechoslovak Academy of Sciences, Prague, Czechoslovakia). This drug was dissolved in PBS prior to intraperitoneal injection. Acyclovir (Wellcome, Basel, Switzerland) was also dissolved in PBS prior to use.

### Superinfection with HSV-1 and treatment with antivirals

Mice at 60–65 days post LP-BM5 infection were infected with HSV-1/MacIntyre by intraperitoneal injection of $5 \times 10^5$ pfu per mouse. The first dose of the drugs was administered 3 h after inoculation with HSV. Deaths were recorded and the data analyzed statistically by Wilcoxon rank analysis using a one-tailed test, comparisons were always made to the immunosuppressed control. Each treatment group consisted of at least 10 mice and experiments were performed at least twice.

## Results and discussion

Figs. 1–6 demonstrate the increased susceptibility of LP-BM5 infected mice to experimental superinfection with HSV-1/MacIntyre. The differences in susceptibility between the experiments presumably reflect slight differences in the degree of immunosuppression within a group of mice, as a delay in superinfection invariably produces greater and more reproducible susceptibility (data not shown). However, if superinfection is delayed much beyond 60–65 days analysis of the data is made more difficult by the occurrence of sporadic deaths due, normally, to respiratory failure caused by the massive lymphadenopathy of the parathymic lymph nodes.

It is apparent (Fig. 1) that even a single dose of MTP-PE/MLV at 1 or 0.1 mg/kg was effective in at least prolonging the survival of the mice, the degree of protection being dose-dependent. Increasing the doses to three (Fig. 2) improved the protection afforded to the extent that the highest dose (1 mg/kg) protected essentially 100% of the animals and even the lowest dose was able to protect 85% of the animals. Increasing the doses to one every second day during the whole course of the experiment (Fig. 3) led to less protection by MTP-PE/MLV while the MLVs themselves appeared to have a beneficial effect on the outcome of the superinfection challenge.

MTP-PE has been shown to be a macrophage activator (Schumann, 1987) and presumably in these experiments acted on the peritoneal macrophages, and thereby prevented the efficient establishment of the infection. We are at present investigating whether intravenous administration of the drug is equally effective in this model.

Fig. 4 demonstrates that rhuIFN$\alpha$B/D was also active in this model at a dose of $5 \times 10^7$ U/kg, the degree of protection afforded being related to the frequency of administration. One dose of rhuIFNαB/D given 3 h after the superinfection was as effective (40% survival) as multiple doses given every second day for 21 days; however, three doses administered at 3, 24 and 48 h after the superinfection afforded protection to 65% of the mice.

Figs. 5 and 6 demonstrate that this model can also be useful for the assessment of chemotherapeutic agents. Acyclovir and PMEA were both effective in at least prolonging survival at the doses used. We are at present investigating the possible benefits of combination therapy in this model.

The model is not limited to HSV as the superinfecting pathogen. Preliminary data suggest that mice immunosuppressed by LP-BM5 are also more susceptible to murine cytomegalovirus (Gangemi, personal communication), and Buller et al. (1987) have demonstrated the increased susceptibility of such mice to mouse pox virus. We are attempting to broaden the application of this model in the search for treatments for opportunistic infections, by investigating the susceptibility of the immunosuppressed mice to bacterial and fungal pathogens.

## References

Blyth, W.A (1980) Effect of immunosuppression on recurrent herpes simplex infection in mice. *Infect. Immunol.* 29, 902–907.

Buller, R.M.L., Yetter, R.A., Fredrickson, T.N. and Morse, H.C. (1987) Abrogation of resistance to severe mousepox in C57Bl/6 mice infected with LP-BM5 murine leukemia viruses. *J. Virol.* 6, 383–387.

De Clercq, E., Holy, A., Rosenberg, I., Sakuma, T., Balzarini, J. and Maudal, P.C. (1986) A novel selective broad-spectrum anti-DNA virus agent. *Nature* 323, 464–467.

De Clercq, E., Sakuma, T., Baba, M., Pauwels, R., Balzarini, J., Rosenberg, I. and Holy, A. (1987) Antiviral activity of phosphonylmethoxyalkyl derivatives of purine and pyrimidines. *Antiviral Res.* 8, 261–272.

Fraser-Smith, E.B., Waters, R.V. and Matthews, T.R. (1982) Correlation between in vivo anti-*Pseudomonas* and anti-*Candida* activities and clearance of carbon by the reticuloendothelial system for various muramyl dipeptide analogs, using normal and immunosuppressed mice. *Infect. Immunol.* 35, 105–110.

Haas, M. and Meshorer, A. (1979) Reticulum cell neoplasms induced in C57B1/6 mice by cultured virus grown in stromal hematopoietic cell lines. *J. Natl. Cancer Inst.* 63, 427–439.

Haas, M. and Reschef, T. (1980) Nonthymic malignant lymphomas induced in C57B1/6 mice by cloned dualtropic viruses. *Eur. J. Cancer* 16, 909–917.

Hahn, H. (1974) Effects of dextran sulfate 500 on cell-mediated resistance to infection with *Listeria monocytogenes* in mice. *Infect. Immunol.* 10, 1105–1109.

Hartley, J.W., Wolford, H.K., Old, L.J. and Rowe, W.P. (1977) A new class of murine leukemia viruses associated with development of spontaneous lymphomas. *Proc. Natl. Acad. Sci. U.S.A.* 74, 789–792.

Klinken, S.P., Fredrickson, T.N., Hartley, J.W., Yetter, R.A. and Morse, H.C. (1988) Evolution of B cell lineage lymphomas in mice with a retrovirus-induced immunodeficiency syndrome, *MAIDS. J. Immunol.* 140, 1123–1131.

Lawson, C.M., Hodgkin, P.D. and Shellam, G.R. (1989) The effect of cyclosporin on major histocompatibility complex-linked resistance to murine cytomegalovirus. *J. Gen. Virol.* 70, 1253–1259.

Mattson, D.M., Howard, R.J. and Balfour, H.H. (1980) Immediate loss of cell-mediated immunity to murine cytomegalovirus upon treatment with immunosuppressive agents. *Infect. Immunol.* 30, 700–708.

Meister, A., Uzé, G., Mogenson, K., Gresser, I., Tovey, M.G., Grütter, M. and Meyer, F. (1986) Biological activities and receptor binding of two human recombinant interferons and their hybrids. *J. Gen. Virol.* 67, 1633–1643.

Mosier, D.E. (1986) Animal models for retrovirus-induced immunodeficiency disease. *Immunol. Invest.* 15, 233–261.

Mosier, D.E., Yetter, R.A. and Morse, H.C. (1985) Retroviral induction of acute lymphoproliferative disease and profound immunosuppression in adult C57B1/6 mice. *J. Exp. Med.* 161, 766–784.

Müller, I., Cobbold, S.P., Waldmann, H. and Kaufmann, S.H.E. (1987) Impaired resistance to *Mycobacterium tuberculosis* infection after selective in vivo depletion of L3T4$^+$ and Lyt-2$^+$ T cells. *Infect. Immunol.* 55, 2037–2041.

Pattengale, P.K., Taylor, C.R., Twomey, P., Hill, S., Jonasson, J., Beardsley, T. and Haas, M. (1982) Immunopathology of B-cell lymphomas induced in C57B1/6 mice by dualtropic murine leukemia virus (MuLV). *Am. J. Pathol.* 107, 362–377.

Schumann, G. (1987) Biological activities of a lipophilic muramylpeptide (MTP-PE). In: I. Azuma and G. Jollès (Eds.), *Immunostimulants: Now and Tomorrow.* Springer Verlag, Berlin, pp. 71–77.

*Eds. H. Schellekens and M.C. Horzinek*
*Animal Models in AIDS*



# 33

# Virus specific cytotoxic T cell response to a neurotropic murine retrovirus

D.S. ROBBINS, S.C. CLABOUGH, J.L. MARTIN and P.M. HOFFMAN

Veterans Administration Medical Center, and University of Maryland at Baltimore, Baltimore, MD, U.S.A.

**Summary**

We detected a murine leukemia virus (MuLV) specific cytotoxic response in vitro in spleen cells from NFS/N mice infected with Cas-Br-M MuLV at 21 days of age. In contrast, this response was greatly diminished in spleens from NFS/N mice infected at 2 days of age even though splenocytes from these mice could mount an allogeneic response. The MuLV specific response was abrogated by anti-Thy1.2 antibody and complement treatment identifying the effector cell as a T lymphocyte. The cytotoxic T lymphocyte (CTL) response was restricted to major histocompatibility complex compatible target cells and was inhibited by unlabeled target cells expressing MuLV viral antigen and appropriate H-2.

In vivo studies showed that immune mediated resistance to Cas-Br-M MuLV induced neurologic disease was T cell mediated and did not require repeated virus exposure. MuLV specific T cells secondarily stimulated in vitro transferred protection against neurologic disease at lower numbers than those required for protection by transfer of unfractionated immune or Ly2.2$^+$ T cell enriched populations.

The dissemination of Cas-Br-M MuLV and neurodegenerative disease that follows neonatal infection occurs in the absence of an effective MuLV specific CTL response but can be prevented by syngeneic transfer of MuLV specific immunocompetent T cells. Therefore, it appears that MuLV specific CTL play an important role in vivo in the age-acquired immunity and prevention of the nervous system effects of Cas-Br-M MuLV infection.

## Introduction

The rapid dissemination of retroviruses at the cellular and organ levels may play an important role in the pathogenesis of lymphomas, leukemia, and neurologic disease resulting from human (HTLV-1) and murine (MuLV) oncornavirus infection (Hoffman and Fleming, 1988). Similarly, rapid dissemination of lentiviruses precedes the lymphoproliferation, immunodeficiency, and neurologic disease that develop during the course of human (HIV-1) and animal (FTLV, SIV, and Visna) lentivirus infection (Hoffman and Panitch, 1988). While recent studies have demonstrated the presence of HIV specific cytotoxic T lymphocytes (CTL) directed against envelope (*env*) and polymerase (*pol*) gene products in HIV seropositive asymptomatic individuals (Walker et al., 1987, 1988), the correlation of an HIV specific CTL response with progression to AIDS related complex (ARC) or acquired immunodeficiency syndrome (AIDS) remains unproven. Because retrovirus infections are highly cell associated, cells that mediate the cellular immune responses are likely to play an important role in viral clearance, lysis of infected cells, and the prevention of persistent infection (Walker et al., 1988). We have investigated a neurotropic MuLV infection in inbred NFS/N mice that offers unique opportunities to evaluate retroviral immunogenicity, the immune interactions that occur during the induction of an MuLV specific CTL response, and the effects of MuLV dissemination to the central nervous system (CNS).

Hind limb paralysis, lymphomas, and high levels of infectious MuLV were described in populations of feral mice in southern California by Gardner et al. (1973). This neurotropic C-type retrovirus from wild mice was capable of inducing a spongiform neurodegenerative disease and lymphomas in NIH Swiss mice (reviewed in Hoffman and Panitch, 1988). Inbred NFS/N mice inoculated by either intraperitoneal (i.p.) or intracerebral (i.c.) injection before 10 days of age with biologically cloned, ecotropic Cas-Br-M MuLV develop neurologic disease as adults while those animals inoculated after 10 days of age do not.

Wild mice that acquire the infection in the neonatal period are viremic through life and have normal immune function (Gardner, 1978). We found that susceptible inbred mouse strains such as NFS/N infected neonatally with Cas-Br-M MuLV had a normal response at both the recognition and killing phases of an allogeneic cytotoxicity assay. Spleen cells from infected, neurologically symptomatic mice were able to respond normally to common mitogens in lymphocyte transformation assays and also were able to generate anti-sheep red blood cell antibodies in vitro (Robbins et al., 1989).

Using cells from hyperimmunized NFS/N mice in syngeneic transfer studies, we previously showed that the age dependent protective immunity was mediated by T cells and not B cells or macrophages (Hoffman et al., 1984). This resistance, complete at 10 days of age, was overcome by treatment with anti-thymocyte serum but not anti-immunoglobulin M antibody and could not be demonstrated in adult nude mice with susceptible genetic backgrounds (Hoffman et al., 1984; Robbins et al., 1989). The fact that all Cas-Br-M MuLV infected NFS/N mice developed significant levels of anti-viral antibody in serum regardless of their neurological status indicated that susceptibility to paralytic disease could not be attributed to a defect in T helper function. In this study, we extend those observations and examine the role of MuLV specific CTL in protective immunity against Cas-Br-M MuLV induced neurodegeneration.

## Results

### CYTOTOXIC T CELL RESPONSE IN CAS-BR-M MULV INFECTED NFS/N MICE

NFS/N mice were infected i.p. with $5 \times 10^3$ pfu of Cas-Br-M MuLV at 2 or 21 days of age. NFS/N mice infected in this manner at 2 days of age developed symptoms of neurologic disease (hind limb weakness and tremor) at 6–8 weeks post infection while those inoculated at 21 days of age remained asymptomatic. Primary in vivo CTL responses to MuLV have been difficult to document possibly because ecotropic MuLV are poor immunogens (reviewed in Robbins et al., 1989). Therefore, we developed an in vitro $^{51}$Cr release assay using splenocytes of NFS/N mice infected in vivo and restimulated in vitro for 5 days with a γ irradiated stimulator cell line. This cell line, NS467, was derived from a pre-B lymphoma that occurred in a Cas-Br-M MuLV infected NFS/N mouse (Mushinski et al., 1987). Similar to other pre-B lymphoma lines, NS467 expresses class I, major histocompatibility complex (MHC), MuLV gp70 and p30, but not Ia antigens. In our assay, NS467 cells were labeled with $^{51}$Cr and used as a syngeneic target cell expressing viral antigen. At a killer to target cell ratio of 20:1 we observed a brisk cytotoxic response directed against NS467 target cells in splenocytes derived from NFS/N mice infected with Cas-Br-M MuLV at 21 days of age (Fig. 1). This response could be detected as early as 1 week post infection and was maintained beyond 20 weeks. In contrast, only low levels of cytotoxicity directed against an MuLV specific target cell were detected in spleens of NFS/N

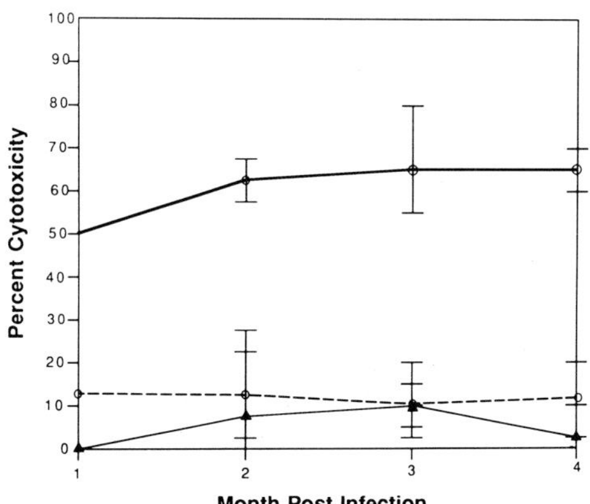


Fig. 1. Spleen cells from NFS/N mice infected with Cas-Br-M MuLV at 2 days of age (--○--) (n = 23) or 21 days of age (–○–) (n = 18) were examined at increasing times post infection for MuLV specific cytotoxicity in a $^{51}$Cr release assay following a secondary in vitro stimulation. NS467, a pre-B lymphoma cell line derived from an NFS/N mouse infected with MuLV and expressing H-$2^{sq4}$ and viral gp70, was used for stimulation and as a labeled target. In contrast to uninfected NFS/N mice (–▲–) (n = 20) and mice infected with Cas-Br-M MuLV at 2 days of age, NFS/N mice infected at 21 days of age developed a brisk MuLV specific CTL response as early as 1 week post infection.

TABLE 1
Ablation of MuLV specific cytotoxicity with anti-Thy1.2 treatment[a]

| Treatment | Percent cytotoxicity [b] |
|---|---|
| None | $66 \pm 1.0$ |
| Complement | $67 \pm 4.0$ |
| Anti-Thy1.2 | $63 \pm 2.0$ |
| Anti-Thy1.2 + complement | $7 \pm 0.2$ |

[a] Effector spleen cells were isolated from an adult NFS/N mouse infected at 21 days of age with Cas-Br-M MuLV and stimulated in vitro with irradiated NS467 cells.

[b] Results from triplicate wells were expressed as percent cytotoxicity ± standard deviation directed against $^{51}Cr$ labeled NS467 cell targets.

mice infected at 2 days of age. This low level of cytotoxic activity was indistinguishable from that observed in NFS/N mice inoculated with medium. However, spleen cells from NFS/N mice infected with Cas-Br-M MuLV at 2 days of age were able to mount an allogeneic cytotoxic response as early as 10 days of age (data not shown).

Anti-Thy1.2 antibody and complement treatment of in vitro stimulated splenocytes from NFS/N mice infected at 21 days of age resulted in abrogation

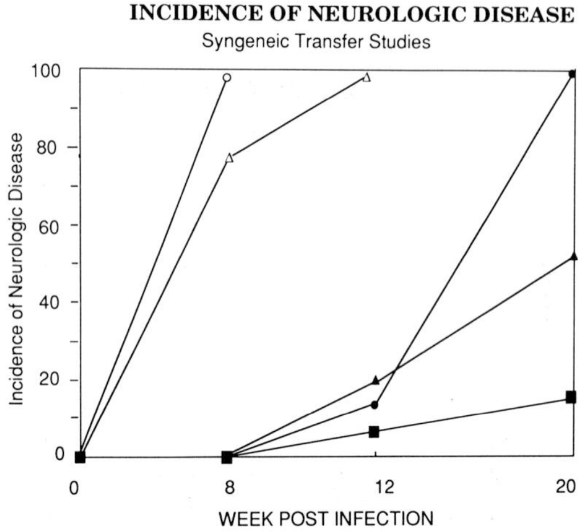

**INCIDENCE OF NEUROLOGIC DISEASE**
Syngeneic Transfer Studies
Incidence of Neurologic Disease
0
20
40
60
80
100
0
8
12
20
WEEK POST INFECTION

Fig. 2. Donor NFS/N mice in syngeneic transfer experiments were inoculated i.p. at 3 weeks of age with 50 $\mu$l of medium or $3 \times 10^4$ pfu of Cas-Br-M MuLV. Twenty recipient NFS/N mice were inoculated with phosphate buffered saline + 1% fetal calf serum at 1 day of age (○). Five NFS/N recipients received $10^6$ T cells from uninfected donors (△), 18 recipient NFS/N mice received $10^6$ MuLV immune T cells (■), 12 NFS/N recipients received $10^5$ MuLV immune T cells (▲), and seven recipient NFS/N mice received $10^4$ MuLV immune T cells (●). T cells were isolated from donor NFS/N mice using panning techniques. All recipient NFS/N mice were 1 day of age at time of cell transfer. All recipients were inoculated i.p. with $3 \times 10^4$ pfu of Cas-Br-M MuLV 24 h after cell transfer.

of MuLV specific cytotoxicity (Table 1) and identified the effector cells as a T lymphocyte. We have further determined that MuLV specific cytotoxicity is restricted to H-2 compatible targets and is inhibited by unlabeled NS467 cells, splenic blasts from Cas-Br-M MuLV infected NFS/N mice, but not by allogeneic cells or by uninfected NFS/N splenic blasts (data not shown).

### Immune mediated resistance in vivo

Experiments reported in an earlier study demonstrated that syngeneic transfers of T cells from NFS/N mice inoculated with three injections of Cas-Br-M MuLV beginning at 21 days of age conferred protection to susceptible neonatal NFS/N mice (Hoffman et al., 1984). In this study, we utilized Cas-Br-M MuLV infected NFS/N mice as cell donors in syngeneic transfer studies following only a single exposure to virus. NFS/N mice were inoculated i.p. at 21 days of age with $3–4 \times 10^4$ pfu of Cas-Br-M MuLV and used as donors of immune T cells at 6–12 weeks post infection. T cells were isolated by negative selection using anti-immunoglobulin coated plates (Hoffman et al., 1984). Graded numbers of T cells (greater than 98% purity as determined by immunofluorescence) were

TABLE 2

Incidence of neurologic disease in MuLV infected mice receiving syngeneic T cell subsets

| Cells transferred | Weeks post infection [c] | | |
|---|---|---|---|
| | 8 | 12 | 20–24 |
| Immune T cells | 0% | 8% | 15% |
| Immune Ly2.2$^{+}$ [a] | | | |
| $10^6$ (n = 13) | 0% | 0% | 0% |
| $10^5$ (n = 7) | 0% | 20% | 20% |
| Immune Ly2.2$^{-}$ [a] | | | |
| $10^6$ (n = 13) | 0% | 11% | 29% |
| $5 \times 10^5$ (n = 4) | 0% | 0% | 33% |
| In vitro stimulated [b] immune T cells (CTL) | | | |
| $3 \times 10^5$ (n = 16) | 0% | 13% | 17% |
| $3 \times 10^4$ (n = 25) | 4% | 21% | 50% |

[a] Ly2.2$^{+}$ cells were isolated from MuLV immune T cells 8–12 weeks post infection using a positive selection on anti-Ly2.2 antibody coated plates. Ly2.2$^{-}$ cells were isolated by negative selection. Purity of Ly2.2$^{-}$ cells ranged from 87 to 92%. Purity of Ly2.2$^{+}$ cells was greater than 96% (as determined by immunofluorescence). Recipient NFS/N mice were inoculated i.p. with T cell subsets at 1 day of age.

[b] Recipient NFS/N mice were inoculated i.p. at 1 day of age with spleen cells from immune donors (8–12 weeks post infection) previously stimulated in vitro for 5 days with irradiated NS467 pre-B lymphoma cells. The proportion of T cells and Ly2.2$^{+}$, Ly2.2$^{-}$ subsets was determined by immunofluorescent techniques.

[c] All recipient NFS/N were inoculated i.p. at 2 days of age with $3 \times 10^4$ pfu of Cas-Br-M MuLV 24 h after cell transfer.

inoculated i.p. into 1 day old NFS/N mice. The recipients were infected with Cas-Br-M MuLV 24 h following cell transfer. The transfer of $10^6$ immune T cells protected 85% of recipient mice from development of neurologic disease while lower numbers of transferred cells afforded less protection (Fig. 2). We then determined whether in vitro stimulated immune spleen cell preparations demonstrating MuLV specific cytotoxicity in vitro could confer protection. Spleen cells from Cas-Br-M MuLV immune donors (8–12 weeks post infection) were stimulated in vitro for 5 days with irradiated NS467 cells and passed over a Ficoll-Isopaque density gradient to remove dead cells (Davidson and Parish, 1975). Thirty percent of the restimulated spleen cells were T cells as determined by immunofluorescence. The ratio of Ly2.2$^+$ to Ly2.2$^-$ T cells was 1.0. These preparations containing MuLV specific T cells effectively protected recipient Cas-Br-M MuLV infected NFS/N mice against the development of neurologic disease at lower numbers than those required for protection by transfer of unfractionated immune T cells or preparations enriched for Ly2.2$^+$ cells (Table 2).

Immunofluorescent microscopy on frozen sections from protected NFS/N mice demonstrated viral antigen in splenic megakaryocytes and lymphoid cells, capillary endothelial cells, and scattered glial cells in the nervous system. The absence of pathology in the brains of protected NFS/N mice differed from symptomatic Cas-Br-M MuLV infected NFS/N mice where more widespread infection of endothelial and glial cells and marked gliosis, vacuolation, and neuronal dropout was apparent (Hoffman et al., 1988).

## Acknowledgement

Supported by the Department of Veterans Affairs, and National Institutes of Health Grant AI25336.

## References

Davidson, W.F. and Parish, C.R. (1975) A procedure for removing red cells and dead cells from lymphoid cell suspensions. *J. Immunol. Methods* 7, 291–300.

Gardner, M.B. (1978) Type C retroviruses of wild mice: characterization and natural history of amphotropic, ecotropic, and xenotropic MuLV. *Curr. Topics Microbiol. Immunol.* 79, 215–259.

Gardner, M.B., Henderson, B.E., Officer, J.E., Rongey, R.W., Parker, J.C., Oliver, C., Estes, J.D. and Heubner, R.J. (1973) A spontaneous lower motor neuron disease apparently caused by indigenous type C RNA virus in wild mice. *J. Natl. Cancer Inst.* 51, 1243–1254.

Hoffman, P.M. and Fleming, J.O. (1989) Neurovirology. In: W.G. Bradley et al. (Eds.), *Clinical Practice,* Chapter 44. Butterworth Publications, Stoneham, MA.

Hoffman, P.M. and Panitch H.S. (1989) Neurologic diseases induced by retroviruses including Visna. In: R.R. McKendall (Ed.), *Handbook of Clinical Neurology. Viral Diseases.* Elsevier, Amsterdam.

Hoffman, P.M., Robbins, D.S. and Morse, H.C. III (1984) Role of immunity in age-related resistance to paralysis after murine leukemia virus infection. *J. Virol.* 52, 734–738.

Hoffman, P.M., Pitts, O.M., Bilello, J.A. and Cimino, E.F. (1988) Retrovirus induced motor degeneration. *Rev. Neurol.* 144, 676–679.

Mushinski, J.F., Davidson, W.F. and Morse, H.C. III (1987) Activation of cellular oncogenes in human and mouse leukemia-lymphomas: spontaneous and induced oncogene expression in murine B lymphocytic neoplasms. *Cancer Invest.* 5, 345–368.

Robbins, D.S., Bilello, J.A. and Hoffman, P.M. (1989) Pathogenesis and treatment of neurotropic murine leukemia virus infections. In: G.C. Roman, J.C. Vernant and M. Osame (Eds.), *HTLV-I and the Nervous System.* Alan R. Liss, New York, NY, pp. 575–587.

Walker, B.D., Chakrabarti, S., Moss, B., Paradis, T.J., Flynn, T., Durno, A.G., Blumberg, R.S., Kaplan, J.C., Hirsch, M.S. and Schooley, R.T. (1987) HIV-specific cytotoxic T lymphocytes in seropositive individuals. *Nature* 328, 345–348.

Walker, B.D., Flexner, C., Paradis, T.J., Fuller, T.C., Hirsch, M.S., Schooley, R.T. and Moss, B. (1988) HIV-1 reverse transcriptase is a target for cytotoxic T lymphocyte in infected individuals. *Science* 240, 64–66.

*Eds. H. Schellekens and M.C. Horzinek*
*Animal Models in AIDS*



# 34

# Effects of sperm and autoimmunity on murine AIDS (MAIDS)

Z. WEISMAN [1], A. MESHORER [2], J. RUBINSTEIN [2], E. MOZES [3] and Z. BENTWICH [1]

[1] R. Ben Ari Institute of Clinical Immunology, Kaplan Medical Center, Hebrew University Medical School, [2] Experimental Animal Unit and [3] Department of Chemical Immunology, The Weizmann Institute of Science, Rehovot, Israel

**Summary**

The purpose of the present study was to determine the effect of sperm and induced autoimmune disease on the generation and course of MAIDS. Disease was induced in male C57Bl/6, B10A, ATL and ATH mice by infection with viruses. Allogeneic sperm cells were injected intravenously prior to and following the viral inoculation. Experimental systemic lupus erythematodes (SLE)-like disease was induced by a human monoclonal anti-DNA antibody (16/6) in Balb/c mice, which were inoculated a month later with the virus. Marked suppression of splenocyte proliferation to mitogen and mild splenomegaly were observed following sperm injections. Sperm significantly enhanced the induction of MAIDS by the virus only in the sensitive strain of mice (C57Bl/6), when animals were infected with a low dose of the virus. Mice injected with the 16/6 antibody and virus expressed enhanced serum IgG, anti-single-stranded DNA, anti-anti-16/6 levels and splenomegaly compared with the 16/6 or virus only injected mice. These results suggest that immunomodulation by sperm and probably by autoimmunity may influence the course of MAIDS and may have direct relevance to their role in the pathogenesis of human AIDS.

## Introduction

The murine acquired immunodeficiency syndrome (MAIDS) is an acute retroviral infection of C57Bl/6 mice characterized by lymphadenopathy, hypergammaglobulinemia, severe immunodeficiency, enhanced susceptibility to infection, and the development of terminal B cell lymphomas (Mosier et al., 1985, 1987; Mosier, 1986; Klinken et al., 1988; Yetter et al., 1988; Klinman and Morse, 1989). The agent that induces the disease is a variable mixtures of C-type B-tropic retroviruses, including ecotropic and mink cell focus-inducing (MCF) murine leukemia viruses (MuLVs) (Pattengale et al., Mosier et al., 1985). This syndrome in mice has many similarities to human AIDS (Lane and Fauci, 1985; Fauci, 1988), particularly to the early stages of the disease, and may thus serve as a useful model for studying the role of various cofactors in the pathogenesis of the disease. As with any infectious disease, it is clear that both the etiologic agent and the host factors determine the outcome of infection and course of the disease. We ourselves have been particularly interested in the role of immune cofactors in human immunodeficiency virus (HIV) infection since we have found that several immune impairments may precede the exposure to HIV and may probably account for the increased susceptibility of all risk groups to HIV infection and AIDS (Bentwich et al., 1987; Sears et al., 1987).

Human spermatozoa and seminal plasma fractions have been shown to inhibit the in vitro proliferation responses of human peripheral blood leukocytes to mitogens (Marcus et al., 1978). Similarly in the mouse, testicular cell suspensions inhibit proliferative responses in vitro (Hurtenbach et al., 1980). Furthermore, it has been shown that a single intravenous injection of syngeneic or allogeneic sperm into mice induced a profound and long-lasting immunosuppression of cellular immune function (Hurtenbach and Shearer, 1982). These observations could possibly have relevance to the increased susceptibility of male homosexuals to HIV infection.

The possibility that autoimmune processes may play an important role in the development and severity of AIDS has also been raised before (Mosier, 1986). Thus, by using an animal model of autoimmune disease the interaction of a retroviral-induced disease with a concomitantly induced autoimmune disease could be explored. An experimental autoimmune disease meeting these requirements could be the one recently reported by Mendelovic et al. (1988) in which induction of experimental systemic lupus erythematodes (SLE) was achieved by immunizing mice with a human monoclonal anti-DNA antibody termed 16/6.

In the present study we have used the murine experimental model of AIDS (MAIDS) to study the effects of immunomodulation caused by either sperm or induction of autoimmunity, on the susceptibility and natural course of the disease.

## Materials and methods

### Mice

Adult male C57Bl/6, ATH, ATL, B10A and female Balb/c mice were obtained from the Jackson Laboratory and were used at the age of 3–6 months.

### Virus

The Laterjet-Duplan isolate (kindly given to us by Dr. N. Haran-Gera, The Weizmann Institute of Science, Rehovot, Israel) and the LP-BM5 MuLV, a freshly thawed suspension of cell free supernatant from the established cell line LP-BM5 Sc-1 (Buller et al., 1987) (kindly given to us by Dr. Morse, NIH, Bethesda, MD, U.S.A.) were used. Volumes of 0.15–0.3 ml of virus suspension were injected intraperitoneally (i.p).

### Sperm

Sperm cells were obtained from the epididymis and vas deferens of 6 month old or older allogeneic strains of mice. The cells were washed and resuspended in phosphate-buffered saline (PBS) at room temperature. $1-2 \times 10^7$ sperm were injected intravenously (i.v.) into the tail vein once or several times at intervals of 10–14 days.

SLE-like disease was induced by the 16/6 antigen which was precipitated from hybridoma culture medium and affinity purified as described (Buller et al., 1987). Blood was collected from all the animals at 3–4 week intervals.

### Immunological assays

Lymphocyte proliferation was determined by plating $2 \times 10^5$ spleen cells in 0.1 ml RPMI 1640 HEPES medium enriched with 5% fetal calf serum, 2 mM glutamine and antibiotics in wells of microtiter plates. Concanavalin A (con A) (0.5, 1, 4 $\mu$g/ml), phytohemagglutinin (PHA-P) (2, 4, 8, 16 $\mu$g/ml) and lipopolysaccharide (LPS) (1, 2, 4, 8 $\mu$g/ml) were added in 0.1 ml volumes into the wells. At the end of 72 h culture the cells were pulsed with [$^3$H]thymidine and harvested. Response was expressed as the stimulation index (SI). Serum immunoglobulin (Ig) levels were determined by enzyme-linked immunosorbent assay (ELISA). Flat bottomed polystyrene plates (Dynatech, Alexandria, VA, U.S.A.) were coated with anti-mouse IgG or IgM (BioMakor, Israel) followed by incubation with the test sera and developing the reaction with alkaline phosphatase-conjugated anti-mouse IgG (BioMakor) or IgM (Sigma, U.S.A.) and Sigma 104 phosphatase substrate. Serum antibodies were determined by antigen specific radioimmunoassay. Flexible plastic microtiter plates were coated with 50 $\mu$l of antigen at 50–100 $\mu$g/ml dissolved in PBS. After 2 h incubation the plates were washed with PBS containing 0.5% bovine serum albumin. Sera diluted 1 : 10–1:1000 were then added and incubated for 4 h. $^{125}$I-labeled goat anti-mouse immunoglobulin ($10^5$ cpm/well) was added to detect bound antibodies using the $\gamma$-counter.

### Histopathology

Samples of spleen, lymph nodes, lungs, liver, thymus and kidney were fixed in Bouin solution, sectioned and stained with hematoxylin and light green.

## Results

### Effects of sperm on the immune system

To verify the immunosuppressive effects of allogeneic sperm, the proliferative responses of spleen cells from mice injected once with $2 \times 10^7$ sperm cells were tested. As shown in Fig. 1, splenocytes obtained from mice of different strains (C57Bl/6, ATH and ATL) showed markedly decreased responses to con A, PHA and LPS 50 days following the injection.

### Effects of sperm immunization on MAIDS

Using the Laterjet-Duplan isolate at first, we found that all C57Bl/6 mice injected with either the virus alone or sperm, 1 month prior to the virus, developed the disease 5–6 months after the infection. In the ATL and ATH resistant mice as well as in the partially resistant B10A strain, sperm injection did not increase the low incidence of the disease (Table 1).

Looking at Ig levels in the sera of the infected animals it was obvious that all C57Bl/6 mice had increased levels which declined with the progression of the disease. However, as shown in Fig. 2, the Ig levels were consistently and significantly higher in mice which were preimmunized with sperm 1 month before virus inoculation. Using LP-BM5 MuLV supernatants, all infected C57Bl/6 mice developed the disease within 1–3 months. Using small volumes of virus preparation (calibrated in preliminary experiments) ensured a slow progress of MAIDS. Such mice were preimmunized with sperm three times before infection and twice

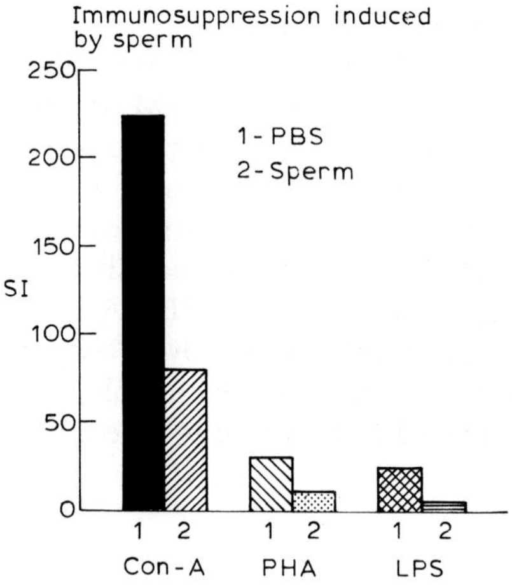


Fig. 1. C57Bl/6, ATL and ATH mice (two of each strain) were injected i.v. with either $1 \times 10^7$ allogeneic sperm cells or PBS. 50 days later the stimulation indices (SI) of their spleen cells to mitogens were determined in a proliferation assay.

TABLE 1
Effect of sperm on MAIDS induction in different strains

| Experiment | Strain | Treatment | Age at inoculation (months) | Spleen weight (mg) [a] | Incidence of splenomegaly [b] |
|---|---|---|---|---|---|
| 1 | C57Bl/6 | Virus | 3 | 200 ± 29 | 5/5 |
| | | Sperm and virus | 3 | 223 ± 11 | 4/4 |
| | ATL and ATH | Virus | 7 | 172 ± 162 | 3/11 |
| | | Sperm and virus | 7 | 125 ± 86 | 2/10 |
| 2 | C57Bl/6 | Virus | 6 | 140 ± 29 | 3/5 |
| | | Sperm and virus | 6 | 236 ± 231 | 3/5 |
| | B10A | Virus | 6 | 110 ± 16 | 1/8 |
| | | Sperm and virus | 6 | 107 ± 20 | 0/9 |

[a] Mean ± SD.
[b] Spleen weight > 130, no. of mice/no. observed.

more thereafter. Animals were killed at intervals of 3 weeks for gross and histopathological observations. As can be seen in Table 2, splenomegaly (an indicator of MAIDS induction) was observed by 12 weeks post infection only in mice which were preimmunized with sperm (5/13) and not at all in mice infected with virus alone (0/14). In animals injected with sperm alone some degree of splenomegaly was also observed a few weeks after sperm injection. By 18 weeks post infection splenomegaly was observed in four additional mice: two virus

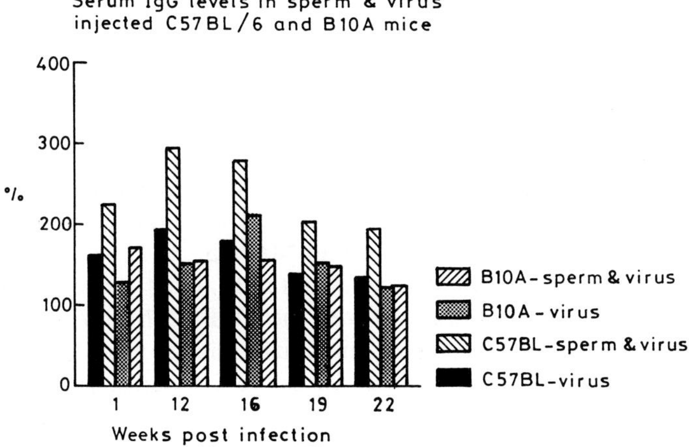


Fig. 2. C57Bl/6 and B10A male mice were injected i.v. with $1 \times 10^7$ allogeneic sperm cells and infected 1 month later with the Laterjet-Duplan isolate MuLV. The results are the mean IgG levels of five or more mice per group expressed as % of IgG levels in age and sex matched untreated animals.

TABLE 2
Development of MAIDS in sperm immunized C57Bl/6 mice infected with LP-BM5 MuLV

| Treatment | Weeks post inoculation | Spleen weight (mg) [a] | Incidence of splenomegaly [b] |
|---|---|---|---|
| LP-BM5 | 3 | 99 ± 6 | 0/4 |
| | 6 | 113 ± 11 | 0/3 |
| | 9 | 120 ± 17 | 0/3 |
| | 12 | 95 ± 6 | 0/4 |
| | 18 | 149 ± 81 | 2/5 |
| Sperm and LP-BM5[c] | 3 | 150 ± 87 | 1/3 |
| | 6 | 226 ± 228 | 1/3 |
| | 9 | 160 ± 58 | 2/3 |
| | 12 | 132 ± 34 | 1/4 |
| | 18 | 303 ± 467 | 2/6 |

[a] Mean ± SD
[b] Spleen weight > 130 mg.
[c] Sperm cells (1–2 × $10^7$) were injected intravenously 5 times at 2 week interval. LP-BM5 was inoculated a week after the third sperm injection.

injected animals (spleen weights 140 and 290 mg) and two sperm and virus injected animals (spleen weights 145 and 1250 mg).

On histopathological examination of the enlarged spleens of LP-BM5 infected mice, advanced disease as defined by Hurtley et al. (1989) was observed only in two animals injected with both sperm and virus while in the other spleens only marked reactive germinal center hyperplasia was seen. The splenomegaly of sperm injected animals was mainly due to red pulp hyperplasia, while a state of red pulp aplasia was prominent in the spleens of such animals examined after a longer interval following sperm injection.

## The interaction of autoimmune disease and LP-BM5 MuLV

Since experimental SLE has been found to be genetically controlled, we used the Balb/c strain that is sensitive to SLE induction but at the same time resistant to MAIDS. Thus we could determine if induction of the autoimmune disease would be able to overcome the resistance to MAIDS.

Female Balb/c mice were immunized with the 16/6 antigen and a month after the boost the animals were inoculated with the LP-BM5 MuLV. Elevated serum Ig levels were observed in all the 16/6 immunized mice as recorded a month after the boost and remained above normal for up to 5 months. However, the IgG levels of mice receiving both the 16/6 and the LP-BM5 MuLV were significantly higher (Fig. 3). The levels of specific antibodies to single-stranded (ss) DNA and to anti-16/6 were similarly affected, being highest in mice injected with 16/6 and LP-BM5 MuLV. The levels of specific antibodies decreased by 28 weeks after the boost almost to normal except in the mice that were also infected by the virus. Mice were killed at 5 and 8 months post virus inoculation. In mice injected with

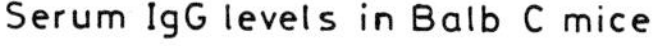


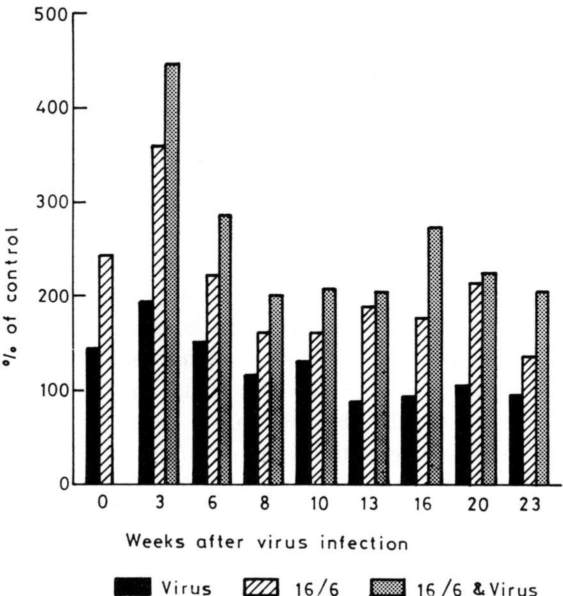


Fig. 3. Balb/c female mice were immunized with the 16/6 antigen and a month after the boost were infected with the LP-BM5 MuLV. The results are the mean IgG levels of at least 10 mice per group expressed as % of IgG levels in age and sex matched untreated animals.

both the 16/6 and the virus, splenomegaly (spleen weight > 130 mg) was found in 8/15 animals whereas in the 16/6 or virus injected animal groups, 5/14 and 2/10 respectively, showed enlarged spleens. This can also be seen in comparing mean spleen weights between these groups (Table 3). On histopathological examination of these enlarged spleens, reactive germinal center hyperplasia was observed mostly in the virus and 16/6 injected group.

TABLE 3

Spleen weight of Balb/c mice immunized with the 16/6 antigen and/or infected with LP-BM5

| Treatment | Mean spleen weight (mg) ± SD<br>Months post virus infection | |
|---|---|---|
| | 5 | 8 |
| None | | 135 ± 29 (5) [a] |
| 16/6 | 118 ± 16 (5) | 123 ± 14 (9) |
| LP-BM5 | 110 ± 26 (5) | 118 ± 20 (6) |
| 16/6 and LP-BM5 | 117 ± 16 (5) | 162 ± 50 (10) |

[a] In parentheses, number of animals.

## Discussion

The role of the host immune system vis-a-vis the role of the viral agent in AIDS is a crucial question which cannot be studied freely and easily in humans and requires an animal model. Furthermore, it is extremely difficult in the human setting to draw the distinction between the possible effect of semen and its different components as immunosuppressive agents "preparing" the ground for several infections and the possible role, especially of sperm, as a vector for virus transmission (Bagasra et al., 1988; Lavitrano et al., 1989).

The MAIDS syndrome in mice (although caused by a C-type retrovirus that is not the causal agent of AIDS) shows striking similarities to the human disease (Lane and Fauci, 1985; Fauci, 1988). It may thus serve as a useful model for studying the role of various cofactors in the pathogenesis of the disease.

In the present study we have tested the immunomodulating effects of sperm cells on the natural course of MAIDS. We first confirmed he observations of Hurtenbach and Shearer (1982), showing that a single intravenous injection of allogeneic sperm causes a long-lasting immunosuppression in various strains of mice. We were then able to show that in the highly MAIDS sensitive C57BL/6 mice, repeated immunization with sperm rendered the mice much more susceptible to the development of MAIDS. This was seen when small doses of virus were used, which in themselves were not sufficient to cause the disease by 3 months post infection, but in combination with sperm generated the disease in 40% (5/13) of the animals. However, a single sperm immunization was not strong enough to overcome the genetic resistance to MAIDS in the resistant strain of mice. The mechanism by which the sperm enhances the virus influence and the relation between this effect and the profound immunosuppression caused by sperm injection are the subjects of ongoing studies in our group.

As has been described (Mosier et al., 1985; Klinman and Morse, 1989), the early stage in MAIDS development is a polyclonal B cell proliferation. A similar process characterizes the early stage in the majority of AIDS cases (Fauci, 1988). Though the causes of such proliferation are as yet poorly understood, it is quite possible that autoimmune processes are operative at this stage and that they could play a major role in the further development of the disease. The interaction of autoimmune processes and retroviral infection was assayed in Balb/c mice, which are resistant to LP-BM5 MuLV. The results so far clearly indicate that such an interaction does exist. While virus infection alone did not affect the animals the combination with the SLE-like induced disease significantly enhanced the Ig secretion, including the generation of specific antibodies. Though splenomegaly was enhanced, no lymphadenopathy was observed 8 months post infection and clear MAIDS has not developed. These results may indicate that there is an interaction between the reaction to the retrovirus and the 16/6 monoclonal antibody. However, these interactions have yet to be further studied and confirmed before final conclusions can be reached.

## References


Bagasra, O., Freund, M., Weidmann, J. and Harley, G. (1988) Interaction of human immunodeficiency virus with human sperm in vitro. *J. AIDS* 1, 431–435.

Bentwich, Z., Saxinger, C., Ben-Ishai, Z., Burstein, R., Berner, Y., Pecht, M., Tranin, N., Levin, S. and Handzel, Z.T. (1987) Immune impairments and antibodies to HTLV-III/LAV in asymptomatic male homosexuals in Israel: relevance to risk of AIDS. *J. Clin. Immunol.* 7, 376–380.

Buller, R.M.L., Yetter, R.A., Fredrikson, T.N. and Morse, H.C. III (1987) Abrogation of resistance to severe mousepox in C57BL/6 mice infected with LP-BM5 murine leukemia viruses. *J. Virol.* 61, 383–387.

Fauci, A.S. (1988) The human immunodeficiency virus: infectivity and mechanisms of pathogenesis. *Science* 239, 617–621.

Hartley, J.W., Fredrikson, T.N., Yetter, R.A., Makino, M. and Morse, H.C. III (1989) Retrovirus-induced murine acquired immunodeficiency syndrome: natural history of infection and differing susceptibility of inbred mouse strains. *J. Virol.* 63, 1223–1231.

Hurtenbach, U. and Shearer, G.M. (1982) Germ cell induced immune suppression in mice. Effect of inoculation of syngeneic spermatozoa on cell-mediated immune responses. *J. Exp. Med.* 155, 1719–1729.

Hurtenbach, U., Morgenstern, F. and Bennett, D. (1980) Induction of tolerance in vitro by autologous murine testicular cells. *J. Exp. Med.* 151, 827.

Klinken, P.S., Fredrikson, T.N., Hartley, J.W., Yetter, R.A. and Morse, H.C. III, (1988) Evolution of B cell lineage lymphomas in mice with a retrovirus-induced immunodeficiency syndrome, MAIDS. *J. Immunol.* 140, 1123–1131.

Klinman, D.M. and Morse, H.C. III, (1989) Characteristics of B cell proliferation and activation in murine AIDS. *J. Immunol.* 142, 1144–1149.

Lane, H.C. and Fauci, A.S. (1985) Immunological abnormalities in the acquired immunodeficiency syndrome. *Annu. Rev. Immunol.* 3, 477.

Lavitrano, M., Camaioni, A., Fazio, V.M., Dolci, S., Farace, M.G. and Spadafora, C. (1989) Sperm cells as vectors for introducing foreign DNA into eggs: genetic transformation of mice. *Cell* 57, 717–723.

Marcus, Z.H., Freishman, I.H., Houk, J.L., Herman, J.H. and Hess, E.V. (1978) In vitro studies in reproductive immunology. 1. Suppression of cell mediated immune response by human spermatozoa and fractions isolated from human seminal plasma. *Clin. Immunol. Immunopathol.* 9, 318.

Mendelovic, S., Brocke, S., Shoenfeld, J., Ben-Bassat, M., Meshorer, A., Bakimer, R. and Mozes, E. (1988) Induction of systemic lupus erythematosus-like disease in mice by a common human anti-DNA idiotype. *Proc. Natl. Acad. Sci. U.S.A.* 85, 2260–2264.

Mosier, D.E. (1986) Animal models for retrovirus-induced immunodeficiency disease. *Immunol. Invest.* 15, 233–261.

Mosier, D.E., Yetter, R.A. and Morse, H.C. III (1985) Retroviral induction of acute lymphoproliferative disease and profound immunosuppression in adult C57BL/6 mice. *J. Exp. Med.* 161, 766–784.

Mosier, D.E., Yetter, R.A. and Morse, H.C. III (1987) Functional T lymphocytes are required for a murine retrovirus-induced immunodeficiency disease (MAIDS). *J. Exp. Med.* 165, 1737–1742.

Pattengale, P.D., Taylor, C.R., Twomey, S., Hill, S., Jonasson, J., Beardsley, T. and Hass, M. (1982) Immunopathology of B cell lymphomas induced in C57BL/6 mice by dualtropic murine leukemia virus (MuLV). *Am. J. Pathol.* 107, 362–377.

Sears, S.D., Fox, R., Brookmeyer, R., Leavitt, R. and Polk, F.B. (1987) Delayed hypersensitivity skin testing and anergy in a population of gay men. *Clin. Immunol. Immunopathol.* 45, 177–183.

Yetter, R.A., Buller, R.M.L., Lee, J.S., Elkins, K.L., Mosier, D.E., Fredrickson, T.N. and Morse, H.C. III (1988) CD4+ T cells are required for development of a murine retrovirus-induced immunodeficiency syndrome, MAIDS. *J. Exp. Med.* 168, 623–635.

# *Outlook*

*Eds. H. Schellekens and M.C. Horzinek*
*Animal Models in AIDS*



# 35

# Perspectives for the chemotherapy of AIDS

E. DE CLERCQ

Rega Institute for Medical Research, Katholieke Universiteit Leuven, B-3000 Leuven, Belgium

## Introduction

The identification of a human retrovirus, HIV (human immunodeficiency virus), as the etiologic agent of acquired immunodeficiency syndrome (AIDS) has prompted the search for inhibitors of HIV replication. To the extent that HIV replication is involved in both the initiation and progression of the disease, one may expect that those compounds that inhibit the replicative cycle of HIV also suppress the pathogenesis of AIDS and its clinical manifestations. Based on this premise, suramin was the first anti-HIV agent to be used in the treatment of AIDS. Suramin had been recognized as a potent inhibitor of retrovirus-associated reverse transcriptase (De Clercq, 1979), which led Mitsuya and his coworkers (1984) to evaluate its inhibitory effect on the infectivity of HIV in vitro. The compound proved inhibitory to the cytopathic effect of HIV at drug concentrations which were not toxic to the host cells (Mitsuya et al., 1984), and this observation has been confirmed in several cell systems (Balzarini et al., 1986a; Baba et al., 1988a). Suramin was also the first anti-HIV agent found to be capable of inhibiting HIV replication in AIDS patients (Broder et al., 1985). However, a short-term (6-week) treatment course with suramin did not lead to either clinical or immunological improvement (Broder et al., 1985), and, upon prolonged treatment, suramin proved rather toxic (Kaplan et al., 1987), so that its use as single-agent therapy for AIDS is not recommended.

Shortly after suramin, 3′-azido-2′,3′-dideoxythymidine (azidothymidine, AzddThd, AZT) was discovered as a selective anti-HIV agent (Mitsuya et al., 1985), and, as AZT appeared to be superior to suramin in both potency and selectivity, it was promptly introduced in the clinic (Yarchoan et al., 1986). A short-term (6-week) treatment of AIDS patients with AZT led to clinical, virological and immunological improvement (Yarchoan et al., 1986) and, consequently, AZT was submitted to a double-blind, placebo-controlled trial, which, in turn, indicated that following a 24-week treatment period with AZT, there was a significant decrease (delay) in mortality and reduction in the frequency of opportunistic infections (Fischl et al., 1987). However, the long-term administration of AZT is associated with severe toxicity, in particular bone marrow suppression (anemia, leukopenia) (Richman et al., 1987), and the initial immunological improvement, i.e., increase in CD4 + cells after the first few weeks of AZT therapy, appears to be transient (Dournon et al., 1988): by 6 months of AZT therapy, CD4 + cell counts have returned to their pretreatment levels and decline further despite continued AZT treatment. The immunologic deterioration of AIDS patients while on AZT therapy may be attributed to various factors: accruing toxicity of the compound for the hemopoietic system, intrinsic inability of AZT to prevent CD4 + cell destruction, and emergence of drug-resistant HIV variants (Larder et al., 1989).

Further search for effective inhibitors of HIV replication has led to the discovery of a variety of 2′,3′-dideoxynucleosides (i.e., 2′,3′-dideoxycytidine (ddCyd), 2′,3′-dideoxyinosine (ddIno) (Mitsuya and Broder, 1986)), 2′,3′-didehydro-2′,3′-dideoxynucleosides (i.e., 2′,3′-didehydro-2′,3′-dideoxycytidine (d4Cyd), 2′,3′-didehydro-2′,3′-dideoxythymidine (d4Thd) (Balzarini et al., 1986b; Baba et al., 1987a; Lin et al., 1987a,b; Hamamoto et al., 1987)), 3′-fluoro-2′,3′-dideoxynucleosides (i.e., 3′-fluoro-2′,3′-dideoxythymidine (FddThd), 3′-fluoro-2′,3′-dideoxy-5-chlorouridine (FddClUrd) (Herdewijn et al., 1987; Balzarini et al., 1988a, 1989a; Bazin et al., 1989; Van Aerschot et al., 1989)) and various 3′-azido-2′,3′-dideoxynucleosides other than AZT (i.e. 3′-azido-2′,3′-dideoxyuridine (AzddUrd), 3′-azido-2′,3′-dideoxy-5-chlorouridine (AzddClUrd) and 3′-azido-2′,3′-dideoxy-2,6-diaminopurineriboside (AzddDAPR) (Balzarini et al., 1988b, 1989b; Robins et al., 1989)). Some of these compounds, i.e. ddCyd (Yarchoan et al., 1988) and ddIno (Yarchoan et al., 1989), have already been submitted to clinical trials. Treatment with ddCyd (for up to 15 weeks) and ddIno (for up to 42 weeks) leads to an improvement of both the immunological (increase in CD4 + cell counts) and virological (decrease in viral p24 antigen levels) parameters. However, the clinical usefulness of ddCyd is limited by peripheral neuropathy, while for ddIno the dose-limiting toxicity still needs to be defined.

Although steady progress has been made in the search for effective chemotherapeutic means against AIDS, it is obvious that our efforts must be continued and even intensified, if we want to prevent initiation or suppress progression of the disease in the patient. To this end, several strategies could be envisaged. They are based on the different targets in the virus replicative cycle with which anti-HIV agents could interact. In addition to the reverse transcriptase, which serves as target for the 2′,3′-dideoxynucleoside analogues, various other targets could serve as sites of chemotherapeutic attack: adsorption of the virus particle to the cell membrane, uncoating of the viral capsid, integration of the proviral DNA into the cellular genome, processing of the viral precursor proteins, and assembly and release ("budding") of the viral progeny particles. Those compounds that interact at different targets may show synergistic activity when combined, and even those compounds that interact with the same target enzyme (i.e., reverse transcriptase) but differ in pharmacological or toxicological behavior may profit from combined or alternating use, and such procedures, while maintaining efficacy, may allow reducing the drug dosage, thus diminishing toxicity.

## Reverse transcriptase inhibitors

AZT, ddCyd and all other 2′,3′-dideoxynucleoside analogues are assumed to be targeted at the reverse transcriptase step where they can act in a dual fashion, that is as either competitive inhibitors with respect to the natural substrates (dTTP, dCTP, dATP, dGTP) or alternate substrates thus leading to the premature termination of the growing DNA chain (Furman et al., 1986; St. Clair et al., 1987). Both processes lead to the shut-off of viral DNA synthesis, but it is not clear which of the two processes is the more important. Whatever the precise mechanism by which 2′,3′-dideoxynucleosides inhibit retroviral DNA synthesis, the 2′,3′-dideoxynucleoside 5′-triphosphates exhibit a much greater affinity for the viral reverse transcriptase than for cellular DNA polymerases $\alpha$ or $\beta$ (Matthes et al., 1987). This differential affinity may obviously contribute to the selectivity of the 2′,3′-dideoxynucleoside analogues as anti-HIV agents, but of equal, if not greater, importance may be the rate and extent by which the 2′,3′-dideoxynucleosides are phosphorylated intracellularly to their 5′-triphosphates (Hao et al., 1988; Balzarini et al., 1989c).

In view of the shortcomings of AZT in the clinical setting (see Introduction), any new candidate anti-AIDS drug that wants to outweigh AZT has to be less toxic and/or more potent; it should be well tolerated, sustain increased CD4 + cell counts and retain activity against AZT-resistant virus mutants (should the latter be responsible for the clinical failure of AZT, which remains to be established). Very few 2′,3′-dideoxynucleoside analogues equal or approach AZT in potency against HIV in vitro (De Clercq, 1989a), and those that do so (for example, FddThd, now also referred to as FLT) are more toxic than AZT, thus achieving a lower selectivity index (Balzarini et al., 1988a). At the other extreme are those 2′,3′-dideoxynucleoside analogues (i.e., d4Thd, FddClUrd) that, while less potent, are much less toxic than AZT. These compounds are also less toxic to the bone marrow, which is the dose-limiting factor in the clinical use of AZT.

The precise reason(s) for the pronounced toxicity of AZT for the bone marrow (Dainiak et al., 1988) have not been elucidated. This myelotoxicity may be related to several factors. A peculiar feature of AZT is that it leads to an accumulation of its 5′-monophosphate (AZT-MP) in cells that have been exposed to the drug. AZT-MP accumulates because it is a potent inhibitor of the enzyme (dTMP kinase) that is needed for its further phosphorylation to AZT-DP. The inhibitory effect of AZT-MP on dTMP kinase also results in an interruption of the dThd salvage pathway, a reduction in the supply of dTTP, and an inhibition of host cell DNA synthesis. Compounds such as FddClUrd and d4Thd are not accumulated in their 5′-monophosphate form. These compounds are virtually not inhibitory to cellular DNA synthesis, and much less toxic to the host cells than AZT. To the extent that inhibition of dTMP kinase is causally related to inhibition of host cell DNA synthesis, accumulation of the 2′,3′-dideoxynucleoside 5′-monophosphate forms may be considered a biochemical parameter of toxicity. It follows that those 2′,3′-dideoxynucleoside analogues that do not inhibit dTMP kinase (and do not accumulate as their 5′-monophosphate forms) may be therapeutically advantageous because of their lesser cytotoxicity.

The emergence of drug-resistant HIV mutants following long-term treatment of AIDS patients with AZT is an important issue that has recently attracted much attention. Larder et al. (1989) described such HIV variants exhibiting decreased sensitivity to AZT. Attempts to obtain AZT-resistant HIV mutants in vitro, i.e., through repeated passage of the virus in the presence of the drug, have not proved successful. Also, the molecular basis of the diminished sensitivity to AZT of the clinical HIV isolates has not been elucidated (Larder et al., 1989). If, however, AZT owes its selective anti-HIV activity to a specific interaction with the viral reverse transcriptase, and if virus resistance to the drug develops, it has to be located at the reverse transcriptase level. Interestingly, the HIV variants that showed diminished sensitivity to AZT also showed reduced susceptibility to AzddUrd, but not d4Thd or ddCyd. This means that, should AZT-resistant HIV strains become a clinical problem, AIDS patients could be effectively treated with other drugs against which the virus has not (yet) developed resistance.

In addition to the 2′,3′-dideoxynucleoside analogues, various acyclic and carbocyclic nucleoside analogues have been described which hold great promise for the treatment of retrovirus infections. Of the carbocyclic derivatives, carbovir (carbocyclic 2′,3′-didehydro-2′,3′-dideoxyguanosine) (Vince et al., 1988) is currently under investigation as a candidate anti-AIDS drug. Among the acyclic nucleoside analogues, adenallene, cytallene (Hayashi et al., 1988) and in particular the phosphonylmethoxyalkyl derivatives PMEA (9-(2-phosphonylmethoxyethyl)adenine) and PMEDAP (9-(2-phosphonylmethoxyethyl)-2,6-diaminopurine) (Pauwels et al., 1988) have been most intensively pursued for their antiretroviral potential. PMEA is presumably targeted at the reverse transcriptase. The compound can as such be taken up by the cells, and then needs two phosphorylation steps (in contrast to all other nucleoside analogues, which require three phosphorylations) to be converted to its active form. PMEA is more efficacious than AZT in the treatment of murine retrovirus infection (Balzarini et al., 1989d). It is also effective in the treatment of simian immunodeficiency virus (SIV) and feline immunodeficiency virus (FIV) infection in monkeys and cats, respectively. A particularly attractive feature of the phosphonylmethoxyethylpurines (PMEA, PMEDAP, etc.) is that they are active against both retroviruses and herpesviruses, which implies that they may be useful in the treatment of both opportunistic herpesvirus infections and the underlying retroviral disease. In fact, experiments with PMEA in the murine AIDS model (LP-BM5 virus-infected mice) have indicated that the drug is at least as efficient as AZT for the treatment of the retrovirus infection and at least as efficient as acyclovir for the treatment of herpes simplex virus infection (Gangemi et al., 1989).

**Inhibitors of virus adsorption**

HIV attachment to the cells requires a specific interaction between the viral glycoprotein gp120 and the host cell CD4 receptor. As a rule, it may be stated that only those cells that contain the CD4 receptor can be infected by HIV. Hence, the gp120-CD4 interaction may be viewed as an attractive target for therapeutic intervention. Any molecules that inhibit this interaction may be expected to block HIV infection at the earliest possible event of the virus replicative cycle, that is the virus adsorption step.

A first class of substances that suppress HIV infectivity through interference with the virus adsorption step are the soluble CD4 derivatives (Smith et al., 1987; Deen et al., 1988; Fisher et al., 1988; Hussey et al., 1988; Traunecker et al., 1988). These molecules can be engineered, i.e., shortened to those peptide fragments that are involved in the binding of gp120 (Lifson et al., 1988) or fused to immunoglobulin portions so as to increase their half-life in the organism (Capon et al., 1989; Traunecker et al., 1989). Soluble CD4 could also be used as a vector for toxins such as ricin (Till et al., 1988). Such ricin-CD4 conjugates may be expected to specifically deliver their toxin to those cells that express gp120 (i.e., cells that have been chronically infected with HIV), and, as a consequence, these cells may be specifically killed upon interaction with the ricin-CD4 conjugates (Till et al., 1988). The therapeutic value of the CD4 derivatives is currently under scrutiny. A general concern applying to all CD4 derivatives is that, in addition to their effects on virus and virus-infected cells, they may also interfere with the natural immunoresponses involving the CD4 ligand, and, hence, exert immunosuppressive effects in vivo. In vitro, soluble CD4 does not appear to inhibit human peripheral blood lymphocyte (PBL) responses to various antigenic stimuli, but this observation is not predictive of what may happen in vivo upon prolonged therapeutic use of CD4 or its derivatives.

A second class of compounds whose anti-HIV activity at least partially resides in the inhibition of virus binding to the cells are the polyanionic compounds represented by suramin, Evans blue, aurintricarboxylic acid, fuchsin acid and glycyrrhizinic acid (De Clercq, 1989a). These compounds may actually act at more than one site of the virus replicative cycle: reverse transcription, protein synthesis, protein kinase C activity (Ito et al., 1988) and virus binding to the cells (Schols et al., 1989a). Aurintricarboxylic acid (ATA) inhibits virus binding to the cells because it specifically interacts with the CD4 receptor (Schols et al., 1989b). This specific affinity of ATA for the CD4 receptor has been recognized based on the use of different monoclonal antibodies (mAb) to cell surface antigens: the anti-CD4 mAb OKT4A/leu-3a is the only monoclonal antibody that ATA competes with. This points to the specificity of its interaction with the CD4 receptor. Thus, ATA can be considered a selective marker for the CD4 receptor and represents a new lead in the development of selective anti-HIV agents.

The third class of compounds that specifically interfere with the virus adsorption process are the sulfated polysaccharides, or sulfated polymers in general. This group contains a number of compounds, i.e., heparin, dextran sulfate (De

Clercq, 1989b), pentosan polysulfate (Baba et al., 1988b; Biesert et al., 1988), λ-, κ-, ι-carrageenans (Baba et al., 1988b), mannan sulfate (Ito et al., 1989), lentinan sulfate (Yoshida et al., 1988), "supersulfated" chondroitin sulfate (Jurkiewicz et al., 1989), sulfated bacterial glycosaminoglycan (Baba et al., 1990a), periodate-treated heparin (Baba et al., 1990a), sulfated polyvinyl alcohol (PVAS) and sulfated co-polymers of acrylic acid with vinyl alcohol (PAVAS) (Baba et al., 1990b), that inhibit HIV replication in vitro at concentrations far below the cytotoxicity threshold. While exquisitely selective as inhibitors of HIV replication in vitro, it is as yet unclear whether these compounds are also effective against HIV replication in vivo. The sole clinical study that has so far been conducted with dextran sulfate (Abrams et al., 1989) did not reveal much benefit, but in this trial dextran sulfate was administered orally, and this is not the ideal route for compounds that are assumed to be poorly absorbed from the gut.

The mechanism of action of the sulfated polysaccharides has been well established. The compounds block virus adsorption to the cells, as has been demonstrated with several techniques using radiolabeled virus particles (Baba et al., 1988c; Mitsuya et al., 1988), a flow cytometric method (Schols et al., 1989a) and a radioimmunoassay (Nakashima et al., 1989). The dose-response curve for inhibition of virus replication by dextran sulfate is virtually identical to its dose-response curve for inhibition of virus adsorption (Schols et al., 1989a). Sulfated polysaccharides are also inhibitory to the reverse transcriptase, but it is unlikely that this effect plays an important role in the anti-HIV activity of the compounds, first because this inhibitory effect is noted only at concentrations that are in excess of those required to inhibit virus binding to the cells, and second, if inhibition of reverse transcriptase were to play a role, it means that the compounds must be taken up by the cells (and be able to reach their target enzyme), and this has not been clearly demonstrated.

Sulfated polysaccharides, and in particular heparin, are used in the clinic to prevent blood coagulation, and hence the question arises whether their usefulness as anti-HIV agents may be endangered by their anticoagulant properties. This anticoagulant activity should not be too great a concern, since all sulfated polysaccharides, including heparin, are active against HIV at concentrations which are well below the anticoagulant threshold (1 heparin unit) (Baba et al., 1988b) and through the appropriate chemical modifications (i.e., following periodate treatment) heparin derivatives can be generated that have virtually lost their anticoagulant (antithrombin) activity, yet remain fully active against HIV (Baba et al., 1990a). Such sulfated polysaccharides would seem prime candidates for further exploration of their therapeutic potential in the treatment of AIDS.

A unique feature of the sulfated polysaccharides (and sulfated polymers in general) is their ability to interfere with giant cell (syncytium) formation, resulting from the fusion between HIV-infected and uninfected cells. Like virus attachment to the cells, this fusion process depends on a specific interaction between the viral gp120 (expressed by the HIV-infected cell) and the CD4 receptor of the uninfected cell. The role of this syncytium formation in the pathogenesis of AIDS has not been unequivocally proven. In vitro fusion of persistently HIV-infected (HUT-78) cells with uninfected CD4 + (Molt-4) cells is accompanied by a selective destruction of the CD4 + Molt-4 cells (Schols et al., 1989c). If this phenomenon also holds in vivo, the selective killing of the target (CD4 + ) cells by the aggressor (gp120 + ) cells may well be an important mechanism that leads to the depletion of CD4 + cells in AIDS patients.

As mentioned above, CD4 + cell counts (after an initial transient rise) progressively decline in AIDS patients while on, and despite of, AZT therapy. If this decrease in CD4 + cell counts indeed ensues from the fusion of persistently HIV-infected cells and uninfected cells, and concomitant destruction of the target CD4 + cells by the HIV-infected "killer" cells, any modalities that block this phenomenon may be of great therapeutic value. AZT is unable to protect the target CD4 + cells against the HIV-infected "killer" cells, and so are all other 2′,3′-dideoxynucleosides that are targeted at the reverse transcriptase. In contrast, the sulfated polysaccharides protect the CD4 + cells against destruction by the gp120 + cells (Baba et al., 1990c), and this protective activity is probably due to the "shielding off" effect of the sulfated polysaccharides on the gp120 glycoprotein (Schols et al., 1989d). Not all sulfated polysaccharides are equally effective in this regard: for example, pentosan polysulfate and dextran sulfate effectively protect the uninfected CD4 + cells against fusion with the HIV-infected cells, whereas heparin fails to do so (Baba et al., 1990c). PVAS and PAVAS have emerged as the most potent inhibitors of syncytium formation (Baba et al., 1990b). These compounds offer unique promise from a therapeutic viewpoint, if, as surmised, syncytium formation, and concomitant destruction of bystander CD4 + cells by persistently HIV-infected cells, plays an important role in the pathogenesis of AIDS.

## Other targets and compounds

In addition to the reverse transcription and virus adsorption step, various other events in the virus replicative cycle have been identified as attractive targets for therapeutic intervention, i.e. virus uncoating (Rossmann, 1988), proviral DNA integration, viral mRNA transcription and translation, and proteolysis and glycosylation of viral proteins (De Clercq, 1989c). In particular, the viral protease, which is autocatalytically cleaved from its (*gag-pol*) precursor protein and then processes the precursor *gag* and *pol* proteins into mature virion components, has received much attention as a target for protease inhibitors. The rationale behind such an approach is that an intact viral protease is required for the maturation of the viral particles and that, if the viral protease is made deficient, i.e., through site-directed mutagenesis, defective virions are formed which are no longer infectious (Kohl et al., 1988). The three-dimensional structure of the HIV-1 protease has been resolved (Navia et al., 1989; Weber et al., 1989), and this information should help in designing specific HIV-1 protease inhibitors. Notwithstanding the specificity of the HIV protease, it may prove a difficult task to develop protease inhibitors that interfere with the HIV protease in its natural habitat, and do so without any harmful effects on host cell proteins.

The development of glycosylation inhibitors as anti-HIV agents faces an even greater problem than that of protease inhibitors, since there are no specific viral enzymes involved in the glycosylation of viral proteins. Hence, the selectivity of glycosylation inhibitors as anti-HIV agents has to be based solely upon quantitative differences in the glycosylation requirements of viral versus cellular glycoproteins. The result of the interaction of glycosylation inhibitors may be similar to that of proteolysis inhibitors, that is the formation of defective virus particles which are no longer infectious. Also, glycosylation inhibitors may interfere with the expression of intact gp120 molecules by chronically HIV-infected cells, and, hence, prevent syncytium formation, and concomitant destruction of target CD4 + cells by HIV-infected aggressor cells. Foremost among the glycosylation inhibitors which have been pursued for their anti-retrovirus activity are castanospermine (Walker et al., 1987; Ruprecht et al., 1989) and *N*-butyldeoxynojirimycin (Fleet et al., 1988; Karpas et al., 1988), and clinical studies have been undertaken with the latter. Whether glycosylation inhibitors may have clinical utility is hard to predict. The compounds are relatively weak inhibitors of HIV replication, thus necessitating the administration of large doses, which, even if tolerated, do not seem practical in the long run.

Another interesting approach in the development of anti-HIV agents is based on the use of so-called "antisense" oligonucleotides, originally referred to as "hybridons" (Zamecnik and Stephenson, 1978). "Antisense" oligonucleotides are complementary to a well-defined portion of the viral genome, hybridize with these target sites and thus block transcription and/or translation of the viral RNA. Experimental evidence suggests that antisense oligodeoxynucleotides are indeed capable of blocking HIV replication in vitro (Zamecnik et al., 1986; Goodchild et al., 1988). Limiting factors in the use of such oligonucleotides are low cellular uptake and rapid degradation by nucleases. To overcome these problems, the phoshodiester linkages can be replaced by methylphosphonate, phosphorothioate or phosphoramidate groups. The resulting oligomers are then termed oligodeoxynucleoside methylphosphonates (Sarin et al., 1988), oligodeoxynucleoside phosphorothioates (Matsukura et al., 1987; Agrawal et al., 1988) and oligodeoxynucleoside phosphoramidates (Agrawal et al., 1988), respectively. As a target for antisense intervention, the regulatory gene, *rev,* of HIV-1 can be chosen, and an antisense oligonucleoside phosphorothioate against *rev* has been found to suppress viral expression in chronically HIV-1-infected T-cells (Matsukura et al., 1989). Sequence specificity and nuclease resistance appeared to be critical for this effect. Antisense molecules thus offer an interesting approach to the chemotherapy of AIDS. It is questionable, however, whether sufficient quantities of these materials could ever be made available to permit efficacy studies in vivo.

In addition to glycyrrhizinic acid (Ito et al., 1988), some other natural products such as the aromatic polycyclic diones hypericin and pseudohypericin (Meruelo et al., 1988) and GLQ223, a basic protein (MW 26,000) isolated from

*Trichosanthes kirilowii* (McGrath et al., 1989), have been described as inhibitors of HIV replication. How these compounds achieve their antiviral action and whether they offer any potential as anti-AIDS drugs is at present unclear. Various other compounds of widely varying structure (i.e. D-penicillamine, amphotericin B methyl ester, peptide T, avarol, avarone, papaverine, somatostatin, fusidic acid, xanthate D609, ansamycin LM 427, etc.) have been reported to inhibit HIV replication in some cell systems, but neither has their mode of anti-HIV action been elucidated nor has their anti-HIV activity been confirmed in other laboratories. In fact, initial clinical studies carried out with some of these compounds (i.e., fusidic acid (Youle et al., 1989), ansamycin LM 427 (Torseth et al., 1989)) failed to demonstrate any anti-retrovirus activity in vivo.

## Combination therapy

Combination therapy is a widely used procedure in the treatment of bacterial infections and malignancies, as it makes higher efficacy and/or lower toxicity possible than when the drugs are used individually; furthermore, it reduces the risk of emergence of drug-resistant microorganisms or cancer cells. Guided by these premises, one may also advocate combination therapy for AIDS. While anti-HIV drugs that interact in a similar fashion with the same target enzyme (i.e., reverse transcriptase) may be expected to show an additive effect when combined, synergism might occur when two drugs are combined that interact at different sites (i.e., reverse transcription and virus adsorption) of the virus replicative cycle. Several combinations of AZT plus other drugs have proved synergistic: for example, AZT with either PMEA (Smith et al., 1989), PFA (phosphonoformate) (Eriksson and Schinazi, 1989; Koshida et al., 1989), castanospermine (Johnson et al., 1989a), recombinant soluble CD4 (Johnson et al., 1989b), recombinant interferon-$\alpha$A (Hartshorn et al., 1987) or granulocyte-macrophage colony-stimulating factor (GM-CSF) (Hammer and Gillis, 1987); and some of these combinations, i.e., AZT plus GM-CSF, have been further explored in the clinic. There is, in fact, a rational basis for combining AZT with GM-CSF, since GM-CSF may be expected to restore the white blood cell counts that are depressed due to the myelotoxicity of AZT, and, moreover, GM-CSF has been shown to potentiate the anti-HIV activity of AZT in macrophages in vitro (Perno et al., 1989).

Not all combinations of AZT act synergistically, however. For example, ribavirin antagonizes the anti-HIV activity of AZT (Baba et al., 1987b; Vogt et al., 1987). Ribavirin also antagonizes the anti-HIV activity of other pyrimidine 2′,3′-dideoxyribosides (i.e., ddCyd, d4Cyd, d4Thd (Baba et al., 1987b)), but potentiates the anti-HIV activity of purine 2′,3′-dideoxyribosides such as ddAdo, ddGuo and AzddDAPR (Baba et al., 1987b; Balzarini et al., 1989e). The antagonistic effect of ribavirin on the anti-HIV activity of AZT may be explained by a reduction in the intracellular phosphorylation of AZT (Vogt et al., 1987). Its potentiating effect on the anti-HIV activity of purine 2′,3′-dideoxyribosides is probably due to an inhibition of the IMP dehydrogenase reaction (IMP → XMP). The latter leads to a shut-off in the supply of the natural substrates dGTP and dATP with which the purine 2′,3′-dideoxyriboside 5′-triphosphates have to compete at the reverse transcriptase level. Thus, an acceptable biochemical explanation can be offered to account for the potentiating effect of ribavirin on the anti-retrovirus activity of the purine 2′,3′-dideoxyribosides. It would seem justified to further explore combinations of ribavirin with purine 2′,3′-dideoxyribosides, i.e., ddIno, ddAdo, AzddDAPR, for their therapeutic potential in the treatment of AIDS.

## Conclusion

AZT was the first and at present is still the only drug that has been formally licensed for the treatment of AIDS patients. This is rather surprising in view of (a) the various deficiencies associated with prolonged AZT treatment (myelotoxicity, progressive fall of CD4 + cell counts, emergence of drug-resistant virus variants) and (b) the abundance of new candidate anti-HIV drugs that have been recently discovered. In fact, these new compounds seem capable of remedying the deficiencies shown by AZT. They either are less toxic for the bone marrow (AzddUrd, d4Thd, FddClUrd), are able to prevent killing of the CD4 + cells (sulfated polymers such as PVAS and PAVAS), or are active against AZT-resistant virus mutants (in principle, all compounds mentioned above, except for the 3′-azido-substituted 2′,3′-dideoxynucleosides).

It would now seem imperative to evaluate these candidate anti-HIV drugs for their effectiveness in the treatment of AIDS patients. These clinical trials should mandatorily be done on a controlled basis, and preferably in comparison with AZT. The outcome of such controlled and comparative studies will not be known until the patients have been followed up for a sufficiently long time. This requires (*i*) a strong commitment of the institutions (i.e., pharmaceutical companies) directing these studies, (*ii*) strict compliance of the patients to their treatment regimen, and (*iii*) careful monitoring of the patients for the clinical, immunological and virological parameters of the disease. In view of the wealth of agents that have been found effective as inhibitors of HIV replication in vitro, the number of possible combinations that could be envisaged with these compounds is gigantic. Most worthy of further investigation would be those combinations that truly act synergistically in several cell culture systems.

It should be emphasized that all anti-HIV agents and all chemotherapeutic approaches that have so far been described or proposed are aimed at suppressing the virus at one or more steps of its replicative cycle. None of these agents or approaches can be expected to eradicate the virus from its reservoir(s). To achieve this goal, which actually implies the elimination of the proviral DNA from the persistently infected cell, more dramatic measures, i.e. antisense oligonucleotides covalently linked to a nucleic acid-cleaving reagent, should be envisaged. Only those devices that succeed in eliminating the viral DNA sequences from the host cells may be assumed to accomplish a real "cure" of the disease. Until such devices are developed, current chemotherapeutic efforts should be directed at keeping the virus under control without harming the host.

## References


Abrams, D.I., Kuno, S., Wong, R., Jeffords, K., Nash, M., Molaghan, J.B., Gorter, R. and Ueno, R. (1989) Oral dextran sulfate (UA001) in the treatment of the acquired immunodeficiency syndrome (AIDS) and AIDS-related complex. *Ann. Intern. Med.* 110, 183–188.

Agrawal, S., Goodchild, J., Civeira, M.P., Thornton, A.H., Sarin, P.S. and Zamecnik, P.C. (1988) Oligodeoxynucleoside phosphoramidates and phosphorothioates as inhibitors of human immunodeficiency virus. *Proc. Natl. Acad. Sci. U.S.A.* 85, 7079–7083.

Baba, M., Pauwels, R., Herdewijn, P., De Clercq, E., Desmyter, J. and Vandeputte, M. (1987a) Both 2′,3′-dideoxythymidine and its 2′,3′-unsaturated derivative (2′,3′-dideoxythymidinene) are potent and selective inhibitors of human immunodeficiency virus replication in vitro. *Biochem. Biophys. Res. Commun.* 142, 128–134.

Baba, M., Pauwels, R., Balzarini, J., Herdewijn, P., De Clercq, E. and Desmyter, J. (1987b) Ribavirin antagonizes inhibitory effects of pyrimidine 2′,3′-dideoxynucleosides but enhances inhibitory effects of purine 2′,3′-dideoxynucleosides on replication of human immunodeficiency virus in vitro. *Antimicrob. Agents Chemother.* 31, 1613–1617.

Baba, M., Schols, D., Pauwels, R., Balzarini, J. and De Clercq, E. (1988a) Fuchsin acid selectively inhibits human immunodeficiency virus (HIV) replication in vitro. *Biochem. Biophys. Res. Commun.* 155, 1404–1411.

Baba, M., Nakajima, M., Schols, D., Pauwels, R., Balzarini, J. and De Clercq, E. (1988b) Pentosan polysulfate, a sulfated oligosaccharide is a potent and selective anti-HIV agent in vitro. *Antiviral Res.* 9, 335–343.

Baba, M., Pauwels, R., Balzarini, J., Arnout, J., Desmyter, J. and De Clercq, E. (1988c) Mechanism of inhibitory effect of dextran sulfate and heparin on replication of human immunodeficiency virus in vitro. *Proc. Natl. Acad. Sci. U.S.A.* 85, 6132–6136.

Baba, M., De Clercq, E., Schols, D., Pauwels, R., Snoeck, R., Van Boeckel, C., Van Dedem, G., Kraaijeveld, N., Hobbelen, P., Ottenheijm, H. and Den Hollander, F. (1990a) Novel sulfated polysaccharides: dissociation of anti-human immunodeficiency virus activity from antithrombin activity. *J. Infect. Dis.* 161, 208–213.

Baba, M., Schols, D., De Clercq, E., Pauwels, R., Nagy, M., Györgyi-Edelényi, J., Löw, M. and Görög, S. (1990b) Novel sulfated polymers as highly potent and selective inhibitors of human immunodeficiency virus (HIV) replication and giant cell formation. *Antimicrob. Agents Chemother.* 34, 134–138.

Baba, M., Schols, D., Pauwels, R., Nakashima, H. and De Clercq, E. (1990c) Sulfated polysaccharides as potent inhibitors of HIV-induced syncytium formation: a new strategy towards AIDS chemotherapy. *J. AIDS* 3, 493–499.

Balzarini, J., Mitsuya, H., De Clercq, E. and Broder, S. (1986a) Comparative inhibitory effects of suramin and other selected compounds on the infectivity and replication of human T-cell lymphotropic virus (HTLV-III)/lymphadenopathy-associated virus (LAV). *Int. J. Cancer* 37, 451–457.

Balzarini, J., Pauwels, R., Herdewijn, P., De Clercq, E., Cooney, D.A., Kang, G.-J., Dalal, M., Johns, D.G. and Broder, S. (1986b) Potent and selective anti-HTLV-III/LAV activity of 2′,3′-dideoxycytidinene, the 2′,3′-unsaturated derivative of 2′,3′-dideoxycytidine. *Biochem. Biophys. Res. Commun.* 140, 735–742.

Balzarini, J., Baba, M., Pauwels, R., Herdewijn, P. and De Clercq, E. (1988a) Anti-retrovirus activity of 3′-fluoro- and 3′-azido-substituted pyrimidine 2′,3′-dideoxynucleoside analogues. *Biochem. Pharmacol.* 37, 2847–2856.

Balzarini, J., Baba, M., Pauwels, R., Herdewijn, P., Wood, S.G., Robins, M.J. and De Clercq, E. (1988b) Potent and selective activity of 3′-azido-2,6-diaminopurine-2′,3′-dideoxyriboside, 3′-fluoro-2,6-diaminopurine-2′,3′-dideoxyriboside, and 3′-fluoro-2′,3′-dideoxyguanosine against human immunodeficiency virus. *Mol. Pharmacol.* 33, 243–249.

Balzarini, J., Van Aerschot, A., Pauwels, R., Baba, M., Schols, D., Herdewijn, P. and De Clercq, E. (1989a) 5-Halogeno-3′-fluoro-2′,3′-dideoxyuridines as inhibitors of human immunodeficiency virus (HIV): potent and selective anti-HIV activity of 3′-fluoro-2′,3′-dideoxy-5-chlorouridine. *Mol. Pharmacol.* 35, 571–577.

Balzarini, J., Van Aerschot, A., Herdewijn, P. and De Clercq, E. (1989b) 5-Chloro-substituted derivatives of 2′,3′-didehydro-2′,3′-dideoxyuridine, 3′-fluoro-2′,3′-dideoxyuridine and 3′-azido-2′,3′-dideoxyuridine as anti-HIV agents. *Biochem. Pharmacol.* 38, 869–874.

Balzarini, J., Herdewijn, P. and De Clercq, E. (1989c) Differential patterns of intracellular metabolism of 2′,3′-didehydro-2′,3′-dideoxythymidine and 3′-azido-2′,3′-dideoxythymidine, two potent anti-human immunodeficiency virus compounds. *J. Biol. Chem.* 264, 6127–6133.

Balzarini, J., Naesens, L., Herdewijn, P., Rosenberg, I., Holy, A., Pauwels, R., Baba, M., Johns, D.G. and De Clercq, E. (1989d) Marked in vivo antiretrovirus activity of 9-(2-phosphonylmethoxyethyl)adenine, a selective anti-human immunodeficiency virus agent. *Proc. Natl. Acad. Sci. U.S.A.* 86, 332–336.

Balzarini, J., Herdewijn, P. and De Clercq, E. (1989e) Potentiating effect of ribavirin on the anti-retrovirus activity of 3′-azido-2,6-diaminopurine-2′,3′-dideoxyriboside in vitro and in vivo. *Antiviral Res.* 11, 161–172.

Bazin, H., Chattopadhyaya, J., Datema, R., Ericson, A.-C., Gilljam, G., Johansson, N.G., Hansen, J., Koshida, R., Moelling, K., Öberg, B., Remaud, G., Stening, G., Vrang, L., Wahren, B. and Wu, J.C. (1989) An analysis of the inhibition of replication of HIV and MULV by some 3′-blocked pyrimidine analogs. *Biochem. Pharmacol.* 38, 109–119.

Biesert, L., Suhartono, H., Winkler, I., Meichsner, C., Helsberg, M., Hewlett, G., Klimetzek, V., Mölling, K., Schlumberger, H.-D., Schrinner, E., Brede, H.-D. and Rübsamen-Waigmann, H. (1988) Inhibition of HIV and virus replication by polysulphated polyxylan: HOE/BAY 946, a new antiviral compound. *AIDS* 2, 449–457.

Broder, S., Yarchoan, R., Collins, J.M., Lane, H.C., Markham, P.D., Klecker, R.W., Redfield, R.R., Mitsuya, H., Hoth, D.F., Gelmann, E., Groopman, J.E., Resnick, L., Gallo, R.C., Myers, C.E. and Fauci, A.S. (1985) Effects of suramin on HTLV-III/LAV infection presenting as Kaposi's sarcoma or AIDS-related complex: clinical pharmacology and suppression of virus replication in vivo. *Lancet* ii, 627–630.

Capon, D.J., Chamow, S.M., Mordenti, J., Marsters, S.A., Gregory, T., Mitsuya, H., Byrn, R.A., Lucas, C., Wurm, F.M., Groopman, J.E., Broder, S. and Smith, D.H. (1989) Designing CD4 immunoadhesins for AIDS therapy. *Nature* 337, 525–531.

Dainiak, N., Worthington, M., Riordan, M.A., Kreczko, S. and Goldman, L. (1988) 3′-Azido-3′-deoxythymidine (AZT) inhibits proliferation in vitro of human haematopoietic progenitor cells. *Br. J. Haematol.* 69, 299–304.

De Clercq, E. (1979) Suramin: a potent inhibitor of the reverse transcriptase of RNA tumor viruses. *Cancer Lett.* 8, 9–22.

De Clercq, E. (1989a) New acquisitions in the development of anti-HIV agents. *Antiviral Res.* 12, 1–20.

De Clercq, E. (1989b) Activity of sulfated polysaccharides against the human immunodeficiency virus. In: H. van der Goot, G. Domány, L. Pallos and H. Timmerman (Eds.), *Trends in Medicinal Chemistry '88.* Elsevier, Amsterdam, pp. 729–742.

De Clercq, E. (1989c) Molecular targets of chemotherapeutic agents against the human immunodeficiency virus. In: G.G. Jackson, H.D. Schlumberger and H.J. Zeiler (Eds.), *Perspectives in Antiinfective Therapy.* Friedrich Vieweg und Sohn, Braunschweig/Wiesbaden, pp. 255–267.

Deen, K.C., McDougal, J.S., Inacker, R., Folena-Wasserman, G., Arthos, J., Rosenberg, J., Maddon, P.J., Axel, R. and Sweet, R.W. (1988) A soluble form of D4T (T4) protein inhibits AIDS virus infection. *Nature* 331, 82–84.

Dournon, E., Matheron, S., Rozenbaum, W., Gharakhanian, S., Michon, C., Girard, P.M., Perronne,

C., Salmon, D., De Truchis, P., Leport, C., Bouvet, E., Dazza, M.C., Levacher, M., Regnier, B. and the Claude Bernard Hospital AZT Study Group (1988) Effects of zidovudine in 365 consecutive patients with AIDS or AIDS-related complex. *Lancet* i, 1297–1302.

Eriksson, B.F.H. and Schinazi, R.F. (1989) Combinations of 3′-azido-3′-deoxythymidine (zidovudine) and phosphonoformate (foscarnet) against human immunodeficiency virus type 1 and cytomegalovirus replication in vitro. *Antimicrob. Agents Chemother.* 33, 663–669.

Fischl, M.A., Richman, D.D., Grieco, M.H., Gottlieb, M.S., Volberding, P.A., Laskin, O.L., Leedom, J.M., Groopman, J.E., Mildvan, D., Schooley, R.T., Jackson, G.G., Durack, D.T., King, D. and the AZT Collaborative Working Group (1987) The efficacy of azidothymidine (AZT) in the treatment of patients with AIDS and AIDS-related complex. *N. Engl. J. Med.* 317, 185–191.

Fisher, R.A., Bertonis, J.M., Meier, W., Johnson, V.A., Costopoulos, D.S., Liu, T., Tizard, R., Walker, B.D., Hirsch, M.S., Schooley, R.T. and Flavell, R.A. (1988) HIV infection is blocked in vitro by recombinant soluble CD4. *Nature* 331, 76–78.

Fleet, G.W.J., Karpas, A., Dwek, R.A., Fellows, L.E., Tyms, A.S., Petursson, S., Namgoong, S.K., Ramsden, N.G., Smith, P.W., Son, J.C., Wilson, F., Witty, D.R., Jacob, G.S. and Rademacher, T.W. (1988) Inhibition of HIV replication by amino-sugar derivatives. *FEBS Lett.* 237, 128–132.

Furman, P.A., Fyfe, J.A., St. Clair, M.H., Weinhold, K., Rideout, J.L., Freeman, G.A., Nusinoff Lehrman, S., Bolognesi, D.P., Broder, S., Mitsuya, H. and Barry, D.W. (1986) Phosphorylation of 3′-azido-3′-deoxythymidine and selective interaction of the 5′-triphosphate with human immunodeficiency virus reverse transcriptase. *Proc. Natl. Acad. Sci. U.S.A.* 83, 8333–8337.

Gangemi, J.D., Cozens, R.M., De Clercq, E., Balzarini, J. and Hochkeppel, H.-K. (1989) 9-(2-Phosphonylmethoxyethyl)adenine in the treatment of murine acquired immunodeficiency disease and opportunistic herpes simplex virus infections. *Antimicrob. Agents Chemother.* 33, 1864–1868.

Goodchild, J., Agrawal, S., Civeira, M.P., Sarin, P.S., Sun, D. and Zamecnik, P.C. (1988) Inhibition of human immunodeficiency virus replication by antisense oligodeoxynucleotides. *Proc. Natl. Acad. Sci. U.S.A.* 85, 5507–5511.

Hamamoto, Y., Nakashima, H., Matsui, T., Matsuda, A., Ueda, T. and Yamamoto, N. (1987) Inhibitory effect of 2′,3′-didehydro-2′,3′-dideoxynucleosides on infectivity, cytopathic effects, and replication of human immunodeficiency virus. *Antimicrob. Agents Chemother.* 31, 907–910.

Hammer, S.M. and Gillis, J.M. (1987) Synergistic activity of granulocyte-macrophage colony-stimulating factor and 3′-azido-3′-deoxythymidine against human immunodeficiency virus in vitro. *Antimicrob. Agents Chemother.* 31, 1046–1050.

Hao, Z., Cooney, D.A., Hartman, N.R., Perno, C.F., Fridland, A., DeVico, A.L., Sarngadharan, M.G., Broder, S. and Johns, D.G. (1988) Factors determining the activity of 2′,3′-dideoxynucleosides in suppressing human immunodeficiency virus in vitro. *Mol. Pharmacol.* 34, 431–435.

Hartshorn, K.L., Vogt, M.W., Chou, T.-C., Blumberg, R.S., Byington, R., Schooley, R.T. and Hirsch, M.S. (1987) Synergistic inhibition of human immunodeficiency virus in vitro by azidothymidine and recombinant alpha A interferon. *Antimicrob. Agents Chemother.* 31, 168–172.

Hayashi, S., Phadtare, S., Zemlicka, J., Matsukura, M., Mitsuya, H. and Broder, S. (1988) Adenallene and cytallene: acyclic nucleoside analogues that inhibit replication and cytopathic effect of human immunodeficiency virus in vitro. *Proc. Natl. Acad. Sci. U.S.A.* 85, 6127–6131.

Herdewijn, P., Balzarini, J., De Clercq, E., Pauwels, R., Baba, M., Broder, S. and Vanderhaeghe, H. (1987) 3′-Substituted 2′,3′-dideoxynucleoside analogues as potential anti-HIV (HTLV-III/LAV) agents. *J. Med. Chem.* 30, 1270–1278.

Hussey, R.E., Richardson, N.E., Kowalski, M., Brown, N.R., Chang, H.-C., Siliciano, R.F., Dorfman, T., Walker, B., Sodroski, J. and Reinherz, E.L. (1988) A soluble CD4 protein selectively inhibits HIV replication and syncytium formation. *Nature* 331, 78–81.

Ito, M., Sato, A., Hirabayashi, K., Tanabe, F., Shigeta, S., Baba, M., De Clercq, E., Nakashima, H. and Yamamoto, N. (1988) Mechanism of inhibitory effect of glycyrrhizin on replication of human immunodeficiency virus (HIV). *Antiviral Res.* 10, 289–298.

Ito, M., Baba, M., Hirabayashi, K., Matsumoto, T., Suzuki, M., Suzuki, S., Shigeta, S. and De Clercq, E. (1989) In vitro activity of mannan sulfate, a novel sulfated polysaccharide, against human immunodeficiency virus type 1 and other enveloped viruses. *Eur. J. Clin. Microbiol. Infect. Dis.* 8, 171–173.

Johnson, V.A., Walker, B.D., Barlow, M.A., Paradis, T.J., Chou, T.-C. and Hirsch, M.S. (1989a) Synergistic inhibition of human immunodeficiency virus type 1 and type 2 replication in vitro by castanospermine and 3′-azido-3′-deoxythymidine. *Antimicrob. Agents Chemother.* 33, 53–57.

Johnson, V.A., Barlow, M.A., Chou, T.-C., Fisher, R.A., Walker, B.D., Hirsch, M.S. and Schooley, R.T. (1989b) Synergistic inhibition of human immunodeficiency virus type 1 (HIV-1) replication in vitro by recombinant soluble CD4 and 3′-azido-3′-deoxythymidine. *J. Infect. Dis.* 159, 837–844.

Jurkiewicz, E., Panse, P., Jentsch, K.-D., Hartmann, H. and Hunsmann, G. (1989) In vitro anti-HIV-1 activity of chondroitin polysulphate. *AIDS* 3, 423–427.

Kaplan, L.D., Wolfe, P.R., Volberding, P.A., Feorino, P., Levy, J.A., Abrams, D.I., Kiprov, D., Wong, R., Kaufman, L. and Gottlieb, M.S. (1987) Lack of response to suramin in patients with AIDS and AIDS-related complex. *Am. J. Med.* 82, 615–620.

Karpas, A., Fleet, G.W.J., Dwek, R.A., Petursson, S., Namgoong, S.K., Ramsden, N.G., Jacob, G.S. and Rademacher, T.W. (1988) Aminosugar derivatives as potential anti-human immunodeficiency virus agents. *Proc. Natl. Acad. Sci. U.S.A.* 85, 9229–9233.

Kohl, N.E., Emini, E.A., Schleif, W.A., Davis, L.J., Heimbach, J.C., Dixon, R.A.F., Scolnick, E.M. and Sigal, I.S. (1988) Active human immunodeficiency virus protease is required for viral infectivity. *Proc. Natl. Acad. Sci. U.S.A.* 85, 4686–4690.

Koshida, R., Vrang, L., Gilljam, G., Harmenberg, J., Öberg, B. and Wahren, B. (1989) Inhibition of human immunodeficiency virus in vitro by combinations of 3′-azido-3′-deoxythymidine and foscarnet. *Antimicrob. Agents Chemother.* 33, 778–780.

Larder, B.A., Darby, G. and Richman, D.D. (1989) HIV with reduced sensitivity to zidovudine (AZT) isolated during prolonged therapy. *Science* 243, 1731–1734.

Lifson, J.D., Hwang, K.M., Nara, P.L., Fraser, B., Padgett, M., Dunlop, N.M. and Eiden, L.E. (1988) Synthetic CD4 peptide derivatives that inhibit HIV infection and cytopathicity. *Science* 241, 712–716.

Lin, T.-S., Schinazi, R.F., Chen, M.S., Kinney-Thomas, E. and Prusoff, W.H. (1987a) Antiviral activity of 2′,3′-dideoxycytidin-2′-ene (2′,3′-dideoxy-2′,3′-didehydrocytidine) against human immunodeficiency virus in vitro. *Biochem. Pharmacol.* 36, 311–316.

Lin, T.-S., Schinazi, R.F. and Prusoff, W.H. (1987b) Potent and selective in vitro activity of 3′-deoxythymidin-2′-ene (3′-deoxy-2′,3′-didehydrothymidine) against human immunodeficiency virus. *Biochem. Pharmacol.* 36, 2713–2718.

Liu, M.A. and Liu, T. (1988) Effect of recombinant soluble CD4 on human peripheral blood lymphocyte responses in vitro. *J. Clin. Invest.* 82, 2176–2180.

Matsukura, M., Shinozuka, K., Zon, G., Mitsuya, H., Reitz, M., Cohen, J.S. and Broder, S. (1987) Phosphorothioate analogs of oligodeoxynucleotides: inhibitors of replication and cytopathic effects of human immunodeficiency virus. *Proc. Natl. Acad. Sci. U.S.A.* 84, 7706–7710.

Matsukura, M., Zon, G., Shinozuka, K., Robert-Guroff, M., Shimada, T., Stein, C.A., Mitsuya, H., Wong-Staal, F., Cohen, J.S. and Broder, S. (1989) Regulation of viral expression of human immunodeficiency virus in vitro by an antisense phosphorothioate oligodeoxynucleotide against *rev* (*art/trs*) in chronically infected cells. *Proc. Natl. Acad. Sci. U.S.A.* 86, 4244–4248.

Matthes, E., Lehmann, Ch., Scholz, D., von Janta-Lipinski, M., Gaertner, K., Rosenthal, H.A. and Langen, P. (1987) Inhibition of HIV-associated reverse transcriptase by sugar-modified derivatives of thymidine 5′-triphosphate in comparison to cellular DNA polymerases $\alpha$ and $\beta$. *Biochem. Biophys. Res. Commun.* 148, 78–85.

McGrath, M.S., Hwang, K.M., Caldwell, S.E., Gaston, I., Luk, K.-C., Wu, P., Ng, V.L., Crowe, S., Daniels, J., Marsh, J., Deinhart, T., Lekas, P.V., Vennari, J.C., Yeung, H.-W. and Lifson, J.D. (1989) GLQ223: an inhibitor of human immunodeficiency virus replication in acutely and chronically infected cells of lymphocyte and mononuclear phagocyte lineage. *Proc. Natl. Acad. Sci. U.S.A.* 86, 2844–2848.

Meruelo, D., Lavie, G. and Lavie, D. (1988) Therapeutic agents with dramatic antiretroviral activity and little toxicity at effective doses: aromatic polycyclic diones hypericin and pseudohypericin. *Proc. Natl. Acad. Sci. U.S.A.* 85, 5230–5234.

Mitsuya, H. and Broder, S. (1986) Inhibition of the in vitro infectivity and cytopathic effect of human

T-lymphotrophic virus type III/lymphadenopathy-associated virus (HTLV-III/LAV) by 2′,3′-dideoxynucleosides. *Proc. Natl. Acad. Sci. U.S.A.* 83, 1911–1915.

Mitsuya, H., Popovic, M., Yarchoan, R., Matsushita, S., Gallo, R.C. and Broder, S. (1984) Suramin protection of T cells in vitro against infectivity and cytopathic effect of HTLV-III. *Science* 226, 172–174.

Mitsuya, H., Weinhold, K.J., Furman, P.A., St. Clair, M.H., Nusinoff-Lehrman, S., Gallo, R.C., Bolognesi, D., Barry, D.W. and Broder, S. (1985) 3′-Azido-3′-deoxythymidine (BW A509U): an antiviral agent that inhibits the infectivity and cytopathic effect of human T-lymphotropic virus type III/lymphadenopathy-associated virus in vitro. *Proc. Natl. Acad. Sci. U.S.A.* 82, 7096–7100.

Mitsuya, H., Looney, D.J., Kuno, S., Ueno, R., Wong-Staal, F. and Broder, S. (1988) Dextran sulfate suppression of viruses in the HIV family: inhibition of virion binding to CD4+ cells. *Science* 240, 646–649.

Nakashima, H., Yoshida, O., Baba, M., De Clercq, E. and Yamamoto, N. (1989) Anti-HIV activity of dextran sulphate as determined under different experimental conditions. *Antiviral Res.* 11, 233–246.

Navia, M.A., Fitzgerald, P.M.D., McKeever, B.M., Leu, C.-T., Heimbach, J.C., Herber, W.K., Sigal, I.S., Darke, P.L. and Springer, J.P. (1989) Three-dimensional structure of aspartyl protease from human immunodeficiency virus HIV-1. *Nature* 337, 615–620.

Pauwels, R., Balzarini, J., Schols, D., Baba, M., Desmyter, J., Rosenberg, I., Holy, A. and De Clercq, E. (1988) Phosphonylmethoxyethyl purine derivatives, a new class of anti-human immunodeficiency virus agents. *Antimicrob. Agents Chemother.* 32, 1025–1030.

Perno, C.-F., Yarchoan, R., Cooney, D.A., Hartman, N.R., Webb, D.S.A., Hao, Z., Mitsuya, H., Johns, D.G. and Broder, S. (1989) Replication of human immunodeficiency virus in monocytes. *J. Exp. Med.* 169, 933–951.

Richman, D.D., Fischl, M.A., Grieco, M.H., Gottlieb, M.S., Volberding, P.A., Laskin, O.L., Leedom, J.M., Groopman, J.E., Mildvan, D., Hirsch, M.S., Jackson, G.G., Durack, D.T., Nusinoff-Lehrman, S. and the AZT Collaborative Working Group (1987) The toxicity of azidothymidine (AZT) in the treatment of patients with AIDS and AIDS-related complex. *N. Engl. J. Med.* 317, 192–197.

Robins, M.J., Wood, S.G., Dalley, N.K., Herdewijn, P., Balzarini, J. and De Clercq, E. (1989) Nucleic acid related compounds. 57. Synthesis, X-ray crystal structure, lipophilic partition properties, and antiretroviral activities of anomeric 3′-azido-2′,3′-dideoxy-2,6-diaminopurine ribosides. *J. Med. Chem.* 32, 1763–1768.

Rossmann, M.G. (1988) Antiviral agents targeted to interact with viral capsid proteins and a possible application to human immunodeficiency virus. *Proc. Natl. Acad. Sci. U.S.A.* 85, 4625–4627.

Ruprecht, R.M., Mullaney, S., Andersen, J. and Bronson, R. (1989) In vivo analysis of castanospermine, a candidate antiretroviral agent. *J. AIDS* 2, 149–157.

Sarin, P.S., Agrawal, S., Civeira, M.P., Goodchild, J., Ikeuchi, T. and Zamecnik, P.C. (1988) Inhibition of acquired immunodeficiency syndrome virus by oligodeoxynucleoside methylphosphonates. *Proc. Natl. Acad. Sci. U.S.A.* 85, 7448–7451.

Schols, D., Baba, M., Pauwels, R. and De Clercq, E. (1989a) Flow cytometric method to demonstrate whether anti-HIV-1 agents inhibit virion binding to T4+ cells. *J. AIDS* 2, 10–15.

Schols, D., Baba, M., Pauwels, R., Desmyter, J. and De Clercq, E. (1989b) Specific interaction of aurintricarboxylic acid with the human immunodeficiency virus/CD4 cell receptor. *Proc. Natl. Acad. Sci. U.S.A.* 86, 3322–3326.

Schols, D., Pauwels, R., Baba, M., Desmyter, J. and De Clercq, E. (1989c) Syncytium formation and destruction of bystander CD4+ cells cocultured with T cells persistently infected with human immunodeficiency virus as demonstrated by flow cytometry. *J. Gen. Virol.* 70, 2397–2408.

Schols, D., Pauwels, R., Desmyter, J. and De Clercq, E. (1989d) Dextran sulfate and other polyanionic anti-HIV compounds specifically interact with the viral gp120 glycoprotein expressed by T-cells persistently infected with HIV-1. *Virology* 175, 556–561.

Smith, D.H., Byrn, R.A., Marsters, S.A., Gregory, T., Groopman, J.E. and Capon, D.J. (1987) Blocking of HIV-1 infectivity by a soluble, secreted form of the CD4 antigen. *Science* 238, 1704–1707.

Smith, M.S., Brian, E.L., De Clercq, E. and Pagano, J.S. (1989) Susceptibility of human immunodeficiency virus type 1 replication in vitro to acyclic adenosine analogs and synergy of the analogs with 3′-azido-3′-deoxythymidine. *Antimicrob. Agents Chemother.* 33, 1482–1486.

St. Clair, M.H., Richards, C.A., Spector, T., Weinhold, K.J., Miller, W.H., Langlois, A.J. and Furman, P.A. (1987) 3′-Azido-3′-deoxythymidine triphosphate as an inhibitor and substrate of purified human immunodeficiency virus reverse transcriptase. *Antimicrob. Agents Chemother.* 31, 1972–1977.

Till, M.A., Ghetie, V., Gregory, T., Patzer, E.J., Porter, J.P., Uhr, J.W., Capon, D.J. and Vitetta, E.S. (1988) HIV-infected cells are killed by rCD4-ricin A chain. *Science* 242, 1166–1168.

Torseth, J., Bhatia, G., Harkonen, S., Child, C., Skinner, M., Robinson, W.S., Blaschke, T.F. and Merigan, T.C. (1989) Evaluation of the antiviral effect of rifabutin in AIDS-related complex. *J. Infect. Dis.* 159, 1115–1118.

Traunecker, A., Lüke, W. and Karjalainen, K. (1988) Soluble CD4 molecules neutralize human immunodeficiency virus type 1. *Nature* 331, 84–86.

Traunecker, A., Schneider, J., Kiefer, H. and Karjalainen, K. (1989) Highly efficient neutralization of HIV with recombinant CD4-immunoglobulin molecules. *Nature* 339, 68–70.

Van Aerschot, A., Herdewijn, P., Balzarini, J., Pauwels, R. and De Clercq, E. (1989) 3′-Fluoro-2′,3′-dideoxy-5-chlorouridine: most selective anti-HIV-1 agent among a series of new 2′- and 3′-fluorinated 2′,3′-dideoxynucleoside analogues. *J. Med. Chem.* 32, 1743–1749.

Vince, R., Hua, M., Brownell, J., Daluge, S., Lee, F., Shannon, W.M., Lavelle, G.C., Qualls, J., Weislow, O.S., Kiser, R., Canonico, R.G., Schultz, R.H., Narayanan, V.L., Mayo, J.G., Shoemaker, R.H. and Boyd, M.R. (1988) Potent and selective activity of a new carbocyclic nucleoside analog (carbovir: NSC 614846) against human immunodeficiency virus in vitro. *Biochem. Biophys. Res. Commun.* 156, 1046–1053.

Vogt, M.W., Hartshorn, K.L., Furman, P.A., Chou, T.-C., Fyfe, J.A., Coleman, L.A., Crumpacker, C., Schooley, R.T. and Hirsch, M.S. (1987) Ribavirin antagonizes the effect of azidothymidine on HIV replication. *Science* 235, 1376–1379.

Walker, B.D., Kowalski, M., Goh, W.C., Kozarsky, K., Krieger, M., Rosen, C., Rohrschneider, L., Haseltine, W.A. and Sodroski, J. (1987) Inhibition of human immunodeficiency virus syncytium formation and virus replication by castanospermine. *Proc. Natl. Acad. Sci. U.S.A.* 84, 8120–8124.

Weber, I.T., Miller, M., Jaskólski, M., Leis, J., Skalka, A.M. and Wlodawer, A. (1989) Molecular modeling of the HIV-1 protease and its substrate binding site. *Science* 243, 928–931.

Yarchoan, R., Klecker, R.W., Weinhold, K.J., Markham, P.D., Lyerly, H.K., Durack, D.T., Gelmann, E., Nusinoff-Lehrman, S., Blum, R.M., Barry, D.W., Shearer, G.M., Fischl, M.A., Mitsuya, H., Gallo, R.C., Collins, J.M., Bolognesi, D.P., Myers, C.E. and Broder, S. (1986) Administration of 3′-azido-3′-deoxythymidine, an inhibitor of HTLV-III/LAV replication, to patients with AIDS or AIDS-related complex. *Lancet* i, 575–580.

Yarchoan, R., Perno, C.F., Thomas, R.V., Klecker, R.W., Allain, J.-P., Wills, R.J., McAtee, N., Fischl, M.A., Dubinsky, R., McNeely, M.C., Mitsuya, H., Pluda, J.M., Lawley, T.J., Leuther, M., Safai, B., Collins, J.M., Myers, C.E. and Broder, S. (1988) Phase I studies of 2′,3′-dideoxycytidine in severe human immunodeficiency virus infection as a single agent and alternating with zidovudine (AZT). *Lancet* i, 76–81.

Yarchoan, R., Mitsuya, H., Thomas, R.V., Pluda, J.M., Hartman, N.R., Perno, C.-F., Marczyk, K.S., Allain, J.-P., Johns, D.G. and Broder, S. (1989) In vivo activity against HIV and favorable toxicity profile of 2′,3′-dideoxyinosine. *Science* 245, 412–415.

Yoshida, O., Nakashima, H., Yoshida, T., Kaneko, Y., Yamamoto, I., Matsuzaki, K., Uryu, T. and Yamamoto, N. (1988) Sulfation of the immunomodulating polysaccharide lentinan: a novel strategy for antivirals to human immunodeficiency virus (HIV). *Biochem. Pharmacol.* 37, 2887–2891.

Youle, M.S., Hawkins, D.A., Lawrence, A.G., Tenant-Flowers, M., Shanson, D.C. and Gazzard, B.G. (1989) Clinical, immunological, and virological effects of sodium fusidate in patients with AIDS or AIDS-related complex (ARC): an open study. *J. AIDS* 2, 59–62.

Zamecnik, P.C. and Stephenson, M.L. (1978) Inhibition of Rous sarcoma virus replication and cell transformation by a specific oligodeoxynucleotide. *Proc. Natl. Acad. Sci. U.S.A.* 75, 280–284.

Zamecnik, P.C., Goodchild, J., Taguchi, Y. and Sarin, P.S. (1986) Inhibition of replication and expression of human T-cell lymphotropic virus type III in cultured cells by exogenous synthetic oligonucleotides complementary to viral RNA. *Proc. Natl. Acad. Sci. U.S.A.* 83, 4143–4146.

*Eds. H. Schellekens and M.C. Horzinek*
*Animal Models in AIDS*



# 36

# Prospects for vaccination against AIDS

ERLING NORRBY

Department of Virology, Karolinska Institute, School of Medicine, Stockholm, Sweden

## Introduction

The development and use of viral vaccines has led to some of the major advances in biomedicine (Norrby, 1987). Smallpox has been eradicated from the world and the occurrence of poliomyelitis and measles has been markedly reduced in industralized countries. The identification of the lentivirus human immunodeficiency virus (HIV) as the etiological agent of acquired immunodeficiency syndrome (AIDS) has opened up possibilities for the development of a vaccine preventing this disease. Within a short time span a remarkably detailed knowledge of the structure of HIV and its immunological as well as replicative characteristics in different cells in vitro and in vivo has accumulated (reviewed in Fauci, 1988; Haseltine, 1988; Levy, 1989). This knowledge has made it clear that attempts to introduce immunoprophylactic measures against HIV infections can be anticipated to be associated with both unique possibilities and unique problems.

## The problem of vaccination against HIV infections

Ideally development of a vaccine against a particular microbial infection should be based of an in depth understanding of the immunobiology and the immunopathogenesis of the infectious agent and the disease. Admittedly such information was not available at the time of the introduction of the vaccines that are successfully used today. As regards HIV we do have an extensive understanding of its biology. This insight has unveiled a wide range of real and potential complications to vaccinations (reviewed in Koff and Hoth, 1988) as listed in Table 1.

There are several possible portals of entry for the HIV infection. In practical terms spread of disease occurs via blood and genital fluids. Only a very low concentration of infectious particles is present in contaminated fluids but these contain in addition virus-infected cells. Therefore it has been suggested that cell-associated virus may be a comparatively more important vehicle for the

TABLE 1
Problems in development of an AIDS vaccine

| |
|---|
| Local immunity required to stop infection at portal of entry |
| Infection transfer may be cell-medicated |
| The infection may evade immune surveillance both when occurring in a latent state and when disseminating by cell-to-cell spread |
| Antigenic variability, especially in the envelope glycoprotein |
| The relative role of B- and T-cell immune responses not clarified |
| Unfavorable immune responses; enhancing antibodies, autoimmune antibodies |
| Availability of an appropriate animal model |

spread of infection than free virus (Levy, 1988). Blocking an attack of virus at mucosal membranes requires the presence of local immunity. Since the immunity may need to handle both virus particles and virus-infected cells it probably will need to include both humoral and cell-mediated defense mechanisms. It will be a tall order to establish a durable local immunity, especially of the latter kind, with these qualities. An additional potential complication is that cells harboring virus upon transfer to a new host may become stimulated by allogenic reactions potentially leading to an amplification of virus replication (Fauci, 1988). Furthermore, virus-infected cells may evade immune surveillance. It has been described that cells of the macrophage/monocyte lineage may allow virus replication without overt exposure of virus-specific antigens. This kind of cell has become increasingly appreciated as an important harbinger of the virus infection. A critical question concerns whether a cell which is immuno-silent with regard to the occurrence of viral antigens may transmit the infection to other cells without giving the immune system an opportunity to interfere.

A key property of HIV is its antigenic variability, especially in the envelope glycoproteins. Like influenza virus HIV has separate surface structures carrying immunodominant properties and mediating virus absorption and penetration. However, whereas influenza virus can only cause acute disease HIV belongs to an RNA virus family which has a unique capacity to persist in a DNA provirus form in cells. As a consequence the antigenic lability can become expressed in an infected individual, similar to the situation in some lentivirus infections in animals, for example visna in sheep and equine infectious anemia in horses.

The relative contribution of dysfunctioning B-cell and T-cell immunity in the failure of the infected individual to handle the HIV infection has not been clarified. It seems likely that both arms of the immune defense are required not only to provide a barrier against viral invasion but also to keep the HIV infection in a suppressed state for variable periods of time. It remains to elucidate the reasons for the eventual emergence of a disseminated infection associated with a general derangement of immune functions. Most likely both changes in the virus and an erosion of the immune defense are decisive factors. In vitro studies have documented the occurrence of enhancing antibodies (Takeda et al., 1988) as well as autoimmune antibodies (Stricker et al., 1987). It is at present a matter of conjecture whether such antibodies may contribute to the pathogenic process.

For a long time the lack of an appropriate animal model has hampered the testing of vaccine products. HIV type 1 can infect chimpanzees and gibbon apes but the virus infection does not lead to disease development. A potentially much more useful model is the infection of macaques with simian immunodeficiency virus (SIV) (for reviews see Desrosiers and Letvin, 1987; Schneider and Hunsman, 1988). The recent finding that not only SIV but also HIV type 2 can infect rhesus and cynomolgus macaques (Dormant et al., 1989; Putkonen et al., 1989b) has further improved possibilities for effective evaluation of vaccine products. Whereas HIV-2-infected animals so far have not displayed any distinct symptoms, SIV gives an immunosuppressive disease remarkably similar to AIDS.

## The immune potential during different phases of HIV infection

Three different phases can be distinguished in HIV infections in man. These are the acute infection, the quiet, retracted infection of varying duration and the expanding immunodeficiency state. During the acute infection influenza- or mononucleosis-like symptoms may develop but as in any other acute virus infection the immune system succeeds in effectively suppressing the replication of virus and in clearing the majority of infected cells. However, a complete clearance of virus is a rarity, if it ever occurs. During the phase of acute infection the immune system appears to function unimpaired. The second phase is the one in which there are no symptoms of disease and no signs of major damage to the immune system as reflected in for example a reduction in the number of circulating CD4 positive T-cells. Still there is evidence that the full range of immune reactions cannot be mobilized. It has been demonstrated that a subset of CD4 positive T-cells that recognizes and responds to soluble antigens is selectively deficient at this stage. A polyclonal stimulation of B-cells is seen and the capacity of the infected individual to mobilize primary immune responses is reduced (Lane et al., 1983; Pahwa et al., 1986). Probably there is also a gradual impairment of cell-mediated immune responses already at this stage presaging the final collapse of the system (Takahashi et al., 1989).

The third phase involves dramatic changes in the immune defense system. There is a progressive reduction of CD4 positive T-helper cells to very low levels. Antibodies against the internal *gag* proteins diminish and are substituted for by reemerging *gag* antigen. The virus infection is allowed to again disseminate in the body.

## The appearance of new virus variants in infected individuals

Selection of new virus variants may be considered in three different contexts. These encompass the emergence of non-neutralizable strains of virus, virus with an altered virulence and virus with a modified cell tropism. The appearance in vivo of neutralization resistant variants has previously been observed in other lentivirus infections such as visna-maedi in sheep and equine infectious anemia in horses. Until recently the situation regarding non-neutralizable virus variants in HIV infections in man was unclear. Originally neutralizing antibodies were described to appear relatively late (Ho et al., 1987). This conclusion was based on tests performed with laboratory-adapted strains and therefore presumably measured mainly cross-reacting antibodies. Studies with serum samples from a laboratory worker accidentally infected with a cell culture-adapted virus strain and experimentally infected chimpanzees have indicated that strain-specific neutralizing antibodies may appear at an earlier stage and that later on more broadly reacting type-specific neutralizing antibodies can be detected (Nara et al., 1987; Blattner et al., 1988; Goudsmidt et al., 1988).

The terminology employed to describe HIV immunological cross-reactions is frequently confusing. In the literature strain-specific and type-specific (cross-reacting) antibodies are relatively often inconsistently referred to as type-specific and group-specific, respectively. Accepting that there are two types of HIV (a distinction based on a non-immunological species definition) antibodies on a scale of increasing cross-neutralizing activity correctly should be referred to as strain-, interstrain-, type- and intertype-specific.

In a recent study including four patients (Albert et al., 1990) the critical examination of longitudinally collected virus isolates and sera was performed. Cross-neutralization tests were performed with all samples collected from each patient. The results (illustrated by data from one of the patients, Fig. 1) provide a new perspective on the synthesis of neutralizing antibodies in HIV-infected individuals. Neutralizing antibodies appeared relatively early and were directed against the first virus isolates. In striking contrast the neutralizing activity of sera in tests with later virus isolates was low or non-detectable, interpreted to mean that these isolates represent immune-selected variants. The poor response to these variants may have different explanations. One possibility is the phenomenon of

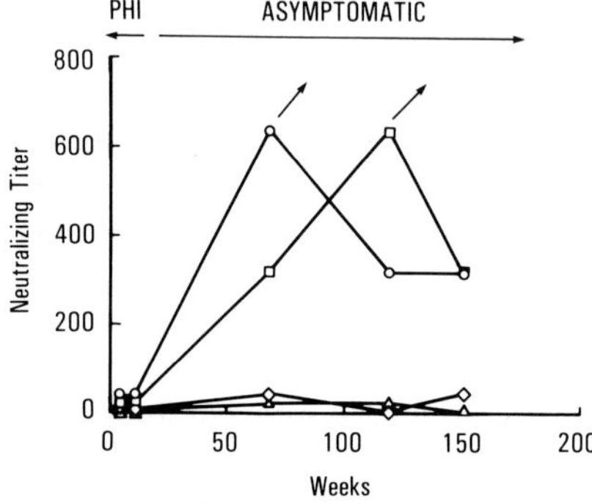


Fig. 1. Neutralizing antibody activity of sera collected at different time intervals after the primary HIV infection (PHI). Virus strains isolated at weeks 2 (□———□), 4 (○———○) and 118 (◇———◇) and as a control HTLV-IIIB virus (△———△) were used in the tests. Data from Albert et al. (1990).

"original antigenic sin", known for example from the field of influenza, meaning that the immune response progressively focuses on antigens which it has encountered during early exposures. The other, and more likely, explanation is that very soon after the acute HIV infection there is a rapidly diminishing capacity to mount primary immune responses even though previously activated antibody responses can be effectively maintained. The contention of emergence of non-neutralizable variants offers a new potential scenario for pathogenic events in HIV infections.

The heterogeneity of HIV is apparent also in the diversification of biological features of virus isolates. Differences in cellular host range, extent and kinetics of virus replication and cytopathology have been observed. Highly replicating cytopathic strains with a broad host range are recovered primarily from patients with clinical disease (Åsjö et al., 1986; Cheng-Mayer et al., 1988; Fenyö et al., 1989). Since individuals producing these so-called rapid/high strains would be expected to be relatively more contagious it is likely that the spread of infection most often occurs by this kind of strain. However rapid/high virus strains are rarely isolated from patients with acute HIV disease (J. Albert, personal communication) inferring a rapid selection in an infected individual of slowly replicating viruses with a narrow host range, slow/low virus strains. Such strains dominate during the asymptomatic phase of HIV infection and appear to associate effectively with macrophage/monocyte cells. Longitudinal characterization of virus strains has shown that rapid/high virus isolates reemerge at the time when the infected individual progresses to the diseased state (Fenyö et al., 1988; Tersmette et al., 1989). It remains to correlate the appearance of non-neutralizable virus strains and the emergence of virulent strains. The non-neutralizable strains identified in the above-mentioned study (Albert et al., 1989) had slow/low characteristics and it is therefore likely that virulent strains, potentially even of a defective nature, are selected from the expanding population of non-neutralizing virus strains.

**Immunological cross-reactions between virus strains**

As mentioned above strain-specific neutralizing antibodies are readily identified. The highly variable V3 site in the extra-membranous glycoprotein (Modrow et al., 1987), also referred to as the "neutralizing loop", is the main target in the envelope for these antibodies (Palker et al., 1988). This site has been extensively characterized by use of peptide antigens, monoclonal antibodies against native protein and peptides etc. The degree of strain specificity of the V3 amino acid sequence was found to vary in different strains. Examples have been given that the change of a single amino acid residue in this part of gp120 may account for a clonal restriction of neutralizing activity (Looney et al., 1988). In contrast V3 peptides representing the MN strain showed relatively extensive interstrain cross-reactivity. In a recent study (Böttiger et al., 1990) cross-neutralization between HIV type 1 and type 2 was examined with human sera. Peptides

```
HIV-1 BRU        C T R P N N N T R K S I R I Q R G P G R A F V T I G K I G – N M R Q A H C
                 |   | |   |   |       |             | |   |           |       | | | |
HIV-2 SBL-6669   C R R P E N K T V V P I T L M S – – G R R F H S Q K I I N K K P R Q A W C
```

Fig. 2. Comparison of the amino acid sequence of the V3 region (Modrow et al., 1987) of HIV-$1_{BRU}$ (residues 301–306) and $HIV_{SBL\text{-}6669}$ (residues 296–330).

mimicking the whole neutralizing loop of both viruses, represented by the strains HTLV-IIIB and $SBL_{6669}$, respectively, were used (Fig. 2). These peptides show some homology in the N-terminal and C-terminal ends but not in their center. Interestingly the amino acid sequence GPGR (glycine, proline, glycine, arginine) which is characteristically conserved in HIV type 1 strains (Goudsmit et al., 1988) has no correspondence in HIV type 2 virus. Enzyme-linked immunosorbent assay (ELISA) with these peptides showed type-specific reactions in as many as 67% (38/57) and 75% (30/40) of HIV type 1 and HIV type 2 positive human sera, respectively. The corresponding figures for cross-reaction with peptides were 23% (13/57) and 33% (13/40), respectively. The capacity of sera to react with the heterotypic peptide was found to correlate with their ability to give cross-neutralization, which was found in 16% of HIV type 1 positive sera and in 22% of HIV type 2 positive sera. According to our present understanding the neutralizing loop may therefore harbor both strain-, interstrain-, type- and intertype-specific determinants. Similar analyses of additional antigenic sites involved in neutralization may show a corresponding situation. Antibodies mediating cellular cytotoxicity have different specificities than neutralizing antibodies. They may show interstrain but not intertype reactivity (Ljunggren et al., 1989). Since individuals concomitantly infected with HIV type 1 and type 2 have been identified, it is obvious that the observed cross-reaction in neutralization tests may not prevent superinfection with the heterologous type of virus. Still the preexisting post-infection immunity may modify the extent of replication of the superinfecting virus. If it is true that HIV type 2 is less pathogenic than HIV type 1 it is possible that in a situation of consecutive infections with first HIV type 2 and then type 1 the pathogenic characteristics of the former type may prevail.

## Infection of cynomolgus macaque monkeys with HIV type 2 protects against pathogenic consequences of a subsequent SIV infection

Infection of macaque monkeys, of the rhesus or cynomolgus kind, with certain strains of simian immunodeficiency virus (SIV) represents an excellent model for HIV infections in man (Desrosier and Letvin, 1987; Putkonen et al., 1989a). The closely related HIV type 2 virus (Hirsch et al., 1989) also infects these primates. Whereas the SIV infection leads to a severe state of immunodeficiency with eventually a fatal outcome for the animals, infection with HIV type 2 has not caused a reduction of CD4 positive T-cells or signs of disease (Dormont et al., 1989; Putkonen et al., 1989b). In a recent study (Putkonen et al., 1990) three cynomolgus monkeys which had been infected with HIV type 2, strain SBL-K135

(Böttiger et al., 1989), were subsequently challenged with about 1000 infectious doses of $SIV_{sm}$ (of sooty mangabey monkey origin, Fultz et al., 1986). A similar dose of virus was given to four monkeys without preexposure immunity. The latter animals showed the expected decline of CD4 positive T-cells to low levels at 6–8 weeks after infection and several distinctly enlarged lymph nodes were palpable. In contrast, after challenge of animals previously infected with HIV type 2 normal levels of CD4 positive T cells were retained and minimal lymph gland enlargements could be detected. However the monkeys became infected, although the replication of virus appeared to be markedly reduced. It remains to follow the superinfected animals for a longer time than the present observation period of 120 days in order to see if prevention against the development of immune suppressive disease will last throughout their life span.

## The approach to vaccination against AIDS

Results of attempts to protect chimpanzees against HIV type 1 infections have been very discouraging. In contrast there are by now four studies showing varying degrees of resistance in infected or immunized macaque monkeys against SIV-related disease. In the study described above replicating virus was used and this was also the case in another study (Marthas et al., 1989). A non-pathogenic infectious clone of $SIV_{mac}$ was used as the primary infection in three rhesus monkeys. After 10 months these animals were challenged with 100–1000 monkey infectious doses but in this case of the homologous type. All three animals became infected but they remained clinically healthy for at least 7 months.

In two of the investigations inactivated homologous antigen was used. In one study (Desrosiers et al., 1989), disrupted whole virus mixed with the adjuvant muramyl dipeptide (MDP) was given as multiple injections to six animals. A challenge of 200–1000 monkey infectious doses was given to the animals. Two monkeys appeared to be completely protected whereas four were partly protected. No disease was observed during an observation time of 435–750 days. The fourth study, finally, used formalin-killed whole virus combined with adjuvant, MDP in some cases combined with aluminum hydroxide. The immunogen was given in multiple injections to nine monkeys and after that, a challenge of 10 monkey infectious doses was given. Eight animals were completely protected during a follow-up time of 9 months. When a preparation of viral glycoprotein was used as immunogen, only partial protection was seen.

The results of these four studies are very encouraging since they clearly demonstrate that immunoprotection against primate lentivirus infections can be obtained. It is now possible to dissect the quality of this immunity, humoral vs. cell-associated etc. Such studies can include both passive and active immunization. Potentially even synthetic immunogens may eventually be tested.

On the basis of the experiences gained it is also possible to discuss potential conditions of immunization and the appropriate goals to be aimed at. One attractive goal would be to establish such an efficient immunity that there is a complete blockage of replication of incoming virus, be it at a mucosal membrane or in the blood. As already emphasized above it may be exceedingly difficult to obtain a durable immunity of this kind. In fact currently employed effective vaccines against poliomyelitis and measles do not provide such a sterilizing immunity. An alternative goal therefore might be to aim at an infection-permissive immunity. In this case a limited replication of virus to which an individual is exposed may be allowed but the impact of the infection should be so limited that no disease would develop during the remaining life span. This approach is based on the assumption that there is a correlation between the extent of virus replication during the acute infection and the incubation time until development of fatal disease. Some data emerging in the literature appear to support this contention. It appears likely that a disease-preventing immunity will require a highly effective preexposure immunization. Because of the projected restriction in capacity to mobilize humoral as well as cellular immunity already early after the acute infection post-exposure immunization of symptom-free individuals would be anticipated not to be an attractive approach.

In summary, studies in primate lentivirus models during the last year have given new encouragement to the development of an AIDS vaccine. However it would seem, for pragmatic reasons, that the aim of this immunization should be to prevent disease but not necessarily to completely block virus replication. The frequently made statement that an AIDS vaccine has to be more effective in inducing the immune system to a specific response than the infection-associated immunization may not be appropriate. Effective sensitization of the immune system prior to exposure to virus may allow it to control the infection not only temporarily but also throughout future host-virus interactions.

## Acknowledgements

The work of the author and colleagues referred to in this review was supported by the Swedish Board of Technical Development under Grants 87-0203P and 87-03356P (G. Biberfeld) and by the U.S. Army Medical Research and Development Command under Grant DAMD 17-89-2-9038.

## References

Albert, J., Abrahamsson, B., Nagy, K., Aurelius, E., Gaines, H., Krook, A., Nyström, G. and Fenyö, E.M. (1990) Rapid development of isolate-specific neutralizing antibodies after primary HIV-1 infection and consequent emergence of virus variants which resist neutralization by autologous sera. *AIDS* 4, 107–112.

Åsjö, B., Albert, J., Karlsson, A., Morfeldt-Månson, L., Biberfeld, G., Lidman K. and Fenyö, E.M. (1986) Replicative capacity of human immunodeficiency virus from patients with varying severity of HIV infection. *Lancet* ii, 660–662.

Blattner, W., Nara, P., Shaw, G., Hahn, B., Kong, L., Matthews, T., Bolognesi, D., Waters, D. and Gallo, R.C. (1989) Prospective clinical, immunological, and virologic follow-up of an infected laboratory worker. *V International Congress of AIDS,* Abstract MC07.

Böttiger, B., Karlsson, A., Andreasson, P.Å., Nauclér, A., Mendes-Costa, C. and Biberfeld, G. (1989) Cross-neutralizing antibodies against HIV-1 (HTLV-IIIB and HTLV-IIIRF) and HIV-2 (SBL-6669 and a new isolate SBL-K135). *AIDS Res. Human Retroviruses* 5, 525–533.

Cheng-Mayer, C., Seto, D., Tatero, M. and Levy, J.A. (1988) Biologic features of HIV-1 that correlate with virulence in the host. *Science* 240, 80–82.

Desrosiers, R.C. and Letvin, N.L. (1987) Animal models for acquired immunodeficiency syndrome. *Rev. Infect. Dis.* 9, 438–446.

Desrosiers, R.C., Wyand, M.S., Kodama, T., Ringler, D.J., Arthur, L.O., Sehgal, P.K., Letvin, N.L., King, N.W. and Daniel, M.D. (1989) Vaccine protection against simian immunodeficiency virus infection. *Proc. Natl. Acad. Sci. U.S.A.* 86, 6353–6357.

Dormont, D., Livartovski, J., Chamaret, S., Guetard, D., Henin, R., Levagueresse, R., Moortelle, P.F., Larke, B., Gourmelon, P., Vazeaux, R., Metivier, H., Flageat, J., Court, L., Hauw, J.J. and Montagnier, L. (1989) HIV-2 in rhesus monkeys: serological, virological and clinical results. *Intervirology* 30 (Suppl. 1), 59–65.

Fauci, A.S. (1988) The human immunodeficiency virus: infectivity and mechanism of pathogenesis. *Science* 239, 617–622.

Fenyö, E.M., Morfeldt-Månson, L., Chiodi, F., Lind, B., von Gegerfeldt, A., Albert, J., Olausson, E. and Åsjö, B. (1988) Distinct replicative and cytopathic characteristic of human immunodeficiency virus isolates. *J. Virol.* 62, 4414–4419.

Fultz, P.N., McClure, H.M., Anderson, D.C., Brent-Svenson, R., Anand, R. and Srinivasan, A. (1986) Isolation of a T-lymphotropic retrovirus from naturally infected sooty mangabey monkeys *(Cercocebus atus). Proc. Natl. Acad. Sci. U.S.A.* 83, 5286–5290.

Goudsmit, J., Debouck, C., Meloen, R.H., Smit, L., Bakker, M., Asher, D.M., Wolff, A.V., Gibbs, C.J. and Carleton, D.C. (1988) Human immunodeficiency virus type 1 neutralizing epitope with conserved architecture elicits early type-specific antibodies in experimentally infected chimpanzees. *Proc. Natl. Acad. Sci. U.S.A.* 85, 4478–4482.

Haseltine, W.A. (1988) Replication and pathogenesis of the AIDS virus. *J. AIDS* 1, 217–240.

Hirsch, V.M., Olmstedt, R.A., Murphey-Corb, M., Purcell, R.H. and Johnson, P.R. (1989) An African primate lentivirus ($SIV_{sm}$) closely related to HIV-2. *Nature* 339, 389–392.

Ho, D.D., Sarngadharan, M.G., Hirsch, M.S., Schooley, R.T., Rota, T.R., Kennedy, R.C., Chank, T.C. and Sato, V.L. (1987) Human immunodeficiency virus neutralizing antibodies recognize several conserved domains of the envelope glycoproteins. *J. Virol.* 61, 2024–2028.

Koff, W.C. and Hoth, D.F. (1988) Development and testing of AIDS vaccines. *Science* 241, 426–432.

Lane, H.C., Masur, H., Edgar, L.C., Whalen, G., Rook, A.H. and Fauci, A.S. (1983) Abnormalities of B-cell activation and immunoregulation in patients with acquired immunodeficiency syndrome. *N. Engl. J. Med.* 309, 453–458.

Levy, J.A. (1989) Human immunodeficiency viruses and the pathogenesis of AIDS. *J. Am. Med. Ass.* 261, 2997–3006.

Ljunggren, K., Biberfeld, G., Jondal, M. and Fenyö, E.M. (1989) Antibody-dependent cellular cytotoxicity detects type- and strain-specific antigens among human immunodeficiency virus types 1 and 2 and simian immunodeficiency virus $SIV_{mac}$ isolates. *J. Virol.* 63, 3376–3381.

Looney, D.J., Fisher, A.G., Putney, S.D., Rusche, J.R., Redfield, R.R., Burke, D.S., Gallo, R.C. and Wong-Staal, F. (1988) Type-restricted neutralization of molecular clones of human immunodeficiency virus. *Science* 241, 357–359.

Marthas, M., Sutjipto, S., Antipa, L., Gettie, A., Higgins, J., Joye, S., Lohman, B., Tosten, J., Luciw, P., Marx, P. and Pedersen, N. (1989) Inoculation with a cloned simian immunodeficiency virus (SIV) prevents acute disease in rhesus macaques challenged with pathogenic SIV. *Symposium on Non-Human Primate Models for AIDS,* Portland, OR, October 11–13, Abstract 82.

Modrow, S., Hahn, B.H., Shaw, G.M., Gallo, R.C., Wong-Staal, F. and Wolf, H. (1987) Computer-assisted analysis of envelope protein sequences of seven human immunodeficiency virus isolates: prediction of antigenic epitopes in conserved and variable regions. *J. Virol.* 61, 570–578.

Murphey-Corb, M., Martin, L., Davison-Fairburn, B., Montelaro, R., West, M. and Miller M. (1989) A formalin-killed whole SIV vaccine, but not DOC-disrupted glycoprotein and *GAG* subunit preparations, protects rhesus monkeys following challenge with a 10 $ID_{50}$ dose of live virus. *Symposium on Non-Human Primate Models for AIDS,* Portland, OR, October 11–13, Abstract 81.

Nara, P.L., Robey, W.G., Arthur, L.O., Asher, D.M., Wolff, A.V., Gibbs, C.J., Gajdusek, D.C. and Fischinger, P.J. (1987) Persistent infection of chimpanzees with human immunodeficiency virus: serological responses and properties of reisolated viruses. *J. Virol.* 61, 3173–3180.

Norrby, E. (1987) Toward new viral vaccines for man. *Adv. Virus Res.* 32, 1–34.

Pahwa, S., Rahwa, R., Good, R.A., Gallo, R.C. and Saxinger, C. (1986) Stimulatory and inhibitory influences of human immunodeficiency virus on normal B lymphocytes. *Proc. Natl. Acad. Sci. U.S.A.* 83, 9124–9128.

Palker, T.J., Clark, M.E., Langlois, A.J., Mathews, T.J., Weinhold, K.J., Randall, R.R., Bolognesi, D.P. and Haynes, B.F. (1988) Type-specific neutralization of the human immunodeficiency virus with antibodies to *env*-encoded synthetic peptides. *Proc. Natl. Acad. Sci. U.S.A.* 85, 1932–1936.

Putkonen, P., Warstedt, K., Thorstensson, R., Bentin, R., Albert, J., Lundgren, B., Öberg, B., Norrby, E. and Biberfeld, G. (1989a) Experimental infection of cynomolgus monkeys (*Macaca fascicularis*) with simian immunodeficiency virus ($SIV_{sm}$). *J. AIDS* 2, 359–365.

Putkonen, P., Böttiger, B., Warstedt, K., Thorstensson, R., Albert, J. and Biberfeld, G. (1989b) Experimental infection of cynomolgus monkeys (*Macaca fascicularis*) with HIV-2. *J. AIDS* 2, 366–373.

Putkonen, P., Thorstensson, R., Albert, J., Hild, K., Norrby, E., Biberfeld, P. and Biberfeld, G. (1990) Infection of cynomolgus monkeys with HIV type 2 protects against pathogenic consequences of a subsequent SIV infection. *AIDS* (in press).

Schneider, J. and Hunsman, G. (1988) Simian lentiviruses—the SIV group. *AIDS* 2, 1–9.

Stricker, R.B., McHugh, T.M., Moody, D.J., Morrow, W.J.W., Stites, D.P., Shuman, M.A. and Levy, J.A. (1987) An AIDS-related cytotoxic autoantibody reacts with a specific antigen on stimulated CD4+ T cells. *Nature* 327, 710–713.

Takahashi, H., Merli, S., Putney, S.D., Houghten, R.A., Moss, B., Germain, R.N. and Berzofsky, J. (1989) A single amino acid interchange yields reciprocal CTL specificities for HIV gp160. *Science* 246, 118–121.

Takeda, A., Tuazon, C.U. and Ennis, F.A. (1988) Antibody-enhanced infection by HIV-1 via Fc-receptor-mediated entry. *Science* 242, 580–583.

Tersmette, M., de Goede, R.E.Y., Winkel, J.N., Gruters, R.A., Cuypers, H.T., Huisman, H.G. and Miedema, F. (1988) Differential syncytium-inducing capacity of human immunodeficiency virus isolates: frequent detection of syncytium-inducing isolates in patients with acquired immunodeficiency syndrome (AIDS) and AIDS-related complex. *J. Virol.* 62, 2026–2032.

# Subject index